RADIATION AND GUT

Dedication

We dedicate this book to the memory of
Professor Laszlo G. Lajtha
CBE, MD, DPhil, FRCP(E), FRCPath
(1920–1995) — mentor, colleague, and friend.

Radiation
and
Gut

edited by
C.S. Potten *and* J. H. Hendry

Patterson Institute for Cancer Research
Manchester, UK

1995
ELSEVIER
AMSTERDAM – LAUSANNE – NEW YORK – OXFORD – SHANNON – TOKYO

ELSEVIER SCIENCE B.V.
Sara Burgerhartstraat 25
P.O. Box 211, 1000 AE Amsterdam, The Netherlands

ISBN 0-444-89053-X

Printed in The Netherlands

Preface

The gut (otherwise referred to generally as the gastrointestinal tract or the alimentary canal) is one of our crucial organs. During evolution it has maintained its basic tubular structure, as in the worm, to become 5 times the body length in man. Although its basic anatomy was described well over 100 years ago, it is only in the last 20 years that a fuller appreciation of its complex proliferative structure has become known. The intestine is one of the most rapidly renewing tissues in the body, and hence it responds rapidly to injury. It is one of the limiting tissues in some radio- and chemotherapy practices. Damage to the gut is of particular concern in cytotoxic therapies involving radiation exposure or chemical agents, and in accidental cases of radiation release, e.g., Chernobyl. Also, cancers of the digestive system account for more than 20% of the total, both in terms of incidence and mortality (Cancer Research Campaign, Facts on Cancer, UK). Notable is the lack of cancer in the small intestine which forms the largest and most rapidly proliferating component of the tract. Reasons for this are only just emerging.

Texts on gut with reference to radiation (or other cytotoxic and carcinogenic agents) consist of primary research papers, review articles, or books which are now very out-of-date. With this in mind, the present book was conceived. Here, with chapters by experts in the field, we cover the basic structure and cell replacement process in the gut, the physical situation relevant for gut radiation exposure and a description of some of the techniques used to study radiation effects, in particular the clonal regeneration assay that assesses stem cell functional capacity. Chapters comprehensively cover the effects of radiation in experimental animal model systems and clinical experiences. The effects of radiation on the supportive tissue of the gut is also reviewed. The special radiation situation involving ingested radionuclides is reviewed and the most important late response — carcinogenesis — within the gut is considered. This book follows a volume on Radiation and Skin (author C.S. Potten, published by Taylor & Francis, London, 1985), and another on Radiation and Bone Marrow is in preparation. The present volume is intended to cover the anatomy and renewal characteristics of the gut, and its response in terms of carcinogenicity and tissue injury in mammalian species including in particular man. The book is expected to be useful to students and teachers in these topics, as well as Clinical Oncologists (Radiotherapists) and Medical Oncologists, and Industrial Health Personnel.

We are grateful to Ann Kaye for her help with the Editorial procedures here in Manchester, and the publishers for producing the book. We are both grateful for support from the Cancer Research Campaign (UK).

Christopher S. Potten
Jolyon H. Hendry
Manchester, UK
February 1995

Contents

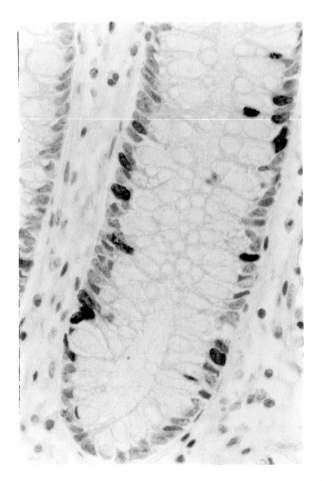

Chapter 1, Fig. 6 (see page 9). Section of a human colonic crypt labelled with bromodeoxyuridine and stained with immunoperoxidase using a monoclonal antibody that recognises the bromodeoxyuridine incorporated into cells in the S phase of the cell cycle.

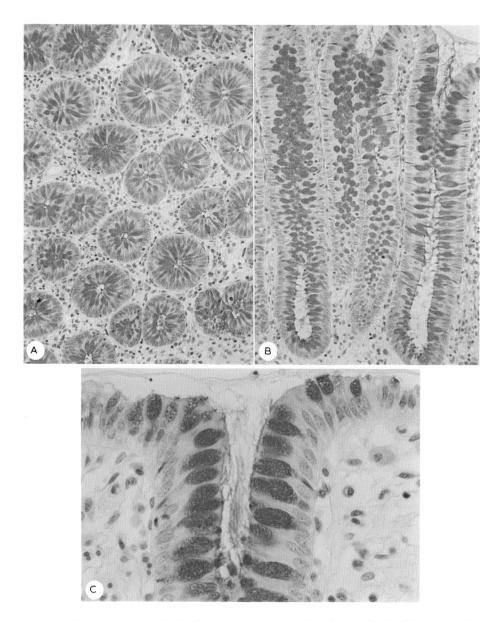

Chapter 1, Fig. 11 (see page 17). Sections cut transversely (A) or longitudinally (B) through the human colonic crypts stained with Alcian blue to show the mucus secreting cells. A high power view (C) showing the typical flash-shape of the goblet cells.

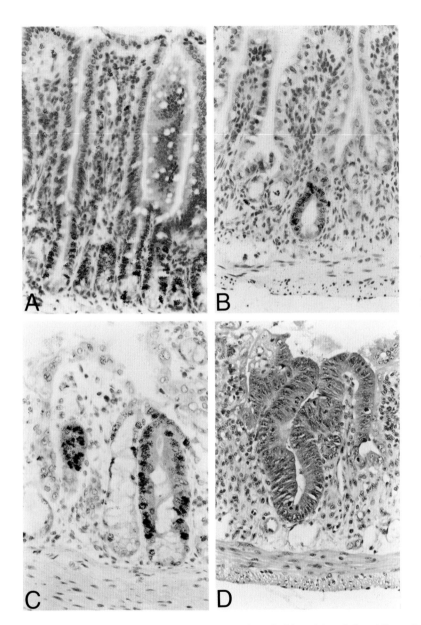

Chapter 3, Fig. 1 (see page 47). Microcolonies identified by tritiated thymidine administration (2 × 925 kBq 6 h apart). A: Unirradiated small intestine showing villi and 7 labelled crypts (3 longitudinally sectioned and 4 tangential). B: 3 days after irradiation a single heavily labelled surviving (regenerating) crypt can be seen in the small intestine. C: 4 days after irradiation of the mid colon an obvious longitudinal sectioned surviving crypt can be seen heavily labelled on the right. A non-surviving relatively unlabelled 'ghost' crypt can be seen in the middle of the picture. A surviving tangentially sectioned and labelled crypt can be seen on the left with more than 14 adjacent labelled cells. D: 5 days after irradiation large expanding foci of regeneration can be seen in the small intestine. Such areas are spreading laterally at the surface and bifurcating near the base.

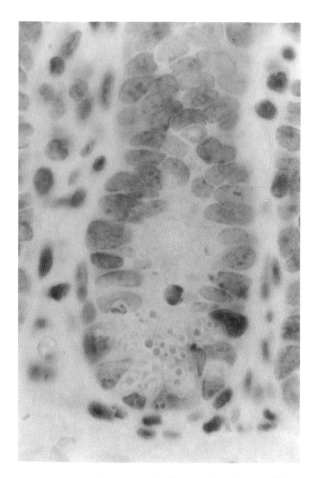

Chapter 4, Fig. 4 (see page 72). Section through a small intestinal crypt 3–4 h after irradiation, stained with an affinity purified polyclonal antibody to p53 gene product. A single positive cell can be seen on the right hand side of the crypt at about cell position 4 immediately above the Paneth cells. A clear apoptotic cell can be seen in the centre of the field. Other apoptotic fragments are recognisable in the section. The function of the single p53 positive cell at the stem cell position remains to be elucidated as does the significance of the fact that the apoptotic cell is p53 negative. I am grateful to Anita Merritt for the section from which this photograph was taken.

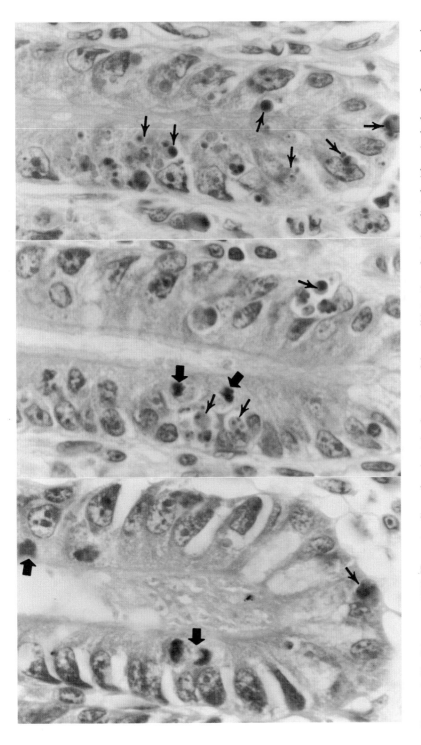

Chapter 5, Fig. 8 (see page 100). Haematoxylin and eosin stained sections of the small intestine of rats irradiated with a single dose of γ rays showing mitotic cells (large arrows) and apoptotic fragments of cells (small arrows). Left hand panel, control unirradiated rats showing a spontaneous apoptotic cell. Middle panel, 6 h after 1 Gy, and right hand panel 6 h after 8 Gy. Many small apoptotic fragments are seen in the right hand panel.

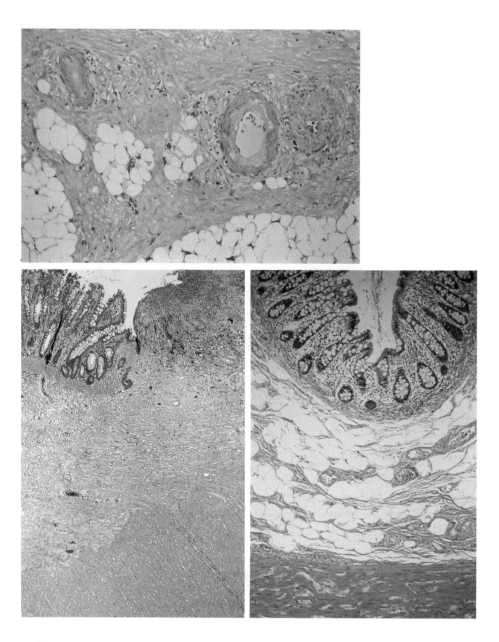

Chapter 8, Fig. 1 (see page 238). Section of normal human bowel (top panel), and irradiated human bowel at 1 year after radiotherapy (bottom 2 panels). The irradiated samples show features of radiation colitis, namely ulceration, submucosal fibrosis, and atypical fibroblasts. Also apparent are vascular changes in the serosal blood vessels. There is marked myointimal thickening with narrowing of the lumina (courtesy of Dr. S. Banerjee, Department of Pathology, Christie Hospital).

C.S. Potten and J.H. Hendry (Eds.), *Radiation and Gut*

CHAPTER 1

Structure, Function and Proliferative Organisation of Mammalian Gut

C.S. Potten

*CRC Department of Epithelial Biology, Paterson Institute for Cancer Research,
Christie Hospital NHS Trust, Wilmslow Road, Manchester M20 9BX, UK*

1. INTRODUCTION

The gastrointestinal (GI) tract is a tubular organ that runs from the mouth to the anus. The primary function of the organ is the processing of food material into its constituent absorbable molecules. It also provides a protective barrier against chemicals and particularly bacteria between the internal organs and the external environment which in this case is the lumen of the gut. The tube is lined by an epithelium with a morphology which changes with position along the gastrointestinal tract. Associated with the GI tract are numerous secondary glandular structures whose responsibility includes the production of the necessary digestive enzymes. The purpose of the epithelium is thus to provide a protective barrier between the body and the food material which may contain noxious organisms, toxins and parasites. By appropriate differentiation of the cells the function also includes the production of saliva, acid in the stomach, enzymes and mucus. Probably the most important function is the transport of water, salts, essential minerals and the degradation products of the enzymatic breakdown of food. This absorption is achieved by an active transport mechanism across the cells of the epithelium and is particularly associated with certain regions of the GI tract. Clearly the upper regions of the GI tract are involved primarily with the manipulation and mechanical breakdown of food material while the lower regions of the tract are involved with the packaging and processing of the indigestible waste material for excretion, and the absorption of water.

In the oral cavity, the oesophagus and parts of the stomach the epithelium in some species is stratified and undergoes a form of keratinisation particularly in the oral cavity where different types of keratinisation are seen. The terminal regions of the stomach contain a columnar epithelium which is folded and organised into long slender glands or crypts which penetrate deep into the connective tissue of the stomach wall with some of these glands containing cells that are responsible for the production of hydrochloric acid.

Beyond the stomach the GI tract consists of a very long narrow tube, the small intestine which in humans is about 20 ft (6–7 m) in length. The first region of this is the duodenum followed shortly by the jejunum and the largest proportion which constitutes the ileum. Here, the simple columnar epithelium covers finger-like projections, the villi, and continues into small flask shaped glands or crypts located at the base of the villi. The villi represent the functional differentiated component of the tissue where cells migrate from the base of the villus to its tip performing their various functions and as they move they become senescent and are shed predominantly from the tip of the villus. This cell loss from the villi is precisely balanced in steady state conditions by cell proliferation that is located in the crypts (see Fig. 1). At the terminal end of the ileum the tube branches in one case to form a small blind sac lined with columnar epithelium, the appendix. The other branch continues as the large bowel. The first part of this is the caecum which is followed by the colon and then the rectum which terminates in the anus. Throughout the entire large bowel the tube is lined by a simple columnar epithelium which is greatly folded into many relatively long or deep crypts. In this region of the intestine there are no villi but between each crypt is a short region of flat epithelium (the table) between crypts. The large intestine in humans is about 5 ft long (1.5 m) and is subdivided into the caecum, the ascending colon, transverse colon, descending colon and finally the sigmoid colon and rectum based mainly on the position of the regions in the abdomen. In rodents these distinctions are not relevant since the large bowel tends to be a straight tube lying close to the spine in the abdomen. Throughout its length the epithelium or mucosa sits upon a connective tissue bed which is rich in blood capillaries (Fig. 2), lymphoid tissue and connective tissue cells (fibroblasts) and is itself surrounded by layers of muscle. The connective tissue core of the villus contains some smooth muscle cells which are involved in the contraction and extension of the villus. The two layers of circumferential striated muscles are involved in peristalsis, the regular 'pumping' action that moves food down the tube.

The size and shape of the villi in the small intestine, the size and number of crypts around each villus and the size of the crypts in the large bowel all vary depending on their location along the length of the tube.

There have been many studies over the last 50 years on the proliferation and differentiation of cells in the small bowel of rodents, particularly mice, somewhat fewer studies on the large bowel of rodents and relatively few studies for obvious technical reasons on the human (for reviews see Refs. [1–4]). This pattern is generally repeated when one considers the effects of radiation on this tissue which have been fairly extensively studied in the small bowel of rodents. For these reasons we shall restrict the contents of this book largely to the rodent systems, providing information on humans where it is available and concentrating mainly on the small and large bowel. Here, I will draw heavily

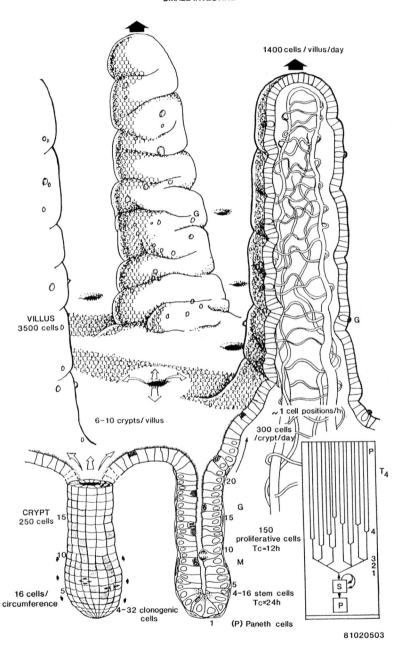

SMALL INTESTINE

Fig. 1. Diagram illustrating the three-dimensional structure, section appearance, cell kinetics and cellular hierarchy for the small intestinal mucosa of the mouse.

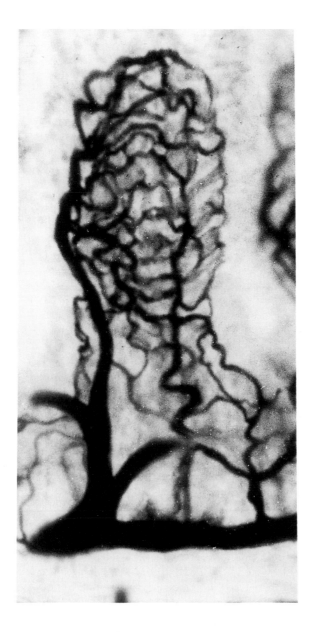

Fig. 2. Indian ink perfusion of the vasculature of a small intestinal villus. I am grateful to Professor Y. Tsuchihashi for this picture.

on data that we have generated ourselves over the years in studying the BDF1 mouse which is a cross between C57Bl6 and DBA2, two inbred strains (see Ref. [5] for review). I will restrict our observations mainly to this experimental animal system since this minimises inter-laboratory, inter-mouse strain and inter-species variability. We have over the past 15 years generated a large data base of both cell kinetic and radiobiological information on young adult, usually male, BDF1 mice bred and housed under controlled laboratory conditions. However, other groups have developed similar large data bases for example the Italian group of Becciolini have for many years acquired data on the effects of radiation on Sprague–Dawley rats and these data will also be reviewed in Chapter 5.

2. BDF1 ILEUM

The villi in this region are simple finger-like projections that taper slightly towards their tip and have a roughly circular cross-sectional profile. Nearer the stomach the villi tend to be more leaf-like in shape tapering towards the tip and having a very oblong cross-sectional profile. In the ileum each one of these villi is covered by approximately 3500 columnar epithelial cells. Scattered amongst these are occasional mucus secreting goblet cells (Fig. 3). Each villus is surrounded at the base by a number of crypts. The precise number per villus varies depending on the position along the small intestine but it generally falls within the range of 6–14 throughout the entire small intestine and between 6–10 in the ileum (Fig. 4). The complete 3-dimensional inter-relationship between crypts and villi is complex with many crypts being positioned in such a way that they can clearly provide cells for more than one villus. Some may be located in such a way that they could serve 3 villi and yet others seem to be positioned in such a way that their cell production is predominantly directed towards only one villus. On average it has been estimated that each crypt in the ileum serves 1.75 villi. In the ileum of BDF1 mice each crypt contains about 250 cells in total with slightly less than 20% of these cells (about 17–18%) being seen in a good longitudinal section cut through the middle of these flask shaped structures, that is about 44 cells per crypt section. Thus, in the crypts that ring the base of the villus there are between 1500 and 2500 cells, say 2000 on average and again on average half of these serve the villus which is located in the centre of this ring of crypts. Thus the relationship between crypt cells and villus cells is approximately 1000:3500. The length of the small intestine in the mouse is about 30 cm in its entirety and this weighs about 1 g. There are about 750 crypts for each milligram of tissue which means that there about 750 000 crypts and about 100 000 villi in the entire small intestine of the mouse. The length of the human ileum is about 500–600 cm (20 ft) and it weighs about 640 g. We have recently estimated that in the human ileum there are almost twice as many cells in each crypt, at 475 per crypt. There are about 1×10^8 villi, about 7×10^{11} villus epithelial cells and probably about 5×10^7 crypts in the small intestine of man. These crypts produce about 2×10^{11} cells per day or about a gram of cells (10^9) every 30–60 min. These figures are all estimates and should be considered with caution.

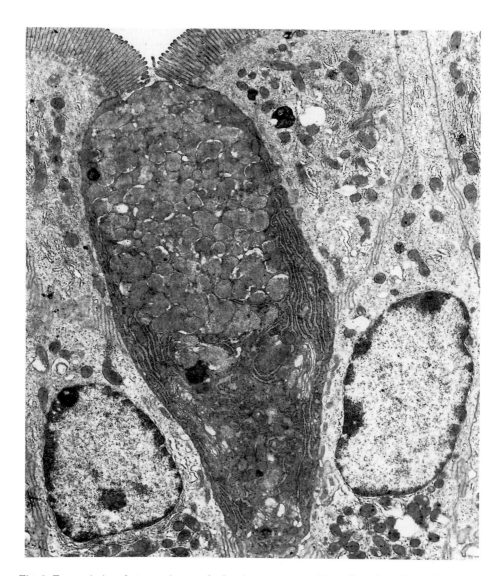

Fig. 3. Transmission electron micrograph showing a mature goblet cell on the villus of the small intestine. I am grateful to Dr. T. Allen for this picture.

About 60% of the 250 crypt cells in the mouse, i.e. about 150 or 160 per crypt, can be shown by appropriate experimental studies to be actively progressing through the cell cycle and can be designated as proliferative cells. Studies using tritiated thymidine or more recently bromodeoxyuridine to label the cells in the S phase of the cell cycle have shown that about half of the proliferative cells, i.e. about 75 cells per crypt, are in the S phase of the cell cycle at any one moment in time (Figs. 5 and 6). Such labelling studies followed by an analysis

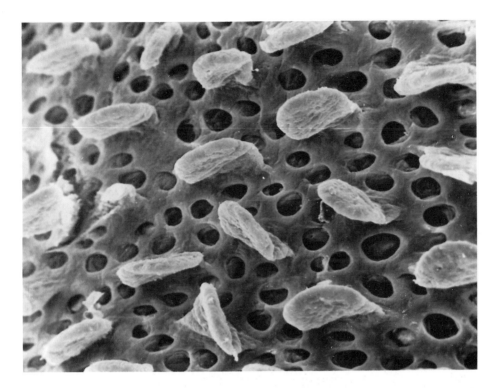

Fig. 4. Scanning electron micrograph showing the relationship between villi and crypts in the murine small intestine. The epithelium has been stripped away using an EDTA approach to reveal the cavities occupied by crypts. The complex three dimensional relationship between the proliferative crypts and the functional villi can be clearly seen. I am grateful to Dr. T. Allen for this picture.

of the percentage of the mitotic figures that are labelled at various times after tritiated thymidine (^{3}HTdR) administration (the PLM technique) show that the average inter-mitotic interval, the *cell cycle time* (T_c) for these proliferating cells in the crypt of a mouse is about 12–13 h. These studies confirm what could already be deduced from the simple observation that half the cells at any one time are ^{3}HTdR labelled, namely that the S phase (T_s) takes about 7 h to complete. Mitosis takes about half an hour for these cells and at any one time 2 or 3 cells will be undergoing mitoses. In fact the general rate of proliferation in the small bowel indicates that a cell divides in every crypt every five minutes and this very dramatically illustrates the highly dynamic nature of this tissue. It is probably the most rapidly proliferating tissue of the entire mammalian body and this high rate of proliferation has a major impact in determining this tissue as being one of the most radio-sensitive tissues of the body. The 150 rapidly proliferating cells are in fact distributed in a band across the middle of the crypt and do not extend right to the base because in the small intestine there are at the very bottom of the crypts up to 30 terminally differentiated

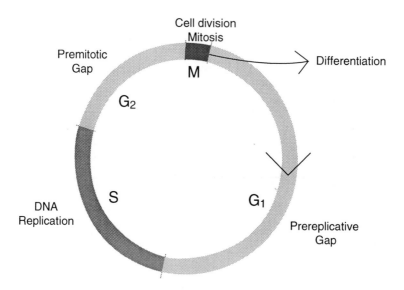

	Small intestine		Large intestine	
	Mouse	Man	Mouse	Man
Cell cycle (T_C)	13.5 (12^c) (13.2^d)	42 (20–36^c) (33^d)	19.2 (24–36^c) (35^d)	69 (36^c) (34^d)
S phase (T_S)*	7.4^a	11	7.8^a	9.3
M phase (T_M)*	0.8^a	2	0.9^a	–
G_1 phase (T_{G1})*	4.7^a	~27	9.1^a	–
G_2 phase (T_{G2})*	1.3^a	1.8	1.3^a	–

From Ref. [1]
[a]Independent estimates, the sum of these does not necessarily add up to T_C.
[b]Approximate values — few estimates.
[c]Our own measurements.
[d]From Ref. [4].

Fig. 5. The cell cycle. The table provides best estimates drawn from the literature for the cell cycle and phase durations for human and mouse small and large bowel.

functional Paneth cells (Fig. 7). These cells contain large secretory granules and do not normally divide. The precise function of these granules remain somewhat obscure but the cells may play an antibacterial role. Within this broad band across the middle of the crypt where rapid proliferation occurs the cell cycle time is fairly uniform, apart from the cells close to, or at, the bottom of this band which appear to be cycling more slowly than the bulk of the proliferative cells and have a cell cycle time of approximately 24 h [6].

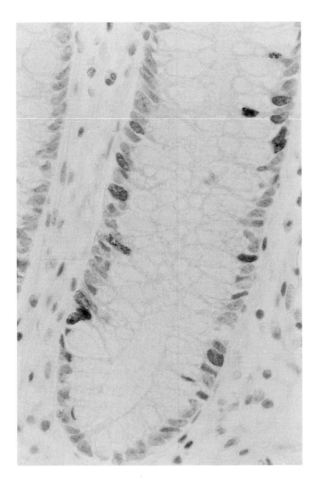

Fig. 6. Section of a human colonic crypt labelled with bromodeoxyuridine and stained with immunoperoxidase using a monoclonal antibody that recognises the bromodeoxyuridine incorporated into cells in the S phase of the cell cycle. (See also colour plate on p. xi.)

Since there are about 150 cells per crypt passing through the cell cycle twice a day this means that each crypt in a mouse will produce per day about 300 cells and since there are about 7.5×10^5 crypts in the entire small intestine this means that in the mouse about 2.25×10^8 cells are produced each day or about a gram of cells (about 10^9 cells) every 5 days (this is equivalent to the mouse producing about 4% of its body weight each day from the lining of the small intestine or replacing a mass equivalent to its entire body weight about 3 times a year). The mouse thus produces about 2×10^{11} cells in the small intestine during its entire 3 year life span under laboratory conditions, i.e., about 200 g or 6–10 times its body weight of small intestinal cells. In the human the crypts are nearly twice as large but the cell cycle time is nearly twice as long and since the total number of crypts may not be very

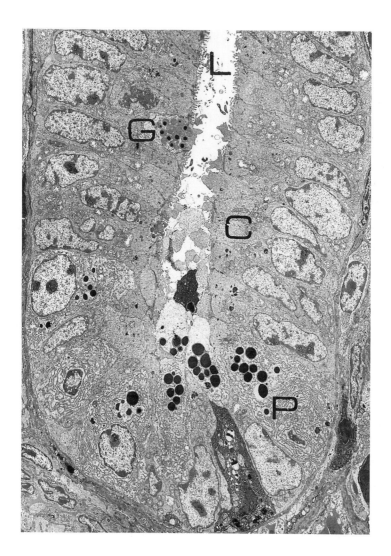

Fig. 7. Transmission electron micrograph of the lower portion of a small intestinal crypt showing typical columnar cells (c), goblet cells (G) and Paneth cells (P). The lumen of crypt (L) can also be seen. I am grateful to Dr. T. Allen for this photograph.

different from that in the mouse the cell production figures for man will be up to about 1000 times greater per day. During a 70 year life span a human may produce and shed a mass of tissue equivalent to about 10 times the body weight and for a mouse the comparable figure is about 40 times its body weight from the small intestine in its 3 year life span. These figures give some idea of the highly dynamic nature of this tissue.

There are about 16 cells in the circumference around each mouse ileal crypt except for the first 3 or 4 positions at the tapering base of the crypt. In longitudinal sections of the crypt one can see about 22 cells in the crypt height, however because of geometric packing problems associated with the cells it is believed that we over-count the number of cells in the vertical column by about 30% which means that there are in reality about 16 cells in the vertical column [7]. The product of the vertical cellularity × the girth cellularity then gives about 250 cells per crypt. With 16 cells in the circumference and about 300 cells per day being produced from the top of the crypt it is clear that cells are being produced at a rate of about 0.78 cells per column per hour out of the top of the crypt. This value is close to the actual cell migration velocities that can be measured experimentally which generally fall within the range 0.5 to a little over 1 cell positions per hour [8]. The experimental observations indicate that this migration velocity increases progressively as the cells move up the some-what tapering villus to reach maximum velocities of close to 2 cell positions per hour in the middle to upper region of the villus. There are about 70 cell positions in the vertical column of cells lining the surface of the villus and if we assume an average migration velocity of around 1 cell position per hour this would mean that a cell that enters the base of the villus will be shed from the tip approximately 3 days later. This time, which is called the villus *transit time* has important implications in understanding the radiobiological response of the tissue since this is the time that it would take for the villus to essentially atrophy if one completely cuts off the flow of cells onto the base of the villus by sterilising the crypt. As each crypt is producing about 300 cells per day and there are about 6–7 crypts surrounding each villus not all of which are produc-ing cells for the central villus, there are between 1000 and 2000 cells entering and leaving each villus per day.

The villus transit time of 72 h mentioned above is likely in fact to be a maximum figure. This is based on the assumption that the velocity remains constant with progression up the villus which is known not to be the case. In reality the transit time from the top of the crypt to the tip of the villus is more likely to be between 48 and 72 h and the migration time from the lower regions of the crypt to the tip of the villus will be something between 100 and 120 h. Thus the total transit time from the crypt base to the villus tip lies between 6 and 8 days. As stated at the beginning of this review the figures that have been quoted here are those that are relevant to the BDF1 adult mouse housed under our laboratory conditions. When comparisons are made between data collected from other laboratories using other strains of animals with possible different housing conditions these numbers may vary by a factor of up to 2 depending somewhat on which particular parameter is being considered.

We have recently made some measurements on some of these parameters in the human ileum from patients that received an intravenous injection of bromodeoxyuridine between 2–16 h prior to surgery. The data are far less precise in their determination but the results indicate that the crypts are almost twice as large as they are in the mouse, containing in the human about 475 cells. Proliferative cells are distributed over a somewhat broader band of cell positions from about the 5th position to about the 30th position from the base of the crypt. The maximum labelling index (fraction of cells in the S phase) is nearly 30%, lower than the 50% in the mouse. This maximum labelling index occurs about the 15th position from the base of the crypt and would be consistent with the average cell cycle time (T_c) of the cells in this region of about 30 h, about 2.5 times longer than it is in the mouse [4].

So far I have discussed the structural and proliferative function of the epithelium that lines the small intestine. It should not be forgotten however, that the small intestine is a composite tissue composed not only of the epithelium but an intricate connective tissue or *lamina propria* which contains connective tissue cells, or fibroblasts, some of which have an intimate proximity with the lining of the crypt and the villus, the pericryptal fibroblasts. Additional fibroblasts and smooth muscle cells are located in the connective tissue matrix which is composed largely of a network of collagen fibres. There is a intricate neural network which again interacts with certain cells within the epithelium. There is a very complex and intricate network of capillaries (Fig. 2) and hence many endothelial cells around the crypts and particularly up the core of the villus. These are clearly of major importance for the function of the tissue in transporting material from the outside of the body (inside the intestinal tube) to inside the body. There is also a complex system of lymph glands and ducts, the most obvious of which are small lymph nodes known as Peyer's patches, over which the epithelium continues but in a specific modified way. There is also a certain amount of trafficking from the lymph system into the epithelium since the epithelium contains under normal circumstances a fairly small number of intra-epithelial lymphocytes. The lymphatic system is clearly involved here, as it is in many sites, with an immunological surveillance and protection of the animal. There is increasing evidence that elements of the stroma, particularly the fibroblasts, but also the lymphocytes are producing growth factor and cytokines that influence the behaviour of the overlying epithelium. Molecules associated with the extracellular matrix at the boundary between the epithelium and the mesenchyme are also probably playing an important role in the overall homeostatic (regulatory) process.

The perimeter of the gut consists of two layers of muscle and the entire structure is connected to the internal abdomen by large blood vessels suspended in a thin membrane or mesentery. All these elements of the tissue will respond to an exposure to radiation and their individual responses will contribute to the overall effects that one sees when the gastrointestinal tract is irradiated. The relative importance of each individual tissue element in the overall radiobiological response remains somewhat unclear. However, it is beyond dispute that the major contributing element to the acute radiobiological response are the proliferative cells of the epithelium which are of course located in the crypts.

3. BDF1 LARGE BOWEL

In the large bowel of BDF1 mice the crypts are generally significantly larger than in the small intestine. We commonly divide the entire length of the large bowel of mice into 3 approximately equal-sized segments. The first of which is at the caecal end and the last third the rectal end. The parameters defining the epithelial structures and their proliferation differ slightly in the three regions. The number of cells per circumference in the crypts in the three regions are 21.2, 20.6 and 19.8 while the number of cells in the vertical column for the three regions are 32.7, 47.4 and 41.7 respectively. The total cellularity of the crypts in these three regions whether determined by the product of the cells per girth × cells per length adjusted for the geometric configuration correction factor (which is related to the packing of the cells) mentioned earlier or whether measured directly from intact crypts optically sectioned in the microscope is around 303, 333 and 450 respectively for the three regions. In the human the mean number of cells per circumference is about 42 in the colon and 46 in the rectum while the number of cells per vertical column is 82 in the colon and 80 in the rectum. These figures suggests that there are about 2000 cells per crypt in the colon and about 2200 cells per crypt in the rectum in man, i.e., the crypts are 2–6 tissues larger in the human large bowel [4]. These figures for the total cellularity in man are similar to values obtained from studies involving whole crypts. The average labelling index in the 3 regions of mouse large bowel are 8.5, 8.2 and 7.7% and the distributions of these S phase cells according to their position in the crypts are somewhat similar for the 3 regions. In all 3 cases the [3]HTdR labelling index figures are high close to the base of the crypt and decline progressively with increasing distance from the base. The maximum labelling index at any given position is 18.2, 19.8 and 21.7 for the 3 positions respectively. These data are consistent with a cell cycle time in the lower regions of the crypt in the mouse large bowel of about 33 h. In the human the curves have a somewhat similar shape to that observed in the human ileum, that is, a clear peak in the labelling index is observed in both the colon and rectum over the range of 10–25 cell positions from the base (Fig. 8). The maximum labelling index in the human is about 29% in the colon and about 22% in the rectum. These figures suggest that in the region of the maximum labelling, the cell cycle time may be of the order of 30 h for the colon and 39 h for the rectum, i.e. values somewhat similar to those in the mouse (Fig. 9).

4. DIFFERENTIATION

Within the epithelium that lines the small and large bowel a variety of different types of epithelial cell can be recognised (different differentiation pathways for the epithelial cells). The bulk of the cells in both the small and large bowel are columnar epithelial cells that are characterised by having a columnar shape with a brush border consisting of micro-villi at the apical surface (Fig. 10) and a nucleus generally located near the basal laminar end of the cell. Generally speaking the nucleus has a spherical to egg-shape or is a flattened oval shape with a smooth surface outline. The cells are relatively rich in mitochondria, possess a good prominent Golgi body, have tight and gap junctions particularly at the apical edge and desmosome and desmosome-like

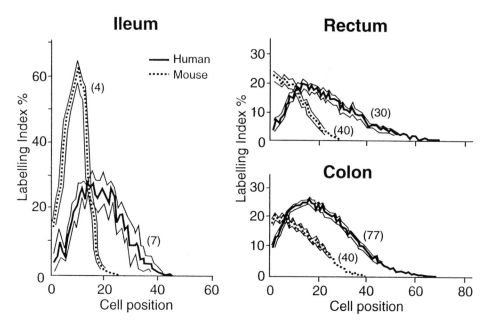

Fig. 8. Cell positional tritiated thymidine (mouse data) and bromodeoxyuridine (human data) labelling index frequency plots for ileum, colon and rectum. (Taken from Ref. [9]).

structures. The second most prominent cell type are the mucus secreting cells or goblet cells (Fig. 3). These are generally flask-shaped cells lacking micro-villi on the surface and having a cytoplasm filled with globular secretory elements. These cells are particularly prominent in the large bowel where their numbers may virtually equal those of the columnar cells (Fig. 11). They secret a range of subtly different types of mucopolysaccharides or mucus. The next most obvious population of cells are the Paneth cells in the small intestine. These are pyramidal shaped cells located in the first 4 or 5 cell positions in the bottom of the small intestinal crypts (Fig. 7). In the mouse they are quite frequent, there may be about 30 of these cells in the base of the crypt [10]. Their numbers per crypt clearly differ from species to species and site to site along the tract and one function that has been attributed to these cells is an antibacterial role. They are characterised by a very prominent endoplasmic reticulum, nuclei that often have indentations and very characteristic granules in the apical regions of the cell that contain lysozyme and are dense to both light and electrons. Scattered amongst the Paneth cells in the base of the crypt are a number of intercalated cells generally of a somewhat spindle shape with long thin nuclei orientated at right angles to the basal membrane. These are either part of the columnar cell population or represent immature stages in the Paneth life history. The final epithelial cell population to be found are the enteroendocrine cells. These are very sparsely distributed with only one or two generally being observed in each longitudinal section through the middle of a crypt. They are

Small Intestine

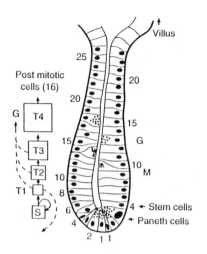

	Mouse	Man
Cells/column	25	34
Cells/circumference	16	22
Cells/crypt	250	450
Cell cycle (h)	12	~33
Stem cell cycle (h)	~24	≥36
Stem cells/crypt	4–16	?
Transit cell generations	4–6	>4–6
Crypts/villus	6–10	~6
Crypts/intestine	$1–3 \times 10^6$	?

Large Intestine

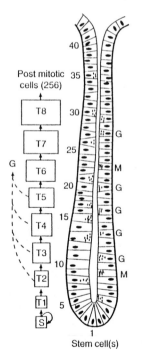

	Mouse	Man
Cells/column	42	82
Cells/circumference	18	46
Cells/crypt	300–450	2250
Cell cycle (h)	~35	~34
Stem cell cycle (h)	≥36	≥36
Stem cells/crypt	1–8?	?
Transit generations	5–9	>5–9

P = Paneth, G = Goblet, M = Mitosis

Fig. 9. Diagram illustrating the section appearance, and cell hierarchy or lineage for small and large intestine together with various numerical parameters taken from a variety of sources (see also Fig. 5).

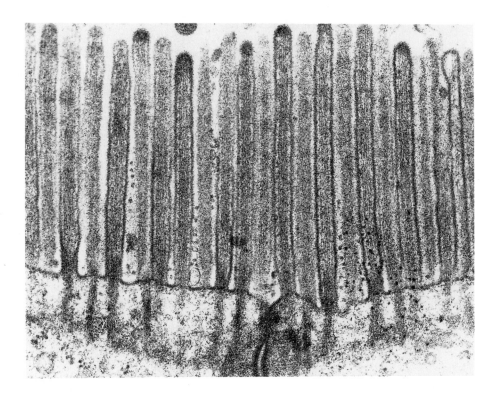

Fig. 10. High power transmission electron micrograph showing the densely packed microvilli on the apical surface of a typical villus epithelial cell. Junctional complexes can be seen in the centre of the base of the picture where two adjacent cells meet. I am grateful to Dr. T. Allen for this picture.

believed to be secretory cells producing a variety of gut hormones, and have an intimate interaction with nerve fibres from outside the crypt. They are believed to secrete a variety of factors or hormones that influence the function and proliferation of the epithelium. Finally as already mentioned the epithelium usually contains a relatively small number of intra-epithelial lymphocytes which tend to be small rounded cells that are insinuated in between the columnar cells generally close to the basal lamina.

5. CIRCADIAN RHYTHMS

As with proliferative cells in most sites of the body those in the intestinal epithelium exhibit daily or circadian (or diurnal) rhythms in proliferative activity (Fig. 12). The consequence of this is that at particular times of day there may be more, or less, cells replicating their DNA or entering mitoses. Throughout the entire gastrointestinal tract from the buccal cavity to the anus the circadian rhythms tend to show their maxima in the early hours of the

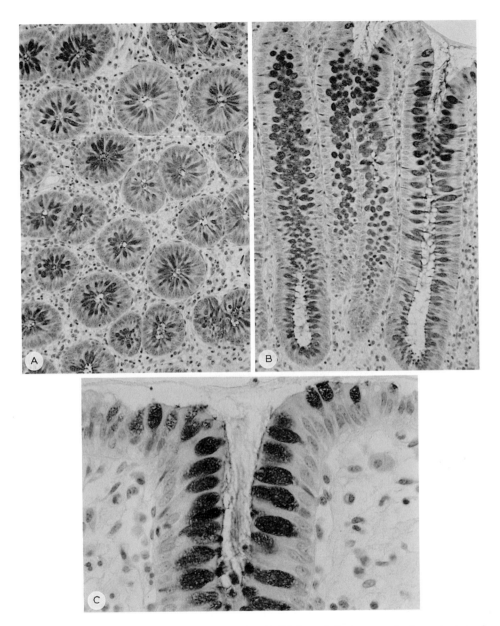

Fig. 11. Sections cut transversely (A) or longitudinally (B) through the human colonic crypts stained with Alcian blue to show the mucus secreting cells. A high power view (C) showing the typical flash-shape of the goblet cells. (See also colour plate on p. xii.)

morning generally between 3 and 6 a.m. In the small intestine the rhythms tend to be very dampened and are sometimes quite hard to detect but in our experience they are a definite phenomenon with the peak in labelling ie, DNA

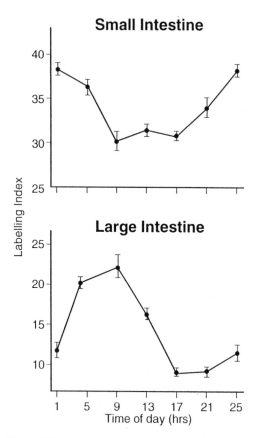

Fig. 12. The circadian rhythm in tritiated thymidine labelling (S phase cells) in the small and large bowel of mice. Peak labelling occurs at about 0100 and 0900 and minimal labelling at about 0900–1700 and 1700–2100 in the small and large bowel respectively. Data from Ref. [8].

synthesis being observed at 3 o'clock with a trough at 1500 hours. The peak in mitotic activity generally follows the peak in labelling by the few hours that represent the G2 phase of the cell cycle. Hence, mitotic peaks in the small bowel tend to be observed between about 4 a.m. and 7 am. However, since mitoses is such a short phase of the cell cycle the rhythms in mitotic activity tend to be more difficult to detect and to precisely define in terms of their peaks and nadirs.

In the large bowel of the mouse the circadian rhythms are much more prominent but the peak and trough times are somewhat similar to those in the small bowel possibly being displaced by up to 3–8 h later in the day. Generally speaking the circadian rhythms show the greatest amplitude when the cells towards the bottom of the crypts are analysed on their own. In regions of the oral cavity some very pronounced circadian rhythms can be detected. An extreme example is the basal cell population at the deepest point in the epithelium lining the dorsal surface of the tongue. Here, the cells are almost totally synchronised by the circadian rhythm with almost all cells in S-phase at 3.00 a.m. and almost non in S-phase at 3.00 p.m. [11].

6. CELL HIERARCHIES AND STEM CELLS

One of the major questions concerning the proliferation and cell replacement processes in the crypt is whether all of the 150 proliferative cells have the same characteristics and perform the same function. Both under normal circumstances and after injury such as radiation. For example, do the cells at the top of the band of proliferation at 15–20 cell positions from the crypt base function in the same manner as those proliferative cells in the first 5 or 6 cell positions; are all of the cells of the crypt proliferative compartment functioning as stem cells or is it only a fraction of the proliferative compartment that functions in this way? It is fairly obvious that the cells at cell position 15–20 under steady state conditions normally will undergo one further mitosis or one more cell cycle before they migrate out of the proliferative compartment. On the other hand cells lower down the crypt may pass through several cell cycles. While cells at the very base of the crypt are unlikely to be in the migratory pathway at all and may divide indefinitely throughout the entire life of the animal. These questions cannot really be considered without first defining what is meant by the term *stem cells*. This is a difficult concept which has been discussed in the literature for a number of years. We have recently reconsidered this whole concept and have reached the following conclusion in terms of the definition [12]. Stem cells are defined by virtue of their functional attributes. This means that one has to look back in the past history of a cell and see what it did in the past or test in some way what its potential might be in the future. This inevitably demands that the cell is manipulated experimentally in order to answer these questions. The second problem with the definition of stem cells is that a variety of adjectives are invariably used to describe the property of these cells and these terms often are open to various interpretations. We would define the stem cell population as relatively undifferentiated cells that are capable of cell cycle progression (proliferation) while at the same time maintaining their own numbers (self-maintenance). They are cells that are capable of producing a large family of more differentiated functional progeny and of regenerating a tissue after injury. Finally, they are clearly cells that have a considerable flexibility from tissue to tissue and context to context in the operation of these functional capabilities. Ideally in order to categorise a cell as a stem cell all of these properties should be satisfied. In practice this is unrealistic and so one tends to rely on some of these attributes in order for identification. This is dangerous because some of these characteristics are much weaker than others. A further point that needs to be borne in mind in relation to defining stem cells is that there may be cells that satisfy some, or many, of these criteria under normal steady state conditions which we would define as *actual* stem cells, however there may be other cells that do not satisfy these criteria under steady state conditions but can assume stem cell properties under abnormal or perturbed situations and we would call these *potential* stem cells. It is fairly clear from the discussion already that the concept, definition and identification of stem cells is likely to be very context dependent — different answers would be obtained to the question of how many stem cells exist in a tissue, depending on whether one is considering: steady state circumstances in different tissues; injured states; *in vivo* situations or *in vitro* situations; one animal system or another animal system, or even plant systems. It is conceivable also that the answer to the question will be strongly influenced by which of the criteria mentioned in the definition of stem cells one accepts under a particular set of circumstances. Proliferation *per se* is probably the weakest of the criteria that can be attributed to stem cells hence the use of this to identify stem cells on its own is not likely to be very effective. Similarly the simple fact of being relatively undifferentiated is also a weak criteria. Differentiation is a qualitative relative term that defines a particular state of genetic expression of a cell relative to another cell. We have defined *differentiation* as a qualitative change in the cellular phenotype that is the consequence of the onset of synthesis of new gene products, i.e. the non-cyclic new changes in gene expression that lead ultimately to functional competence. It is often recognised by a change in morphology of the cell or by the appearance of, or changes in, enzyme activity or protein composition. Since it is qualitative a cell can only be said to be differentiated relative to another and may be capable of undergoing many differentiated events. It is commonly identified by the detection of novel proteins (these days usually utilising monoclonal antibodies) and the ability therefore to detect a cell as differentiated clearly depends on the sensitivity of the detection procedures. Although a detection approach may ultimately be capable of identifying the first few differentiation molecules synthesised the theoretical initial step in the differentiation process involved mRNA synthesis (translation) and even earlier DNA repression and transcription. In this connection it is probably worth noting that an alternative term "maturation" is commonly used in a somewhat interchangeable way with differentiation. However, we have recently defined *maturation* more strictly as being a quantitative change in the cellular phenotype or the cellular constituent proteins that lead to functional competence. The degree of maturation could therefore in principle be measured on a quantitative scale for example, the weight of a specific protein per cell. So a differentiated cell matures with the passage of time to form a functionally competent cell and during its maturation new differentiation events could occur.

    The strongest terms that define and characterise stem cells are self-maintenance, the ability to vary self-maintenance, the ability to produce a large family of differentiated descendants and the ability to regenerate the tissue or elements of the tissue following injury (by extensive cell division often from an isolated surviving stem cell which means that the progeny represent a clone and the parent cell can be called a clonogenic cell). These terms are amenable to experimental analyses. One can test a cell (or more correctly a group of cells) to see whether it, or they, are capable of maintaining its or their own numbers over a period of time by asking the question, have more cells like the parent cell been made by a subcloning experiment *in vitro* or a repeated insult experiment *in vivo*. Similarly one can test to see whether a particular cell is capable of producing a large progeny of differentiated cells or even a range of differentiated cell types. The question of whether a cell is capable of regenerating a tissue after injury involves somewhat similar experimental situations. Self-maintenance means to keep the population at an existing state or level in terms of cell numbers and it is common practice to consider the stem cell population in terms of the probability of self-maintenance P_{sm}. Stem cells make up a populations of cells with P_{sm} values that are either constantly greater than 0.5 in which case the population is expanding in size or have a P_{sm} value that is equal to 0.5 as observed in steady state circumstances. Clearly if the population of stem cells increases in size to a situation that represents an excess of cells to requirements for a particular tissue the P_{sm} value for the population may temporarily reduce to less than 0.5 in which case some stem cells die or leave or are forced out of the stem cell compartment which shrinks back to the required numbers.

For a system like the intestinal crypt it is clear that cells in the upper region of the crypt neither satisfy the requirements for self-maintenance nor do they satisfy the requirements for producing a large progeny of differentiated cells and therefore are poor candidates to be considered as stem cells. However, they are clearly cells that are capable of division. They are cells also that are obviously in transit from the proliferative state to the functional state and physically in transit from the crypt to the villus and therefore can be referred to as transit cells. Since they are capable of division they can be called *dividing transit cells*. We can ask one further question about these cells and that is whether they are capable of regenerating the tissue after injury. This can be done by appropriately designed radiation or drug experiments. The results of these experiments will be discussed in greater detail in other parts of this text (Chapter 3) but suffice to say here that the experimental data indicate that the bulk of these cells do not possess the ability to regenerate the epithelium after injury.

There is one final complication in terms of stem cell concepts and that refers to the frame size that is being considered either in terms of number of cells or in terms of time. Questions regarding stem cells are more easily dealt with on a population basis than an individual cell basis. An individual cell may divide to produce two cells and the answer as to whether self-maintenance has been achieved may require the identification of which of the two new cells represents the maintenance of the original cell — a difficult concept. It is also intimately linked with questions involving the mode of differentiation and whether stem cells divide symmetrically or asymmetrically and whether differentiation occurs at random within the population or is intrinsically controlled. Similar problems arise with regard to the size of the time frame being considered. A cell may divide asymmetrically and maintain its number for one division but at the next division both daughters may differentiate. If the time frame involved in analyses in only the first division a different answer is obtained to that when two divisions are considered. As a consequence of this it is easier to consider the stem cell question in relation to populations of cells and long time scales.

One of the properties of stem cells is that they can produce progeny that undergo differentiation events and eventually become functionally competent cells within a tissue. Most tissues contain a range of differentiated cell types which may originate from a common compartment of stem cells. The limit to the differentiation potential for individual stem cells is at present unclear and may well differ from tissue to tissue. The ability to produce progeny that differentiate down various different lineages (pluripotency) is not necessarily a property of stem cells *per se* although it does appear that many stem cells possess this capability. The precise mechanisms that initiate differentiation remain obscure. It is unclear whether cell divisions are needed in order for sequential differentiation events to be expressed. However, we have recently suggested that the larger (longer) the dividing transit population the more differentiation options may be open. Thus in a tissue like bone marrow a large degree of pluripotency exists and this may be related to the large number of divisions in the transit population.

One further question that is often raised with regard to stem cells is the question of their rate of progression through the cell cycle: their cell cycle time. There is no reason *per se* why stem cells should cycle more slowly than their transit progeny, but in practice this is often the case. There are some arguments in favour of slow cycling as a method of minimising the genetic risks associated with DNA replication and mitosis. In the intestine the data available suggest that the stem cells have a cell cycle time approximately twice as long as the dividing transit cells [6]. In one site in the oral cavity, the tongue, the stem cells and the transit cells have the same cell cycle time.

Having discussed these problems associated with the concept of stem cells one must now address the question of how this relates to the gastrointestinal tract. Most work here has been done on small intestinal crypts with some studies in colonic epithelium. However, if we consider the stratified epithelium in the mouth and oesophagus it is clear that the proliferative cells reside somewhere in the lowest stratum, the basal layer but, with the exception of the dorsal surface of the tongue, little information is available concerning the question of whether all cells in the basal layer are proliferative and whether all are stem cells. In the dorsal surface of the tongue the basal layer undulates and the migration pathways of cells along and away from the basal layer have been mapped. Such studies allow one to identify the cells at the origin of the migratory pathways namely the cells that satisfy the criteria of self-maintenance and the criteria of the production of a long number of progeny over a large period of time. Such cells are few in number and are located in the lower regions of the epidermal projection into the dermis [13]. Such studies suggest that stratified epithelia are heterogeneous and that the stem cell population makes up only a small fraction (probably about 10%) of the basal cells. A conclusion that has also been drawn for another epithelial region the epidermis of skin. It would seem reasonable to assume that a similar type of proliferative organisation or heterogeneity exists in those areas where migration pathways have not yet been, or cannot be, mapped in the same fashion, for example, oesophagus.

In the long thin glandular structures in the stomach limited studies have indicated that the cells from which the rest of the gland is replaced are located at a particular position along the length of the gland. The precise position varies somewhat depending on the location in the stomach but tends to be towards the middle of the gland or nearer the surface. This indicates that in this region of the epithelium there is considerable movement of cells and differentiation down the gland towards its base and that there must be senescent cell death and cell loss from the lower regions of the crypt/gland as well as up the gland towards the surface.

Considerable work has been done over the last 50 years studying cell replacement in the small intestinal crypt particularly in the mouse. The conclusions reached by most workers is that a hierarchy with stem cells and dividing transit cells most effectively explains all the data on cell proliferation and cell replacement. The earliest evidence for such an hierarchy derived from ingenious experiments where phagosomes of ingested fragments of dead cells labelled with tritiated thymidine were initially observed near the crypt base and these phagosomes were then used as a cytoplasmic marker to track the differentiation and turnover (replacement time) of the various crypt cell populations [14].

The first four or five cell positions from the base of the flask-shaped crypt contain a mixture of about 30 Paneth cells and 10–15 thin columnar intercalated (or crypt base columnar) cells and a circumferential ring of about 16 columnar cells sitting on top of the highest Paneth cells. It is clear that the Paneth cells satisfy none of the criteria for stem cells but it has been suggested that the intercalated cells may perform a stem cell function. However, in our view the biggest problem with the idea that the intercalated cells are the actual stem cells of the crypt concerns the geometric and spatial organisation of cells in this region of the crypt. The Paneth cells tend to be large pyramid shaped cells with a large surface area attached to the basal lamina. If the intercalated cells divide to produce progeny that ultimately are going to migrate up the crypt their daughters would have to undergo some complex migratory patterns to circumvent the Paneth cells. Two other minor pieces of evidence argue against this concept. Firstly, it is extremely rare to see a pair of adjacent intercalated cells or non-Paneth cells and finally, division of intercalated cells does not result in the vertical displacement of the Paneth cells. Although far from conclusive, these arguments do suggest that whatever the function of the intercalated cells they do not constitute the actual stem cells of the crypt. In our view it is more likely that they are part of the Paneth cell lineage or serve some other function. They are unlikely to be a reserve population of quiescent stem cells since they are clearly in the process of cell cycle progression, ie, can be labelled with [3]HTdR [10].

A range of cell kinetic studies including detailed cell migration pathway analyses [8] suggests that the cells from which all other upper crypt and villus cells are derived are located at about the 4th position from the base of the crypt in the small intestine and at the very base of the crypt in the mid-colon, that is, the position immediately above the highest Paneth cell in the small intestine. Detailed mathematical modelling of the three-dimensional architecture and temporal patterns of cell replacement also suggest that the crypt is ultimately dependent upon a few cells near the crypt base. Such studies suggest that the actual stem cells are located within the ring of about 16 circumferential cells that are positioned, on average, 4 cells from the base of the crypt. It is not entirely clear whether all 16 of these cells represent stem cells or whether it is only some fraction of the 16 that satisfy all the criteria of stemness. In principle the number of stem cells at this 4th position could be anything from 1–16. For various reasons that are discussed below our current view is that the most likely number of stem cells per crypt is about 4 and that these are situated in the ring of 16 cells at cell position 4.

It is important to realise that this 4th position is an average value and not a simple ring circumventing the crypt at that position. It is determined by the Paneth cell distribution and this distribution is quite irregular. In some sections through the crypt the highest Paneth cell might be at the second position while in other sections the highest Paneth cell might be at the 5th or 6th position or even the 7th cell position. In these cases the stem cells will be located at the 3rd or the 6–8th respectively. Thus the stem cell position 4 is an irregular ring that waves between about the 3rd and 8th position as it goes round the crypt.

Studies with mouse embryo aggregation chimeras and *Dolichos biflorus* lectin binding to visualise a mosaic staining pattern [15,16] and similar studies using F1 mice that are heterozygous for the alleles that determine this lectin binding in conjunction with the application of various mutagens [17,18] have led to the suggestion that the crypts might contain a single actual stem cell. Although this is still a possible scenario for the crypt its confirmation awaits further experimental analyses [19]. The idea that the crypt contains a single stem cell poses certain problems. Firstly, there is the topographical question of where such a stem cell should be located. If it is placed near the base of the crypt amongst the Paneth cells the same considerations arise that were discussed in relation to the intercalated cells. Namely why are doublets and runs of intercalated cells not observed and why are Paneth cells not displaced and how do the stem cell progeny migrate between the Paneth cell population? If the single stem cell is placed in the ring of cells at the 4th position it is hard to see how an asymmetry in overall cell proliferation within the crypt is avoided. Since the progeny from that stem cell would have to spread both laterally and vertically. This could not be achieved without asymmetry of proliferation if there are a fixed number of dividing transit cells or a precise cut-off point in the crypt in terms of cell proliferation. However, it could be compensated for by having a flexible number of dividing transit cells. These points have to be considered in relation to the observed patterns of distribution of labelled cells within the crypt as a whole. These distributions tend to have a relatively steep leading edge and one of the possible consequences of having a single stem cell per crypt is that the leading edge of these distributions would be considerably more spread than is actually observed. The final problem associated with a single stem cell concerns the question of how rapidly it proliferates. Part of the explanation for the chimaeric mouse and mutation studies with lectin binding requires that the stem cell has an extremely long cell cycle. This is hard to reconcile with the observed cell cycle data for the crypt. Unless some unusual cell kinetic characteristics are attributed to the early part of the cell lineage a single slow cycling stem cell would result in large fluctuations in the proliferative compartment of the crypt which is not observed. Finally, mathematical modelling studies have shown that the lectin binding results can in fact be quite adequately explained on the basis of mutations occurring in one out of a population of several stem cells which usually divide asymmetrically but occasionally divide symmetrically [20]. Thus, although the idea of a single stem cell cannot be rejected at the moment our view is that it is less likely than the existence of a few (say four) actual stem cells per crypt.

There are indications from a variety of different experiments that the actual stem cells of the crypt are capable of producing all four differentiated cell lineages within the crypt (columnar, goblet, Paneth and enteroendocrine cells), i.e. they possess an element of pluripotency for differentiation. The evidence comes from detailed histological studies of radioactively marked cells and a knowledge of the turnover time of the four cell lineages [14] and from irradiation studies where all four differentiated cell lineages are observed in clones derived from a single surviving potential stem cell [21]. In some cases here the clonality can be confirmed by using appropriate X-linked enzyme markers in heterozygous F1 mice and by the use of appropriate transgenic animals.

The final evidence concerning stem cells in the crypt comes from radiation studies. These will be presented in detail in subsequent sections of this report. However, they are summarised here in the context of the stem cell question. It is possible using irradiation to reproducibly sterilise all the cells but one in a crypt. If the last surviving cell has the ability to produce a large number of progeny and maintain the life of the crypt for a significant period of time the cell can be considered as satisfying the stem cell criteria. Since the surviving crypt in this case derives from a single surviving (stem) cell the crypt can be regarded as a clone of cells (see Fig. 13) and the originator cell as a clonogenic cell. Such experiments can be done and the number of crypts surviving a given treatment with radiation or drugs counted on the 3rd or 4th day after treatment. This is a time sufficient for crypts with no surviving regenerative cells to disappear but those with one or more surviving regenerative cells to form a recognisable focus of regeneration. These foci have a crypt morphology (Fig. 13) and the technique has become known as the *microcolony* or crypt survival assay [22,23]. An alternative assay involves waiting for a longer period of time 14–20 days when the foci of regeneration grow even bigger and become visible to the naked eye and this has become known as the *macrocolony* assay [24,25]. The latter is technically much more restrictive and so many experiments have been done using the microcolony approach. The number of microcolonies can be counted following various doses of radiation to generate a crypt survival curve (Fig. 14) which, using Poisson statistics, can be converted to a regenerative cell, or clonogenic cell, or potential stem cell survival curve (Fig. 14 and Ref. [30]).

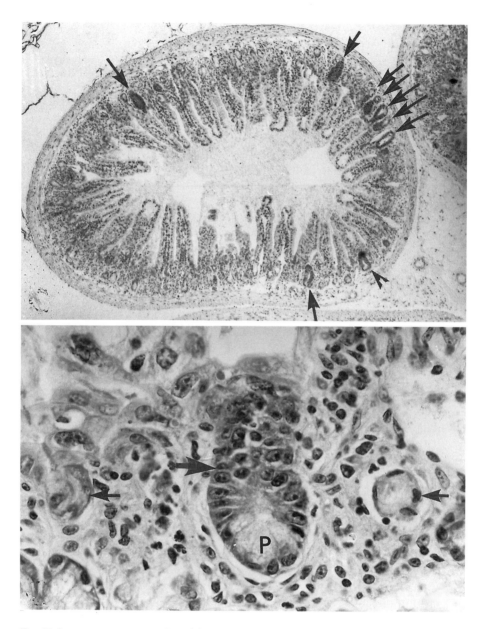

Fig. 13. Lower power cross section of the small bowel (upper panel) three days after a high dose of radiation. Regenerative foci (arrows) can be seen. The lower panel shows a higher power view of one regenerative focus (crypt, large arrow) and various degenerating crypts (small arrows).

An analysis of the shoulder of the crypt survival curve or more recently a comparison of the survival ratios after one or two doses of radiation have been used to provide information on the number of clonogenic or potential stem cells

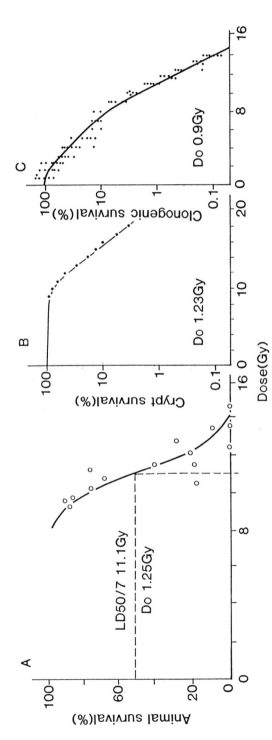

Fig. 14. A typical crypt survival curve (panel B) is shown together with the survival curve for the clonogenic cells (panel C) derived from the crypt survival data using Poisson statistics [33]. Panel A shows the survival curve for mice assessed on the 7th day after irradiation. Animal survival depends on crypt survival which is determined by clonogenic cell survival.

per crypt (see Chapter 3). Initially these studies indicated that less than half of the proliferative cells possessed a clonogenic potential. However, using the two-dose approach this estimate of the number of clonogenic cells per crypt is lower. In 1987 the results of a series of experiments suggested that the number of clonogenic cells per crypt may be about 32 which represents two annuli of cells in the circumference [26]. This concept was biologically acceptable since it implied that the actual stem cells which may occupy one annulus and the daughters of these actual stem cells, the first dividing transit populations which would be located in the immediately adjacent distal annulus may also function as stem cells when the tissue is severely damaged. Recent estimates using low energy beta irradiation at the bases of the crypts showed that clonogenic cells are not likely to be located in the upper crypt region [27]. The crypt can be sterilised merely by irradiating the lower regions of the crypt. These studies provided dose response curves that are most compatible with a model assuming a very small number of clonogenic cells (about three per crypt, ie, essentially the same number as the number of actual stem cells). Analyses of various drug dose response curves also suggest very few clonogenic cells per crypt, perhaps as few as one per crypt [28,29] However, there are questions relating to the validity of applying the same assumptions and interpretation to

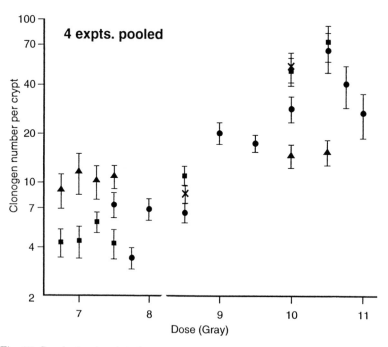

Fig. 15. Graph showing data from 4 experiments where the variation in the number of clonogenic cells per crypt with increasing radiation dose (level of cytotoxic damage) have been estimated using the split dose technique [32]. The data fall into 2 distinct categories: estimates determined with doses below 9 Gy and those using dose of 9 Gy or above. Taken from Ref. [31].

drugs as to the radiation experiments. More recent analyses of new experiments using split doses of radiation of various sizes suggested that the number of clonogens per crypt may be influenced by the dose of radiation used to assay the clonogens. The higher the dose the greater the number of clonogens that are estimated. The actual data suggested that for doses less than 9 Gy the number of clonogenic cells per crypt is about 6 (very similar to the estimates of the number of actual steady-state stem cells) while using doses greater than 9 Gy provided values of up to 30–40 clonogenic cells per crypt (Fig. 15 and Ref. [31]). The explanation for this might be that with increasing levels of damage more and more cells are forced or recruited into the clonogenic compartment. Such studies would suggest that if the true number of *potential* stem cells per crypt is to be determined then the answer should be calculated from experiments where the highest dose of radiation has been delivered while if the number of *actual* or *functional* stem cells is to be estimated the best approach would be to use small doses of radiation. All of these calculations have been performed using some fairly basic assumptions and a simple mathematical approach. They result in a series of independent estimates each of which tends to have a fairly large error limit and when the means of these individual estimates are determined the error limits are still quite large.

In conclusion, the studies on the number of clonogens have provided estimates of their numbers per crypt that have been steadily declining with increasing years concomitant with the use of more appropriate techniques and analyses. The best estimate to date is that the number of clonogens per crypt is small probably comparable to our estimate of the number of actual stem cells when low levels of injury are induced (small doses), but that up to about 30–40 cells can be recruited into the clonogenic pool when the level of injury is high. If the number of potential stem cells or clonogens equals the number of actual stem cells then there is no distinction between these two categories of cells.

The situation in the colon is far less clear. Radiation survival curves suggest from their shape that the number of stem cells per crypt is likely to be small. Topographical considerations would permit a single stem cell, or a small number of stem cells, to be located at the base of each individual colonic crypt since there are no Paneth cells complicating the migration pathway. Whether topographical considerations could distinguish between a single apical stem cell at the base of the crypt and approximately four apical stem cells is unlikely. There are mutation assays that have been performed in the colon using X-linked enzyme markers in female F1 mice which indicated that a mutation in the single allele on the X chromosome resulted over a period of about 14 days in a crypt that uniformly expressed the changed pattern i.e. a monophenotypic or monoclonal crypt [32]. This observation has been interpreted as indicating that each crypt is derived from a single cell, i.e. there is one stem cell per crypt, but this may not be conclusive for the reasons discussed earlier.

Mathematical modelling has shown that the patterns of labelling and mitoses in the colonic crypt could be explained on the basis of a single stem cell with about eight generations of dividing transit cells, in contrast to the four stem cells and six generations observed in the small intestine. However, such modelling exercises do not prove that the number of stem cells per crypt is one because the data could equally be modelled with several stem cells. Split-dose clonogenic assays in the colon have provided estimates for the number of potential stem cells or clonogenic cells at around 8–10 per crypt. In summary (see Fig. 9), it looks as if the colonic crypts although larger in both size and the number of proliferative cells may have about the same number of actual and potential stem cells, or perhaps even slightly fewer than occur in the small intestine.

References

1. Wright, N. and Alison, M. (1984) The Biology of Epithelial Cell Populations, Vol. 2. Clarendon Press, Oxford, pp. 537–870.
2. Potten, C.S. and Hendry, J.H. (1983) Stem cells in murine small intestine. In: C.S. Potten (Ed.), Stem Cells: Their Identification and Characterisation. Churchill Livingstone, Edinburgh, pp. 155–199.
3. Potten, C.S., Hendry, J.H., Moore, J.V. and Chwalinski, S. (1983) Cytotoxic effects in gastrointestinal epithelium (as exemplified by small intestine). In: C.S. Potten and J.H. Hendry (Eds.), Cytotoxic Insult to Tissue. Churchill Livingstone, Edinburgh, pp. 105–152.
4. Kellett, M., Potten, C.S. and Rew, D.A. (1992) A comparison of in vivo cell proliferation measurements in the intestine of mouse and man. Epithel. Cell Biol. 1: 147–155.
5. Potten, C.S. (1990) A comprehensive study of the radiobiological response of the murine (BDF1) small intestine. Int. J. Radiat. Biol. 58: 925–974.
6. Potten, C.S. (1986) Cell cycles in cell hierarchies. Int. J. Radiat. Biol. 49: 257–278.
7. Potten, C.S., Roberts, S.A., Chwalinski, S., Loeffler, M. and Paulus, U. (1988) The reliability in scoring mitotic activity in longitudinal crypts of the small sections of intestine. Cell. Tissue Kinet. 21: 231–246.
8. Qiu, J.M., Roberts, S.A. and Potten, C.S. (1994) Cell migration in the small and large bowel shows a strong circadian rhythm. Epith. Cell Biol. 3: 138–148.
9. Potten, C.S., Kellett, M., Roberts, S.A. and Rew, D.A. (1992) The measurement of *in vivo* proliferation in human gastrointestinal epithelium using bromodeoxyuridine: data on different sites, proximity to a tumour and polyposis coli patients. Gut 33: 524–529.
10. Chwalinski, S. and Potten, C.S. (1989) Crypt base columnar cells: their numbers and cell kinetics in BDF1 male mice. Am. J. Anat. 186: 397–406.
11. Hume, W.J. and Potten, C.S. (1976) The ordered columnar structure of mouse filiform papillae. J. Cell Sci. 22: 149–160.
12. Potten, C.S. and Loeffler, M. (1990) Stem cells: attributes, cycles, spirals, uncertainties and pitfalls: lessons for and from the crypt. Development 110: 1001–1019.
13. Miller, S.J., Lavker, R.M. and Sun, T.T. (1993) Keratinocyte stem cells of cornea, skin and hair follicles: common and distinguishing features. Sem. Develop. Biol. 4: 217–240.
14. Cheng, H. and Leblond, C.P. (1974) Origin, differentiation and renewal of the four main epithelial cell types in the mouse small intestine. V. Unitarian theory of the origin of the four epithelial cell types. Am. J. Anat. 141: 537–562.
15. Ponder, B.A.J., Schmidt, G.H., Wilkinson, M.M., Wood, M.J., Monk, M. and Reid,

A. (1985) Derivation of mouse intenstinal crypts from single progenitor cells. Nature 313: 689–691.

16. Schmidt, G.H., Winton, D.J. and Ponder, B.A.J. (1988) Development of the pattern of cell renewal in the crypt villus unit of chimaeric mouse small intestine. Development 103: 785–790.

17. Winton, D.J., Blount, M.A. and Ponder, B.A.J. (1988) A clonal marker induced by mutation in mouse intestinal epithelium. Nature, 33: 463–466.

18. Winton, D.J. and Ponder, B.A.J. (1990) Stem cell organisation in mouse small intestine. Proc. Roy. Soc. London, 241: 13–18.

19. Winton, D.J. (1993) Mutation induced clonal markers from polymorphia loci: application to stem cell organisation in the mouse intestine. Sem. Develop. Biol. 4, 293–302.

20. Loeffler, M., Birke, A., Winton, D. and Potten, C.S. (1993) Somatic mutation, monoclonality and stochastic models of stem cell organisation in the intestinal crypt. J. Theoret. Biol., 160: 471–491.

21. Inoue, M., Imada, M., Fukushima, Y., Matsumura, N., Shiozaki, H., Mori, T., Kitamura, Y. and Fujita, H. (1988) Macroscopic intestinal colonies of mice as a tool for studying differentiation of multipotential intestinal stem cells. Am. J. Path. 132: 49–58.

22. Withers and Elkind, M.M. (1970) Microcolony survival assay for cells of mouse intestinal mucosa exposed to irradiation. Int. J. Radiat. Biol., 17: 261–267.

23. Potten, C.S. and Hendry, J.H. (1985) Introduction. In: C.S. Potten and J.H. Hendry (Eds.), Cell Clones: Manual of Mammalian Cell Techniques. Churchill Livingstone, Edinburgh. pp. ix–xi.

24. Withers, H.R. and Elkind, M.M. (1968) Dose survival characteristics of epithelial cells of mouse intestinal mucosa. Radiology 91: 998–1000.

25. Withers, H.R. and Elkind, M.M. (1969) Radiosensitivity and fractionation response of crypt cells in mouse jejunal. Radiat. Res. 38: 598–613.

26. Potten, C.S., Hendry, J.H. and Moore, J.V. (1987) New estimates of the number of clonogenic cells in crypts of murine small intestine. Virchow Arch. B Cell Path. 53: 227–234.

27. Hendry, J.H., Potten, C.S., Ghafoor, A. and Moore, J.V. (1989) The response of murine crypts to inhomogeneous [147]Pm-irradiation: deductions of clonogenic cell numbers and positions. Radiat. Res. 118: 364–374.

28. Moore, J.V. (1979) Ablation of murine jejunal crypts by alkylating agents. Br. J. Cancer 39: 175–181.

29. Moore, J.V. and Broadbent, D.A. (1980) Survival of intestinal crypts after treatment by adriamycin alone or with radiation. Br. J. Cancer 42: 692–696.

30. Hendry, J.H., Potten, C.S. and Roberts, N.P. (1983) The gastrointestinal syndrome and mucosal clonogenic cells relationship between target cell sensitivities, LD_{50} and cell survival, and their modification by antibodies. Radiat. Res. 96: 100–112.

31. Hendry, J.H., Roberts, S.A. and Potten, C.S. (1992) The clonogen content of murine intestinal crypts: dependence on radiation dose used in its determination. Radiat. Res. 132: 115–119.

32. Griffiths, D.F.R., Davies, S.J., Williams, D., Williams, G.T. and Williams, E.D. (1988) Demonstration of somatic mutation and colonic crypt clonality by x-linked enzyme histochemistry. Nature 333: 461–463.

33. Hendry, J.H. (1979) A new derivation, from split-dose data, of the complete survival curve for clonogenic normal cells *in vivo*. Radiat. Res. 78: 404–414.

C.S. Potten and J.H. Hendry (Eds.), *Radiation and Gut*

CHAPTER 2

Radiation Sources, Geometry, Exposure Schedules, and Effect Quantitation for Irradiation of the Gut

J.H. Hendry

CRC Department of Experimental Radiation Oncology, Paterson Institute for Cancer Research, Christie Hospital NHS Trust, Wilmslow Road, Manchester M20 9BX, UK

1. RADIATION SOURCES

Radiations which damage the gastrointestinal tract comprise those which penetrate from outside the body, and those which are emitted from ingested radionuclides. The former comprise photon beams in the form of γ-rays (emitted from decaying radio-isotopes) and X-rays (their machine-made equivalent) which have photon energies greater than around 30 keV, as well as high energy particulate radiations in the form of electrons, protons, or neutrons. Ingested radionuclides may emit γ-rays, β-particles (electrons) or α-particles with characteristic energies. β particles have short ranges and hence they have to be fairly well dispersed in high activity around the serosal surfaces in order to damage regions of the GI tract. Further details of the physics of ionizing radiation in relation to biological systems can be found in other texts (e.g., see Ref. [1]).

In radiotherapy, external exposures are usually delivered using megavoltage X-rays, as well as γ-rays, electrons and occasionally protons or neutrons. High energy X-rays have the advantage of deep penetration as well as a build-up region giving 'skin sparing'. Electrons do not show the latter and hence are used generally for specific skin treatments. High energy protons have the characteristic of a 'Bragg peak', so that their energy deposition is concentrated at a particular depth of penetration. Neutrons do not show 'skin sparing' nor a 'Bragg peak'. They were used in radiotherapy to provide a more-densely ionising form of radiation, where the biological effects were less influenced by the chemical and biological milieu of the irradiated cells. However, their use has declined because of the lack of evidence of their expected benefits compared to photons. The density of ionisations is usually quantified using the term linear energy transfer (LET), which is the rate of deposition of energy per unit length of track, usually expressed as keV per μm.

Doses are quantified in terms of absorbed energy per unit mass, and 1 joule per kg is the unit called the gray (Gy). The official "Systeme Internationale" of Units (SI) recognises Gy and mGy, but cGy is a very commonly used alternative because it is identical to the old unit, the rad. When different qualities of radiation are used, i.e., radiations with different values of LET, they often have different efficiencies in causing biological damage. This is described by their RBE (relative biological effectiveness), which is the ratio of the doses of low and high LET radiation causing the same effect. For radiation protection purposes the RBE is taken into account using a Quality Factor (QF) so that doses in Gy are converted into biologically equivalent doses (in Sievert, Sv) of another radiation type using $Sv = QF \times Gy$.

Following any build-up region, photons, electrons, and neutrons are attenuated in tissues in an approximately exponential fashion due to scattering interactions which are characteristic of the energies of the beam and the scattering medium.

Depth dose distributions are shown in Fig. 1 for a variety of radiation qualities. These are expressed as percentages of maximum tissue–air ratios, independent of the inverse-square law, and measured for large radiotherapy fields (>20 cm × 20 cm) and source-to-surface distances (SSD) greater than or equal to 40 cm. No ideal comparison exists wherein a full range of radiation qualities has been used with the same large field size and the same SSD. Hence the curves shown in Fig. 1 would change slightly, depending on the particular irradiation set-up. For 3 MV X-rays, the highest energy considered, the surface dose for well-collimated beams and short SSD is between 40 and 50% of the maximum dose. For low energies and non-collimated beams, the surface dose is a greater percentage of the maximum dose. With non-collimated beams and very long SSD, the surface dose may be equal to the maximum dose. For fission neutrons, a significant build-up effect would be unlikely. For experimental purposes, small animals are usually irradiated under conditions of full build-up, i.e., full secondary charged particle equilibrium. Guidelines for such exposures are available, e.g., EULEP [2].

2. EXPOSURE GEOMETRY

Doses to the GI tract depend upon the direction of the beam with respect to the body, because of the exponential decline in dose with depth in tissue. Hence, doses to the gut of large animals will be less in those accidental situations where exposure is from the top of the head downwards rather than from the side of the body. Calculations have been made of the dose in the human abdomen when radiation of different energy is delivered from the back, the front, or all round [3]. These intestinal doses are shown in Fig. 2. Such doses may not accurately predict the overall response of the gut, for several reasons. Firstly, because of the approximate exponential relationship between cell survival and dose, irradiation of a cell population with a non-uniform dose is

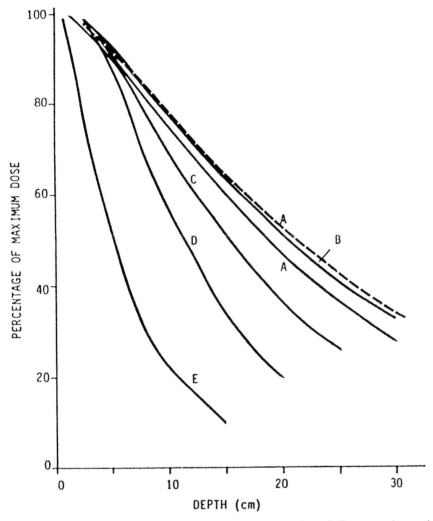

Fig. 1. Depth dose curves for different radiation qualities [24,25]. Data are tissue–air ratios (corrected for the inverse-square law) expressed as a percent of the maximum dose:

	Radiation type	SSD (cm)	Field size (cm × cm)
Curve A	^{60}Co γ rays	80	20 × 20 and 35 × 35
Curve B	4 MV X-rays	Infinite	20 × 20 or 35 × 35
Curve C	^{137}Cs γ rays	40	20 × 20
Curve D	230 kVp X-rays	50	20 × 20
Curve E	^{235}U fission neutrons	500	6 × 8

always less effective than a homogeneous irradiation with the average dose of the distribution [4]. Secondly, early reactions depend on the area of intestinal mucosa irradiated to varying doses, but for late reactions a high dose to a short segment may produce a fistula or stenosis [5], probably irrespective of the dose

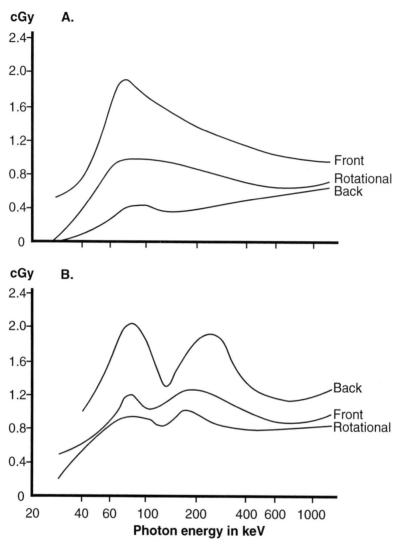

Fig. 2. (A) The dose to the human intestine from an exposure in air of 2.58×10^{-4} C kg^{-1} (previously = 1 röentgen) when exposed from the front, the back, or from all sides (rotational). Doses measured at 3 cm depth from the front body surface, and at 18 cm from the back body surface of a phantom. (B) Doses measured similarly for the same exposure level at the usual film body site on the front surface of the trunk. Redrawn from Ref. [3].

to the remainder. Thirdly, with neutron irradiation, a large part of the dose to small animals from neutrons is from charged particles, whereas with large body masses neutron capture reactions dilute the dose from charged particles with dose from less-efficient knock-on protons.

The calculation of doses delivered at low dose rate from ingested or injected radionuclides which emit short-range irradiation has the additional difficulty of estimating the distance of the isotopes from the target cells. Experiments in dogs indicated a value of $LD_{50/8}$ (death of 50% in 8 days) corresponding, to 130 MBq per kg body weight of [106]Ru-[106]Rh, which delivered approximately 40 Gy to the mucosa over about 18 hours [6]. Comparisons were made of doses from [147]Pm or [106]Ru-[106]Rh resulting in death from GI injury. These isotopes have widely differing β energies, and it was calculated that a dose of 35 Gy of either isotope to the crypt cells resulted in the death of 50% of the dogs [7]. Values of 35 up to 40 Gy in these experiments with dogs are compatible with similar doses of multifractionated external irradiations in man considered to be tolerance doses [8]. Also in a detailed study of short range [147]Pm irradiation from an isotopic plaque placed against the intestinal wall, it was shown that the crypt survival curve was compatible with the low LET response of around 3 stem cells per crypt situated at cell position 4 from the crypt base [9].

3. EXPOSURE SCHEDULES

Doses received in accidents can be due either to single acute or protracted exposures. Doses from the A-bombs at Hiroshima and Nagasaki in World War II were almost totally γ-rays delivered acutely. The Marshall Islanders received fall-out irradiation from the late A-bomb tests amounting to about 1.75 Gy, delivered at about 0.055 Gy per hour at the start of irradiation declining to about 0.016 Gy per hour after 50 hours [10].

Some other accidents have been more protracted. For example in the radiation accident in Mexico City in 1962, the highest exposed individual received 3 Gy per day for 2 days, and 0.25 Gy per day for a further 17 days [11]. The lowest exposed individual received 1 Gy over 106 days at 0.09–0.16 Gy per day.

In the radiotherapy of abdominal malignancies the doses and schedules are very varied. Examples are 15–20 Gy delivered in daily fractions of 1–2 Gy [12], 30–40 Gy in daily fractions of 1–1.5 Gy over 5 weeks [13] or 2 Gy fractions to a total of 45–55 Gy midline dose [14]. In earlier total body radiotherapy for disseminated disease, some treatments were delivered as 0.015–0.20 Gy per day (at the stomach) for 30 days or more [15].

4. EFFECT QUANTITATION

In order to calculate what doses delivered singly at high-dose-rate, fractionated, or at low-dose-rate are equivalent in terms of effect, the biologically-based linear quadratic model is now generally preferred compared to earlier more empirical models [16]. This model has a foundation in cellular radiobiology. It is generally recognised that the response of a tissue is some function of the response of particular target-cell populations responsible for recovery of the tissue. Target-cell responses can be described simply in terms of a quadratic dependence of cell survival (S) on dose (D), such that $S = \exp-(\alpha D + \beta D^2)$ where

α and β are constants which differ between cell types. This equation describes a sensitivity (α) to low doses, with sensitivity increasing with increasing dose due to the β component. The latter describes the ability of the cells to accumulate damage before it is lethal, and recovery from this damage can be demonstrated using fractionated doses or at low dose rate when recovery occurs during the radiation exposure and β tends to zero. Before the linear quadratic model was widely introduced, sensitivity was quantified using the parameter D_0, and this is still used fairly widely. The simplest equivalent equation using this parameterisation is

$$S = N\exp(-D/D_0)$$

where N is a constant to denote the presence of a threshold effect before the exponential decline in survival takes effect with increasing dose. It can be deduced that at high dose

$$D_0 = 1/(\alpha + 2\beta D).$$

Hence D_0 is the reciprocal of the sensitivity measured at a particular dose D. Also, when $\beta = 0$, $D_0 = 1/\alpha$. D_0 can be described as the mean lethal dose, such that if survival declines exponentially with increasing dose then if one lethal event is delivered *on average* to each cell, by statistical random events e^{-1} or 37% of the cells will survive. (A different parameter, $\bar{D}$, called rather confusingly the mean inactivation dose, has been introduced in recent years. This is the integral of the whole cell survival curve using linear co-ordinates for survival and dose.) A diagrammatic representation of the different parameters used to describe cell survival curves is shown in Fig. 3.

The linear quadratic model for cell survival has been translated into tissue dose-responses by proposing that a given effect (E) in a tissue corresponds to a given level of cell survival. Hence:

$$E = -\ln S = \alpha D + \beta D^2$$

When doses are fractionated into n fractions of dose d,

$$E = n(\alpha d + \beta d^2)$$

where α (Gy^{-1}) and β(Gy^{-2}) are constants.

When n and d are changed from n_1 and d_1 to n_2 and d_2, the total doses D_1 and D_2 resulting in the same effect E are related by $D_2/D_1 = n_2d_2/n_1d_1 = (\alpha/\beta + d_1)/(\alpha/\beta + d_2)$.

The ratio α/β is specific for a given end point in a particular tissue. In general, lower values of α/β indicate that there will be a greater sparing of damage using dose fractionation particularly for later reacting tissues. The values of α/β for various early and late reactions in human intestine are not

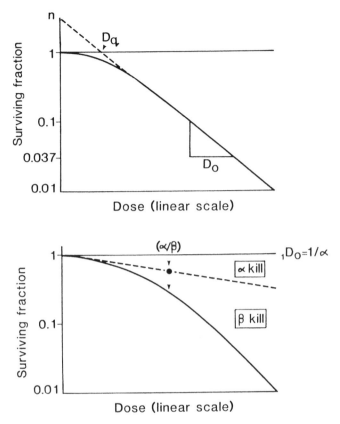

Fig. 3. Top panel: Cell survival curve representation in terms of the mean lethal dose parameter (D_0), the extrapolation (n) of the y-axis, and the intercept D_q on the x-axis. D_q is known as the quasi-threshold dose. Bottom panel: Cell survival curve representation in terms of the initial sensitivity parameter α (= 1/(initial D_0)), and the increasing sensitivity at higher doses due to the presence of the β parameter. (α/β) is the dose at which the amounts of cell kill due to α and β components are equal. Note that the top curve has an exponential final portion, whereas the bottom curve is continuously bending with increasing dose. See text for further description.

known accurately. In animal experiments, the α/β ratio is generally greater than 13 Gy for early reactions such as weight loss and death before 2 months [17]. For late reactions the α/β ratio is lower at between 4 and 7 Gy. The available human data are also compatible with an α/β ratio less than 7 Gy for late reactions [17]. These authors recommended the use of 3 Gy as an α/β ratio when calculating equivalent effects in man over a range of large dose fractions, and 6 Gy in the case of a range of small dose fractions. When the interval between fractions is less than that required for full intracellular repair in surviving cells, another factor has to be introduced into the equation, so that d is replaced by $d(1 + h_M)$. Values of h_M are given in Table 1 [16]. When irradiations are delivered continuously, but at low dose rate, another factor is used in the equation, so that d is replaced by $d \times g$. Values of g are given in Table 2 [16].

TABLE 1

Incomplete-repair factors h_M for multiple fractions per day

Repair halftime (h)	Interval (h)				
	3	4	5	6	8
0.5*	0.0156	0.0039	0.0010	0.0002	–
	0.0210	0.0052	0.0013	0.0003	–
0.75	0.0625	0.0248	0.0098	0.0039	0.0006
	0.0859	0.0335	0.0132	0.0052	0.0008
1.0	0.1250	0.0625	0.0312	0.0156	0.0039
	0.1771	0.0859	0.0423	0.0210	0.0052
1.25	0.1895	0.1088	0.0625	0.0359	0.0118
	0.2766	0.1530	0.0859	0.0487	0.0159
1.5	0.2500	0.1575	0.0992	0.0625	0.0248
	0.3750	0.2265	0.1388	0.0859	0.0335
2.0	0.3536	0.2500	0.1768	0.1250	0.0625
	0.5547	0.3750	0.2565	0.1771	0.0859
2.5	0.4353	0.3299	0.2500	0.1895	0.1088
	0.7067	0.5124	0.3750	0.2766	0.1530
3.0	0.5000	0.3969	0.3150	0.2500	0.1575
	0.8333	0.6341	0.4861	0.3750	0.2265
4.0	0.5946	0.5000	0.4204	0.3536	0.2500
	1.0285	0.8333	0.6784	0.5547	0.3750

*For each half-time, upper number applies for 2 fractions per day, lower number for 3 fractions per day.

The above considerations apply to the biological equivalence of different dose delivery patterns. The degree of non-equivalence can be calculated if the steepness of the dose–response curve is known. The latter can be described in a number of empirical ways, for example using probit or logit functions. A probit function has been used to linearize the sigmoid curve of the incidence of tissue failure versus dose shown in the two left panels of Fig. 4. One of the biologically-based approaches is to propose that the effect (E) will not occur if 1 or more of K tissue-rescuing units (TRU) survives in the organism [18,19]. Hence the probability (P) of the effect occurring $= \exp(-KS)$ where S is the survival function for the TRU. If S is described by the linear-quadratic model, then

$$P = \exp(-K \cdot \exp[-\alpha D + \beta D^2])$$

Hence for given values of K, α and β, this describes the dependence of S on the dose D. The function can be linearised by taking logs twice, and this is shown in the two right panels in Fig. 4, where for simplicity the linear quadratic model has been reduced to a linear (D_0 type) formulation. Note that the original linear-scale sigmoid curve has a slightly different shape to that describing the

TABLE 2

Continuous repair factors (g) for irradiations at low dose-rate

Repair halftime (h)	Exposure time (h)						Exposure time (days)						
	1	2	3	4	8	12	1	1.5	2	2.5	3	3.5	4
0.5	0.6622	0.4774	0.3671	0.2959	0.1641	0.1130	0.0583	0.0393	0.0296	0.0238	0.0198	0.0170	0.0149
0.75	0.7517	0.5888	0.4774	0.3983	0.2339	0.1641	0.0861	0.0583	0.0441	0.0354	0.0296	0.0254	0.0223
1	0.8040	0.6622	0.5571	0.4774	0.2959	0.2115	0.1130	0.0769	0.0583	0.0469	0.0393	0.0338	0.0296
1.25	0.8382	0.7137	0.6165	0.5394	0.3504	0.2555	0.1390	0.0952	0.0723	0.0583	0.0488	0.0420	0.0369
1.5	0.8622	0.7517	0.6622	0.5888	0.3983	0.2959	0.1641	0.1130	0.0861	0.0695	0.0583	0.0502	0.0441
2	0.8938	0.8040	0.7276	0.6622	0.4774	0.3671	0.2115	0.1475	0.1130	0.0916	0.0769	0.0663	0.0583
2.5	0.9136	0.8382	0.7720	0.7137	0.5394	0.4269	0.2555	0.1803	0.1390	0.1130	0.0952	0.0822	0.0723
3	0.9272	0.8622	0.8040	0.7517	0.5888	0.4774	0.2959	0.2115	0.1641	0.1339	0.1130	0.0977	0.0861
4	0.9447	0.8938	0.8471	0.8040	0.6622	0.5571	0.3671	0.2693	0.2115	0.1739	0.1475	0.1280	0.1130

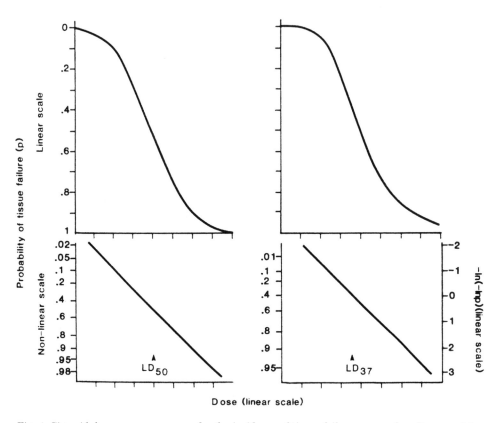

Fig. 4. Sigmoid dose–response curves for the incidence of tissue failure versus dose (top panels), linearised in the bottom panels. Left two panels: probit function linearised with LD_{50} at the midpoint. Right two panels: double log function (see text) linearised with LD_{37} corresponding to zero on the y-axis.

probit formulation. Also, that when 1 TRU survives on average among a number of organisms, tissue failure will occur in 37% of cases.

This model has been used to describe dose–response curves for tissues, and in particular it has been found that dose–response curves are very steep for late reactions in tissues [20]. A contributory factor in this steepness is the structured arrangement of functional units in the tissue or organ concerned [21,22]. With tissue sub-units arranged in "parallel" and operating almost independently of their neighbours (e.g., nephrons in the kidney, alveoli in the lung), depletion of these units will parallel functional damage in the organ as a whole. With critical tissue elements arranged in "series" and exemplified by the spinal cord, (and circumferential lesions in the intestine), severe damage will be expressed if any one element is inactivated. The latter arrangement would result in a very steep dose–response curve, and also the response would be very dependent on the volume of tissue irradiated. The effect of combinations of these two basic structural arrangements have also been described [23].

References

1. Potten, C.S. (1985) Radiation and Skin. Taylor & Francis, London.
2. Zoetelief, J., Broerse, J.J. and Davies, R.W. (1985) Protocol for X-ray dosimetry: EULEP. Commission of the European Communities, Project Group Report, Luxembourg, 1985.
3. Jones, A.R. (1966) Proposed calibration factors for various dosimeters at different energies. Health Phys. 12, 663–671.
4. Bond, V.P. and Robinson, C.V. (1967) Bone marrow stem cell survival in the non-uniformly exposed mammal. In: Effects of Ionising Radiations on the Haematopoietic Tissue. IAEA, Vienna.
5. Withers, H.R., Taylor, J.M.G. and Maciejewski, B. (1988) Treatment volume and tissue tolerance. Int. J. Radiat. Oncol. Biol. Phys. 14, 751–759.
6. Cross, F.T., Endres, G.W.R. and Sullivan, M.F. (1978) Dose to the GI tract from ingested insoluble beta emitters. Radiat. Res. 73, 37–50.
7. Sullivan, M.F., Ruemmber, P.S., Beamer, J.L., et al. (1978) Acute toxicity of Beta-emitting radionuclides that may be released in a reactor accident and ingested. Radiat. Res. 73, 21–36.
8. Roswit, B., Malsky, S.J. and Reid, C.B. (1972) Radiation tolerance of the gastrointestinal tract. Front. Radiat. Oncol. 6, 160–181.
9. Hendry, J.H., Potten, C.S., Ghafoor, A., Moore, J.V., Roberts, S.A. and Williams, P.C. (1989) The response of murine intestinal crypts to short-range ^{147}Pm β-irradiation: deductions concerning clonogenic cell numbers and positions. Rad. Res. 118, 364–374.
10. Cronkite, E. Bond, V.P. and Dunham, C.L. (1956) Some effects of ionising radiation on human beings: A report on the Marshallese and Americans exposed to radiation from fallout and a discussion of radiation injury in the human being. AEC-TID 5385. (Effect of ionising radiation on the human organism: Report on the injuries sustained by the inhabitants of the Marshall Islands. E.P. Cronkite et al. (Eds.), Moscow, Medgiz, 1960.
11. Martinez, G.R., Cassab, H.G., Ganem, G.G., et al. (1964) Observations of the accidental exposure of a family to a source of cobalt-60. Rev. Med. Inst. Mex. Seguro. Social 3, Suppl. 1, 14–68.
12. Trier, J.S., Browning, T.H. and Foroozan, P. (1968) The effect of x-ray therapy on the morphology of the mucosa of the human small intestine. In: M.F. Sullivan (Ed.), Gastrointestinal Radiation Injury. Excerpta Medica Foundation, Amsterdam, pp. 57–81.
13. Palma, L.D. (1968) Intestinal malabsorption in patients undergoing abdominal radiation therapy. In: M.F. Sullivan (Ed.), Gastrointestinal Radiation Injury. Excerpta Medica Foundation, Amsterdam, pp. 261–274.
14. Becciolini, A. (1987) Relative radiosensitivities of the small and large intestine. In: Relative radiation sensitivities of human organ systems. Adv. Radiat. Biol. 12, 83–128.
15. Lushbaugh, C.C. (1982) The impact of estimates of human radiation tolerance upon radiation emergency management. In: The control of exposure of the public to ionising radiation in the event of accident or attack. Proceedings of a symposium held in April 1982, NCRP, pp. 46–57.
16. Thames, H.D. and Hendry, J.H. (1987) Fractionation in radiotherapy. Taylor & Francis Ltd.

17. Dubray, B.M., Thames, H.D., Terry, N.H.A., Gaskinska, A., van der Kogel, A.J., Breitner, N., Dewit, L. and Bentzen, S.M. (1995) Fractionation sensitivity of the rectum: review of human and rodent data with emphasis on α/β ratios. In preparation.

18. Hendry, J.H., Potten, C.S. and Roberts, N.P. (1983) The gastrointestinal syndrome and mucosal clonogenic cells: relationship between cell sensitivities, LD_{50} and cell survival, and their modification by antibiotic. Radiat. Res. 96, 100–112.

19. Hendry, J.H. and Thames, H.D. (1986) The tissue-rescuing unit. Br. J. Radiol. 59, 628–630.

20. Thames, H.D., Hendry, J.H., Moore, J.V., et al (1989) The high steepness of dose-response curves for late-responding normal tissues. Radiother. Oncol. 15, 49–53.

21. Yaes, R.J. and Kalend, A. (1988) Local stem cell depletion model for radiation myelitis. Int. J. Radiat. Oncol. Biol. Phys. 14, 1247–1259.

22. Withers, H.R., Taylor, J.M.G. and Maciejewski, B. (1988) Treatment volume and tissue tolerance. Int. J. Radiat. Oncol. Biol. Phys. 14, 751–759.

23. Kallman, P., Agren, A. and Brahme, A. (1992) Tumour and normal tissue responses to fractionated non-uniform dose delivery. Int. J. Radiat. Biol. 62, 249–262.

24. British Journal of Radiology, Supplement 17 (1983) Central axis depth dose data for use in radiotherapy.

25. Schraube, H., Koester, L. and Briet, A. (1981) Status report on neutron treatment planning for the RENT-project. In: G. Burger (Ed.), Treatment planning for external beam therapy with neutrons. Supplement to Strahlentherapie, Vol. 77, Urban and Schwarzenberg, Munich-Wein-Baltimore, pp. 238.

C.S. Potten and J.H. Hendry (Eds.), *Radiation and Gut*

CHAPTER 3

Clonal Regeneration Studies

C.S. Potten[1] and J.H. Hendry[2]

[1]CRC Department of Epithelial Biology, [2]CRC Department of Experimental Radiation Oncology, Paterson Institute for Cancer Research, Christie Hospital NHS Trust, Wilmslow Road, Manchester M20 9BX, UK

1. CLONOGENIC CELLS AND THE MICROCOLONY ASSAY

Acute doses of radiation kill some cells in the crypt directly and this can be seen in histological preparations by the occurrence of apoptotic figures. However, these doses also have an effect on the ability of cells to progress through successive rounds of cell division (see Chapter 4). This is known as impairment of reproductive activity or potential, or the reproductive sterilisation of cells. Cells damaged in this way survive long enough to repair certain types of sublethal damage but sustain other forms of irreparable damage some of which are chromosomal rearrangements. With this type of damage, some cells are capable of undergoing 1 or a few rounds of cell cycle activity culminating in mitosis, but they either die or cease dividing at the first attempted mitosis (mitotic death) or struggle through and succumb at the second or third mitosis. These doomed cells in the crypt clearly are capable of producing some daughter cells and they themselves persist as cellular entities and will continue to migrate from the crypt onto the villus. In one sense, all dividing transit cells in unirradiated crypts can be similarly regarded as doomed since they also have a limited division potential.

As we have seen, the cells that die rapidly via apoptosis tend to be located in the lower regions of the crypt (see Figs. 1 and 2, Chapter 4) and, therefore, this form of death or damage expression has been linked to cells early in the proliferative hierarchy, if not to the stem cells themselves. Following a moderate dose of irradiation (5–8 Gy for example), many of these more primitive cells will also be reproductively impaired. However, these doses are insufficient to reproductively sterilise all the cells in the crypt that make up the actual or potential stem cells (see earlier discussion). These stem cell or early transit cells find themselves in a heavily damaged and rapidly depopulating crypt and as a consequence receive strong signals for rapid proliferation, regeneration of the crypt, and re-epithelialisation of the entire mucosa. As a consequence of this, they start rapid divisions with shortened cell cycle times and altered (raised) self-maintenance probabilities. The raised self-maintenance probability re-establishes first the stem cell population and then the crypt populations over a period of about 72 hours. Following these moderate doses, virtually all crypts undergo this process. So, although the crypt cellularity may fall on days 1 and 2, it is generally re-established by day 3.

As the dose of radiation increases above these levels, more and more of the potential regenerative cells are reproductively sterilised until a point is reached when on average each crypt contains only a single surviving regenerative cell. This point is probably reached at about 9 Gy for many strains of mice. Here, the single surviving regenerative cell divides rapidly, regenerates first the stem cell compartment, then the crypt cellularity and then cells are produced for the villus. Since there is no possibility of cells moving into a crypt from outside, for example from another crypt, and after such a dose each crypt is re-established from a single cell, the regenerated crypt that appears by the third day can be regarded as a clone of cells and the surviving regenerative cell as a clonogenic cell (see Refs. [1–4]).

As the dose of radiation considered increases above this, more and more of the crypts have all the clonogenic cells sterilised and fewer and fewer crypts survive. Those crypts that are completely reproductively sterilised disappear as a consequence of some acute cell death and continued emigration of remaining cells onto the villus over the first 48 hours. Thus, by day 3 in the small intestine only crypts derived from surviving clonogenic cells are present (Fig 1 and see Fig. 13 in Chapter 1). These clones (crypts) continue to expand in size over the next 2 or 3 days and as a consequence exceed the size of normal crypts in control unirradiated animals by about day 3.5–4.0. Because of the increased size of the regenerating clones (crypts) at times in excess of 3 days counts of the number of these structures have to be adjusted for their size and subsequent over-scoring when the data are to be compared with other experimental groups [3,5]. In some experimental cases the crypts might be smaller (e.g. after some drug treatments) and here the counts have to be corrected for under-scoring. With the further passage of time, the clones enlarge further, the crypts then split or bud into 2 or several crypts [6] and by 14–21 days, the regenerating clones reach a size that can be seen as a nodule by the naked eye in appropriately fixed and prepared material [1,7]. The colonies or clones observed at 3 days have been termed 'microcolonies' since they have to be visualised through the microscope while those observed at 2–3 weeks have been referred to as 'macrocolonies'. As a generalised term, 'colonies' is probably preferable to 'clones' since these regenerating foci are only true clones following high doses when all but one of the clonogenic cells per crypt have been sterilised. At lower doses, several clonogenic cells may survive in each crypt and so here the regenerated crypt is not a clone.

By varying the dose of radiation given to mice and sampling either at about 3 days or between 2–3 weeks, the relationship between the number of surviving colonies and dose can be determined for the microcolonies or the macrocolonies,

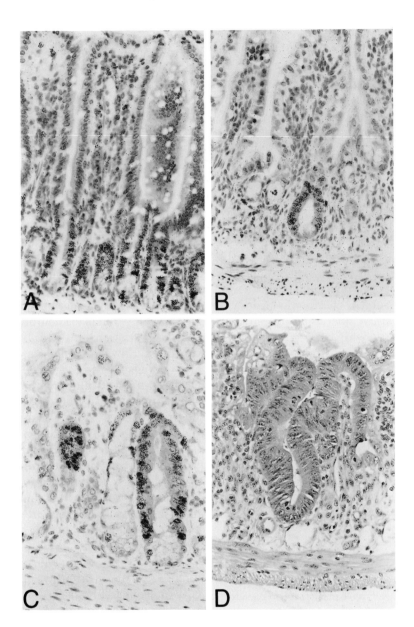

Fig. 1. Microcolonies identified by tritiated thymidine administration (2 × 925 kBq 6 h apart). A: Unirradiated small intestine showing villi and 7 labelled crypts (3 longitudinally sectioned and 4 tangential). B: 3 days after irradiation a single heavily labelled surviving (regenerating) crypt can be seen in the small intestine. C: 4 days after irradiation of the mid colon an obvious longitudinal sectioned surviving crypt can be seen heavily labelled on the right. A non-surviving relatively unlabelled 'ghost' crypt can be seen in the middle of the picture. A surviving tangentially sectioned and labelled crypt can be seen on the left with more than 14 adjacent labelled cells. D: 5 days after irradiation large expanding foci of regeneration can be seen in the small intestine. Such areas are spreading laterally at the surface and bifurcating near the base. (See also colour plate on p. xiii.)

thus generating survival curves for the crypt clonogen units. The survival curves for macrocolonies can be shown to be the high dose extension of the microcolonies survival curve [2,4]. For practical reasons, the macrocolony technique is firstly very technically limiting, and secondly, can only be performed following high doses of radiation. As a consequence of the latter, the survival curve generated approximates well to the true survival curve for individual clonogenic cells since at these doses, each crypt clonogen unit that survives will only be derived from a single clonogenic cell. Because of the technical limitations, most workers have adopted the microcolony approach and there have been many papers published (see review Ref. [8]) since its original description by Withers and Elkind in 1969/70 [1,2]. The survival curves that are produced using this approach are usually referred to as crypt survival curves since this is essentially what is scored (see Fig. 2 and Chapter 2). These crypt survival curves are characterised by an extremely broad shoulder region where there is little change in the survival of crypts until a break point in the curve at around 8 or 9 Gy. As mentioned above, this is the point at which on average each crypt that is going to survive now only contains a single surviving cell (the actual number of cells will be distributed amongst the crypts according to Poisson statistics). Thereafter, the survival curve for crypts tends to show an exponential relationship between surviving fraction and radiation dose. This is one mathematical approximation to describe the data. However, it is also possible that the shape of the curve is continuously bending on a semi-logarithmic plot instead of a straight line as determined by an exponential relationship. If it is continuously bending a different mathematical approximation has to be applied. This comprises an initial exponential region, together with a dose-squared parameter which increases the steepness gradually at higher doses. For the exponential curve, the sensitivity of the cells is defined by the reciprocal of the slope on the exponential region, the D_0. For the continuously bending curve, the sensitivity is defined by the parameters α and β (see Chapter 2).

Clonogen sensitivity parameters can be derived from crypt survival curves by various ways. Originally a Poisson correction was applied to deduce the

---

Opposite: Fig. 2. Crypt survival curves obtained for various regions of the small intestine 3 days after irradiation (upper panel) and for various regions of the large intestine 4 days after irradiation (lower panel). The parameters that define these curves are as follows:

	Duodenum	Jejunum	Upper ileum	Lower ileum
D_0 (cGy)	144±24	145±27	1357±8	179±8
n	773±1016	945±1380	1765±863	215±52

	Caecum	Mid Colon	Rectum
D_0 (cGy)	225±12	228±9	228±16
n	71±18	83±16	52±14

We are grateful to Weibo Cai for these data.

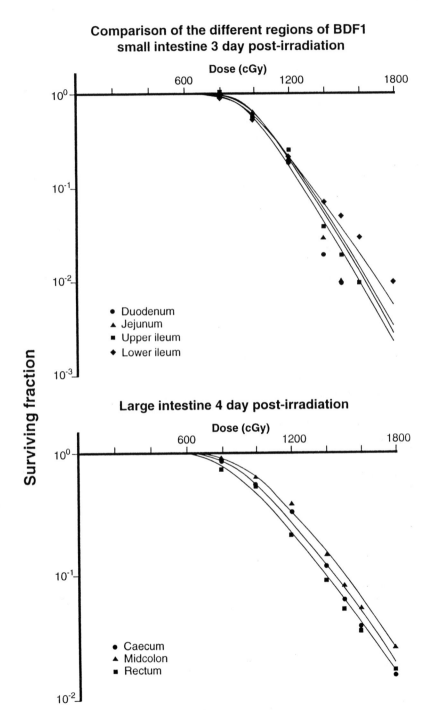

Fig. 2. Caption opposite.

average number of surviving clonogens at each dose, and these data were then plotted on semi-logarithmic paper (see Fig. 14 in Chapter 1). The D_0 was determined from a line drawn through the data on such a plot [2]. Alternatively a double-logarithmic transformation can be applied to the crypt surviving fractions so that the transformed data are plotted on a linear graph to deduce D_0 [9]. The latter computations can now be done very easily using a computer program [10]. Another method, using another option in the same program is to analyse the data in terms of the response of identical groups of cells [11]. The number of cells becomes a part of the "extrapolation number" describing the width of the "shoulder" of the exponential survival curve (see Chapter 2), or becomes a third parameter (γ) in the linear quadratic model:

Crypt surviving fraction = $1 - (1 - [\exp(-\alpha D - \beta D^2)])^\gamma$

The relationship between crypt survival and cell survival is given diagrammatically in Fig. 3.

A large number of experiments using the microcolony technique have been reported in the literature. In 1983, we reviewed 23 examples for the small intestine, two for the colon and one for the stomach in rats and mice [8]. The feature of all of these curves was that broadly speaking, they had a similar slope, ie, could be defined by roughly the same D_0 value. What was somewhat surprising and remains largely unexplained is the fact that these curves in their extremes showed differences of a factor of about 20 in the level of survival of crypts for a particular dose. This can be partly explained by either differences in the biological effectiveness of the radiation (i.e., LET), differences between strains of mice and animals and finally, differences in technical approach and scoring procedures. It is in fact likely that all three of these factors contribute to this variability.

This review of microcolony assay data indicated that (1) colon and stomach do not differ strikingly from the small intestine in radiosensitivity; (2) the macrocolony data can generally be regarded as part of the same survival curve as the microcolony data; (3) there is some tendency for the survival curves even from within one laboratory to drift with time; and (4) the D_0 values lie between about 1.2 and 1.4 Gy. Generally speaking all subsequent microcolony data would fall within the range of survival curves that we analysed in 1983.

In the colon the time course for both regeneration of crypts and for the removal of dead crypts, which fortuitously coincided at day 3 in the small intestine, differs. Here the optimum time for analysis is about day 4. In the small intestine the regenerated surviving crypts tend to be easily recognised in well fixed haematoxylin and eosin (H & E) stained sections. The criterion used as the threshold for detection is 10 or more chromophilic adjacent, healthy non-Paneth cells. There is some difference in the survival curves if this critical number is increased or decreased slightly [12]. There is no difference when tritiated thymidine (^{3}HTdR) is used to mark the S phase cells in the crypt as an indicator of active cell proliferation.

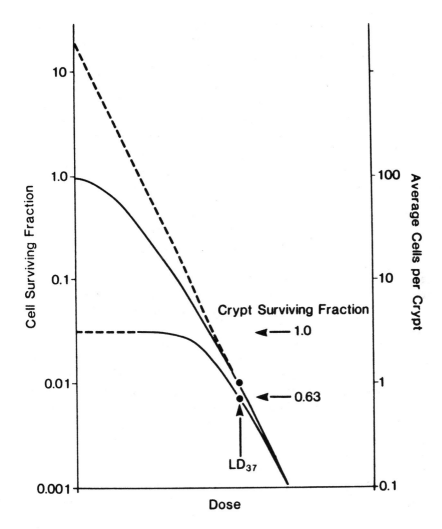

Fig. 3. Cell surviving fraction (left ordinate and continuous curve) or average cells surviving per crypt (right ordinate. For simplicity, 100 clonogens per crypt were assumed, with a "shouldered" survival curve (N = 20) and an exponential terminal portion. The crypt surviving fraction (bottom curve) shows a long threshold region (dashed) before decreasing with increasing dose to an asymptote to the cell survival curve. Hence at high dose the crypt survival curve and the clonogen survival curve are coincident, because the crypts then act as single-cell units. At LD_{37}, 37% of the crypts are sterilised, and this corresponds to an average of 1.0 surviving cells in all original crypt structures, and 1.6 [ie 1/(1 - 0.37)] surviving cells on average in each of the 63% of surviving crypt structures. (Taken from Ref. [13]).

We have found it difficult to transfer these scoring criteria directly to the large intestine. In H & E stained sections it is much more difficult to distinguish regenerating from dying crypts or cells. However, using [3]HTdR and a threshold of 10 adjacent labelled cells in autoradiographs prepared after two

[3]HTdR injections 6 h apart it is believed surviving crypts can be identified. Figure 1 shows examples of the microcolony assay in the small and large bowel and Fig. 2 some survival curves for various regions in the small and large intestine.

The regenerated crypts that are obtained beyond 3 days after irradiation are characterised by possessing Goblet cells and Paneth cells as well as the predominant columnar cells. These crypts also contain the minority class of enteroendocrine cells. This indicates that the surviving clonogenic cells possess the potential to produce daughters that differentiate down all these lineages (see also Ref. [14].

Following doses such as 12 Gy which result in up to about 80% kill or 20% survival of crypts, about half the animals will survive beyond a 6–7 day period. In other words, this dose is close to the $LD_{50\ (6/7)}$ (the dose for 50% kill as measured on days 6 or 7). This means that the 20% surviving crypts, each one of which contained only a single surviving clonogenic cell, eventually re-epithelialises the entire mucosa and maintains some animals potentially for the rest of their life. In practice, if the animals had been whole body irradiated, bone marrow damage would result in death within a 30 day period since the $LD_{50\ (30)}$ which measures haematopoietic death is lower than $LD_{50\ (6/7)}$. However, if only the abdomen, or the intestine, was irradiated, some animals would have the potential to survive a near normal life span. This means that the clonogenic cells have a very large division potential and are capable of producing all the differentiated elements of the tissue and, therefore, these cells satisfy two of the strongest elements in the stem cell definition (cells having a large division potential and producing daughter cells that differentiate to produce all the cell types that characterise the tissue) and hence these clonogenic cells can be regarded as stem cells.

2. THE NUMBER OF CLONOGENIC CELLS PER CRYPT

One of the questions that interested workers in this field, as well as stem cell biologists, is the question of whether such data can be interpreted to provide an answer to the question of how many stem cells or clonogenic cells exist in an unirradiated normal crypt. In principle, the answer is yes, the data should be able to provide this information. In practice it has been quite difficult to extract good well defined answers. The general principle is based on the fact that the very broad shoulder that typifies a crypt survival curve after irradiation at high dose-rate should depend on two interacting elements. Firstly, the number of clonogenic cells in a crypt, and secondly, the efficiency with which each individual clonogenic cell can repair sublethal damage [9,15]. The product of these should explain the width of the shoulder (Dq) or the extrapolation number (n) which is another measure of the size of the shoulder. If a dose of radiation, for example 12 Gy is split into 2 equal fractions of 6 Gy and these fractions are separated by variable time intervals and the level of crypt survival is determined at these intervals of time and compared with the level of survival obtained by 12 Gy delivered as a single dose, the efficiency of the repair process of the cells can be measured. When such an experiment is performed and the interval of time between the two fractions is 4–8 h the survival levels remain roughly constant throughout this time and the survival levels are dramatically (perhaps 20-fold) higher than the survival after a single dose of 12 Gy. In this way, the repair efficiency or repair capacity of the clonogenic cells can be measured and hence, the number of clonogenic cells can be deduced from the extrapolation number by dividing it by the repair capacity. Initially this approach was adopted and a variety of experiments were performed, all of which suggested that the number of clonogenic cells per crypt (about 80) was significantly less than the number of proliferative cells (about 150) [9,15]. In these experiments it was recognised that it was important to correct for sampling frequency of surviving crypts in histological sections, which depends on crypt size. This procedure has been consistently adopted by the Manchester group but not all investigators do this. These studies indicated that the crypt contained at least two types of proliferating cells — those that could regenerate a crypt and those that could not and the initial estimates suggested that about half the proliferative cells could be regarded as clonogenic. Subsequent refinements in the technique and the adoption of a simplified two dose approach has allowed us to refine these estimates considerably in the intervening years (Potten et al. concluded that the number of clonogens per crypt was about 32 [16]). The two dose method requires that two equal doses are chosen so that the level of survival after the first dose can be measured, as well as the level after the first plus the second dose [17,18]. Hence, the full response to only the second dose can be calculated since the starting point in terms of clonogen number is known — it is the survival level after the first dose. The assumption is that the first dose and the second dose which are equal in size each kill the same proportion of clonogens. If the crypt survival fractions are converted into clonogen surviving fractions using Poisson statistics we have a measured number of clonogens after the first dose but an unknown number of clonogens as the starting point in the unirradiated crypt. All the data are available for the second dose, the starting value and the surviving value and hence a true surviving fraction can be calculated and then this can be used to calculate the unknown starting value for the first dose — the initial number of clonogens in unirradiated crypts. The number of surviving clonogenic cells/crypts after the first dose N_1 can be deduced from the surviving fraction of crypts, SF_1, using Poisson statistics.

$$N_1 = -\log_e(1 - SF_1)$$

Similarly for the second dose $N_2 = -\log_e(1 - SF_2)$. After the second dose the fraction of clonogenic cells surviving $F_2 = N_2/N_1$.

Assuming the same fractional survival after the first dose then

$$F_1 = N_2/N_1 = N_1/N_0.$$

This can be solved for N_0, the number of clonogenic cells at the start of the experiment, i.e., the number in an unirradiated crypt,

$$N_0 = \frac{N_1}{(N_2/N_1)} = (N_1)^2 / N_2.$$

The advantage of this method [17,18] over curve fitting procedures [9,15] and parameter estimations is that systematic uncertainties due to the particular choice of the model to fit are eliminated as sources of uncertainty. We believe that criticisms [21] of the two-dose method on the basis of using the extremes of the range of survival in the calculations are not well founded.

Our most recent experiments using the two-dose technique have indicated that the number of cells that can be demonstrated to display clonogenic capacity seems to depend on the level of dose that is used to make the measurement of the number of clonogenic cells (Fig. 15 in Chapter 1 and Ref. [22,23]). Biologically this implies that the more severe the damage to the crypt, the more cells are recruited into the clonogenic or potential stem cell compartment. When low doses are used to damage the system, the current estimate for the number of clonogenic cells is about 6 per crypt which is essentially the same as our estimate of the number of actual stem cells in a steady-state crypt which is about 4. If larger doses (<9 Gy) are used to damage the system, the estimates for the number of clonogenic cells are about 30–40 per crypt [22]. This is also consistent with estimates from the back-extrapolates of survival curves obtained using low-dose-rate irradiation. These have an exponential tail characterised by the α component (see Fig. 4) and since there is no curvature ($\beta = 0$), the extrapolation number is comprised solely of the cell multiplicity term. Of course such a survival curve is dominated by the higher-dose data where the two-dose data would also indicate higher clonogen numbers. This would suggest that under these severe damage situations, the clonogenic compartment is comprised of not only the 4 stem cells, but also the 16 or so cells that would be expected in the T_1–T_3 dividing transit compartments while the 120 or so cells that would be expected in the T_4–T_6 compartment would not be part of the clonogenic compartment and not be capable of regeneration phenomena. This implies that the hierarchical system has a certain degree of flexibility in it and that up to the T_2 or T_3 transit generation, cells still have the capability of functioning as clonogenic stem cells under severely perturbed conditions. Studies using promethium as a low penetration radiation source applied to the surface of the intestine showed that the clonogens are located at the crypt base. The cells higher up the crypt could not repopulate the crypt [24]. Taking the data described above on clonogen numbers per crypt, together with the steady state estimate of about 4 actual stem cells, and the data that suggested about 6 cells at the stem cell position in murine small intestinal crypts are very radiosensitive and die via apoptosis, this would all suggest that the stem cell compartment in the small intestinal crypts is itself hierarchical (as outlined in Table 1).

Many experiments have been performed by other workers concerning fractionated irradiation, to determine clonogen numbers, and fractionation parameters for clinical application. This situation becomes quite complex when irradiations are protracted over many days because cell-cycle-related changes

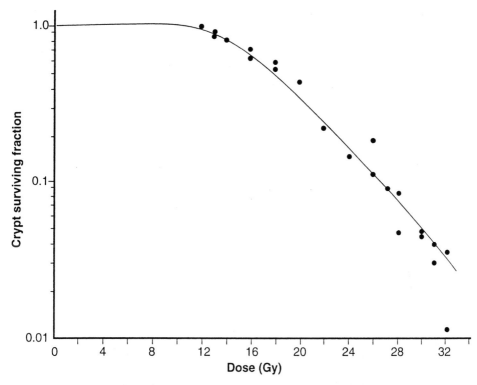

Fig. 4. The response of mouse intestinal crypts to low dose rate γ-irradiation (0.97 Gy/min). the curve is characterised by $D_0 = 4.6 \pm 0.2$ Gy and n = 34 ± 6. The back extrapolate (n) of the curve on the y-axis is representative of the number of clonogens at risk at zero dose (taken from Ref. [19]).

in sensitivity can begin to play a role. This is shown by the generally higher values of fractionation sensitivity (β/α) when the latter is calculated from two-dose compared to multifraction data [20]. Also, induced heterogeneity in cell-cycle-phase distribution should tend to flatten dose–response curves and give low effective clonogen numbers at risk. This does not appear to happen, as clonogen numbers tend to be higher when calculated using multifraction rather than two-dose data, but the lack of use of a sampling size correction procedure might also be a confounding factor.

3. REGENERATION OF CLONOGENIC CELLS

A number of methods have been used to study the regeneration of clonogens following high-dose irradiation. These consist of either the use of a single second dose to test the residual survival at different times after a first dose, or a double second dose to eliminate any problem of possible changes in sensitivity following the first dose. Many of the published data are summarised in Fig. 5.

TABLE 1

Possible crypt stem cell hierarchy

Up to 6	Very radiosensitive ultimate stem cells (accounts for the apoptotic response). No repair capability, very efficient self-regulatory mechanisms if numbers change up or down	Actual steady-state stem cells
About 6	More resistant clonogenic cells (good repair capacity). Replace stem cell compartment after low level injury i.e. when all 6 actual stem cells are killed.	Low level injury clonogens. Potential stem cells
Up to about 24	Resistant clonogenic cells (includes low level injury clonogens). Very good repair.	High level injury. Potential stem cells.
~36 per crypt	Total stem cells including clonogens.	

Besides these there are about 124 dividing transit non-stem cells.

A consistent feature in many of the experiments, where changes in sensitivity have been allowed for, is a doubling time of around 20–24 h. The regeneration of the number of clonogens over the period of 4 days post-irradiation has been measured using the split-dose technique. These studies provided a clonogen repopulation doubling time of 22 h (Ref. [25] and Fig. 5). This of course is longer than the regenerating stem cell cycle time because of concomitant differentiation at each cell division in a proportion of the cells (i.e. a self-maintenance probability of less than 1.0). The doubling time is similar to that in bone marrow stem cells (and in epidermis) where the value can be reconciled with a 6-h cycle time during early regeneration and a 40% loss of cells to differentiation pathways at each division. Hence, this percentage appears to be an optimal and common rate in the regenerative states of several renewing tissues.

Following repeated irradiation, with recovery allowed between each treatment, surviving crypts become permanently enlarged [8] and the surviving fraction never completely rejoins its control value. Presumably there is insufficient stromal damage so preventing the budding and repopulation of neighbouring denuded crypts in this situation, as occurs early after a single dose. Interestingly, in the larger crypts there is a smaller complement of clonogens, but they cycle more rapidly probably with extra amplification divisions to maintain the required output of cells for the villi. A second feature of such multiple or repeated exposure experiments is the fact that when the epithelium is re-established between exposures, or even at late times after a single exposure the crypt density never returns to the full control value: usually it plateaus at about 75% of the control value for crypts per unit length (i.e., crypts per circumference).

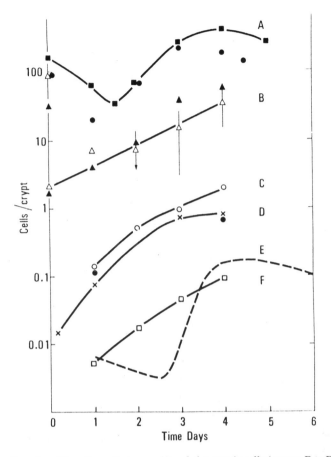

Fig. 5. Regeneration of proliferative cells (curve A) and clonogenic cells (curves B to F) in the crypt after irradiation. Curve A and closed circles, labelled nuclei per crypt after 9 Gy (900 R) *partial-body* irradiation to the abdomen [26]. Virtually identical data were reported after 1000 R *whole-body* irradiation [26], except at day 1 when the level was higher by a factor of 2. Curve A and closed squares, cell numbers in the crypt proliferation zone after 9 Gy [14]. Curve B and open triangles, clonogenic cells per crypt after 9 Gy. At zero time upper symbol refers to control crypts, and lower symbol refers to cell number per *surviving* crypt immediately after 9 Gy [14]. Curve B and closed triangles, clonogenic cells per crypt after 9 Gy, calculated using a common D_0 for the survival curves measured at all times after the priming dose [14]. Curve C and open circles, clonogenic cells per crypt surviving a test dose of 9 Gy delivered at different times after the priming dose of 9 Gy ie, not corrected for any changes in survival curve shape with tie [14]. Curve D and crosses, other data similar to curve C [28]. Curve D and closed circles, other data similar to curve C using a test dose of 12 Gy (1200 R) [29]. Curve E shown dashed, clonogenic cells surviving a test dose of 14.15 Gy given at varying times after a priming dose of 6.6 Gy, positioned as described in the text [1]. Curve F and open squares, clonogenic cells per crypt surviving a test dose of 14 Gy given at varying times after a priming dose of 9 Gy, extrapolated from data at lower doses assuming a common D_0 at all times [14]. Figure reproduced from Ref. [16] with permission from the Japanese Association for Radiation Research.

Clonal Regeneration Studies

References

1. Withers, H.R. and Elkind, M. (1969) Radiosensitivity and fractionation response of crypt cells of mouse jejunum. Radiat. Res. 38, 598–613.
2. Withers, H.R. and Elkind, M. (1970) Microcolony survival assay for cells of mouse intestinal mucosa exposed to radiation. Int. J. Radiat. Biol. 17, 261–268.
3. Potten, C.S. and Hendry, J.H. (1985) The microcolony assay in mouse small intestine. In: C.S. Potten and J.H. Hendry (Eds.), Cell Clones: Manual of Mammalian Cell Techniques. Churchill-Livingstone, Edinburgh, pp. 50–60.
4. Hornsey, S. (1985) The macrocolony assay in small intestine. In: In: C.S. Potten and J.H. Hendry (Eds.), Cell Clones: Manual of Mammalian Cell Techniques. Churchill-Livingstone, Edinburgh, pp. 44–49.
5. Potten, C.S., Rezvani, M., Hendry, J.H., Moore, J.V. and Major, D. (1981) The correction of the intestinal microcolony counts for variation in size. Int. J. Radiat. Biol. 40, 217–225.
6. Cairnie, A.B. and Millen, B.H. (1975) Fission of crypts in the small intestine of the irradiated mouse. Cell Tissue Kinet. 8, 189–196.
7. Withers, H.R. and Elkind, M. (1968) Dose-survival characteristics of epithelial cells of mouse intestinal mucosa. Radiol. 91, 998–1000.
8. Potten, C.S., Hendry, J.H., Moore, J.V. and Chwalinski, S. (1983) Cytotoxic effects in gastrointestinal epithelium (as exemplified by small intestine). In: C.S. Potten and J.H. Hendry (Eds.), Cytotoxic Insult to Tissue: Effects on Cell Lineages. Churchill-Livingstone, Edinburgh, pp. 105–152.
9. Hendry, J.H. and Potten, C.S. (1974) Cryptogenic cells and proliferative cells in intestinal epithelium. Int. J. Rad. Biol. 25, 583–588.
10. Roberts, S.A. (1990) DRFIT: A program for fitting radiation survival models. Int. J. Radiat. Biol. 57, 1243–1246.
11. Yau, H.C., and Cairnie, A.B. (1979) Cell survival characteristics of intestinal stem cells and crypts of γ-irradiated mice. Radiat. Res. 80, 92–107.
12. Hendry, J.H. (1994) Quantitation of intestinal clonogens by regeneration following cytotoxicity. Seminars in Developmental Biology 4, 303–312.
13. Potten, C.S. and Hendry, J.H. (1983) Stem cells in murine small intestine. In: C.S. Potten (Eds.), Stem Cells: Their Identification and Characterisation. Churchill-Livingstone, Edinburgh, pp. 155–199.
14. Inoue, M., Imada, M., Fukushima, Y., Matsumara, N., Shiozaki, H., Mori, T., Kitamura, Y. and Fujita, H. (1988) Macroscopic intestinal colonies of mice as a tool for studying differentiation of multipotential intestinal stem cells. Am. J. Path. 132, 49–58.
15. Potten, C.S. and Hendry, J.H. (1975) Differential regeneration of intestinal proliferative cells and cryptogenic cells after irradiation. Int. J. Rad. Biol. 27, 413–424.
16. Potten, C.S., Hendry, J.H. and Moore, J.V. (1987) New estimates of the number of clonogenic cells in crypts of murine small intestine. Virchow Arch. B Cell Path. 53, 227–234.
17. Hendry, J.H. (1979) Regeneration of stem-cells in intestinal epithelium after irradiation. In: S. Okada, M. Imamura, T. Terasima and H. Yamaguchi, H. (Eds.), Proceedings of the 6th International Congress of Radiation Research, Tokyo, Jpn. Assoc. Radiat. Res., Tokyo, p. 665.
18. Hendry J.H. (1978) A new derivation from split-dose data of the complete survival curve for clonogenic normal cells in vivo. Rad. Res. 78, 404-414.

19. Rezvani, M. (1980) The response of mouse intestine and spleen to low dose rate radiation. MSc thesis, University of Manchester, UK.

20. Hendry, J.H. and Potten, C.S. (1988) α/β ratios and the cycling status of tissue target cells. Letter to Editor. Radiother. Oncol. 12, 79–83.

21. Withers, H.R., Mason, K.A. and Taylor, J.M.G. (1993) The number of clonogenic cells in a mouse jejunal crypt. Radiother. Oncol. 26, 238–243.

22. Hendry, J.H., Roberts, S.A. and Potten, C.S. (1992) The clonogen content of murine intestinal crypts: dependence on radiation dose used in its determination. Radiat. Res. 132, 115–119.

23. Roberts, S.A., Hendry, J.H. and Potten, C.S. (1995) The deduction of the clonogen content of intestinal crypts: a direct comparison of fractionated-dose and graded-dose methodologies. Radiat Res, in press.

24. Hendry, J.H., Potten, C.S., Ghafoor, A., Moore, J.V., Roberts, S.A. and Williams, P.C. (1989) The response of murine intestinal crypts to short-range [147]Pm β-irradiation: deductions concerning clonogenic cell numbers and positions. Rad. Res. 118, 364–374.

25. Potten, C.S., Hendry, J.H. and Taylor, Y. (1988) The doubling time of regenerating clonogenic cells in the crypts of the small intestine. Int. J. Radiat. Biol. 54, 1041–1051.

26. Lesher, J. and Lesher S. (1974) Radiat. Res. 57, 148.

27. Hagemann, R.F. and Lesher, S. (1971) Irradiation of the GI tract: compensatory response of stomach, jejunum and colon. Br. J. Radiol. 44, 599.

28. Potten, C.S. (1978) Small intestinal cryptogenic cells in W/W[v] mutant mice. Radiat. Res. 74, 139.

29. Hagemann, R.F., Sigdestad, C.P. and Lesher, S. (1972) Intestinal crypt survival and total and per crypt levels of proliferative cellularity following irradiation: role of crypt cellularity. Radiat. Res. 50, 583.

C.S. Potten and J.H. Hendry (Eds.), *Radiation and Gut*

CHAPTER 4

Effects of Radiation on Murine Gastrointestinal Cell Proliferation

C.S. Potten

CRC Department of Epithelial Biology, Paterson Institute for Cancer Research, Christie Hospital NHS Trust, Wilmslow Road, Manchester M20 9BX, UK

1. INTRODUCTION

A considerable amount of quantitate data on the changes in various parameters associated with proliferation have been obtained by us over the last 15–20 years on one strain of BDF1 mice housed under standard laboratory conditions (reviewed in Ref. [1]). There have been a number of other studies in the literature and wherever possible the present data will be compared with those studies. However, there are few, if any, sets of accumulated data that are as extensive as those generated in Manchester. For this reason we shall concentrate mainly on describing these experiments. Most of these studies have involved the small intestine and hence we will use the small intestine as an example to display the general trends that can be expected when a rapidly proliferating tissue is exposed to radiation. Over a similar time period an extensive series of investigations have been performed in the Sprague–Dawley rat by the group in Florence and these experiments are reviewed in Chapter 5. These studies have had a particular interest in radiation induced changes in proliferative parameters in relation to the daily or circadian cycles of proliferation and also to the expression of various differentiation markers in the intestine, such as the brush border enzymes.

2. INDUCTION OF CELL DEATH

One of the first and most easily observed effects of irradiation on the small intestine is the appearance in the crypts of cells with abnormal morphological appearances. These changes in appearance suggest that the cells are dying or dead. The changes can be observed in routine histological sections and are characterised by a range of alterations that are for the most part consistent

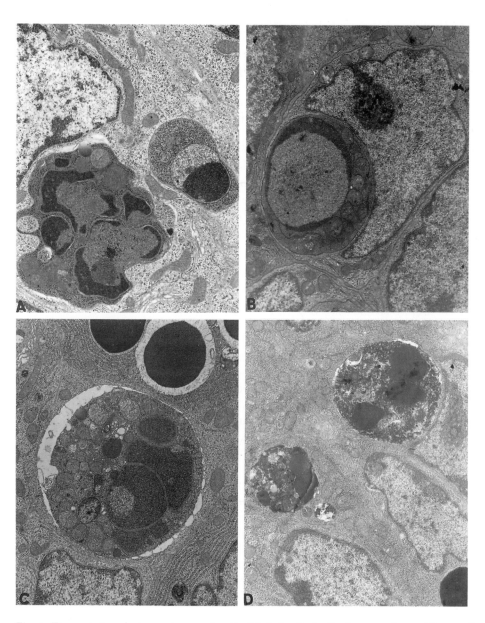

Fig. 1. Transmission electron micrographs of epithelial cells in the lower regions of the small intestinal crypt exhibiting various stages of the apoptotic sequence. (A) shows the nucleus of a normal healthy cell (top left), and beneath this a cell in the early stages of apoptosis exhibiting the condensed cytoplasm, chromatin condensation at the margins of the nucleus and the beginnings of the fragmentation process for the nucleus. To the right of this is what is probably an apoptotic fragment from another cell. (B) shows an apoptotic fragment enclosed in a phagosome of a normal healthy epithelial cell. The apoptotic fragment shows the condensed cytoplasm, mitochondria with intact internal structures and a fragment of the nucleus showing condensation at the margins with

with the changes described for a mode of cell death called *apoptosis* [2,8]. These include a shrinkage of the cell away from its neighbours, i.e., a rounding-up of the cell and a condensation of the chromatin material in the nucleus particularly at the nuclear membrane. With the shrinkage in the total volume of the cell, the cytoplasm also becomes more condensed. The chromatin condensation continues often producing characteristic crescent shaped areas that take up stain intensely. Both the nucleus and the body of the cell then begin to break up into a number of fragments. Some of these fragments may contain parts of the nucleus, others not. These apoptotic fragments or bodies are generally ingested by the process of phagocytosis by neighbouring healthy epithelial cells in the gut or by migrating macrophages in other tissues. If these cells are in the mid or upper crypt region, they will be migrating along the crypt to villus axis and hence, the fragments that they carry will appear to migrate as well. The fragments are gradually absorbed by the host cell and it is believed that they ultimately result in structures called residual bodies (the 'indigestible residues'). These processes can all be readily recognised in the electron microscope, but once their general appearance is appreciated, they can be recognised in well-fixed, thin, well-stained, light microscopic sections. There have been several examples of the EM and light microscope appearance of these apoptotic cells in normal and damaged intestinal epithelium published [3–6] and examples are shown in Figs. 1 and 2.

The process of apoptosis is believed to represent a form of programmed, or genetically determined, self-deletion or suicide involving individual cells. While undergoing apoptosis, the cells remain metabolically active and can be influenced by protein synthesis and RNA synthesis inhibitors [7], the cytoplasmic organelles remain intact, for example the mitochondria are still easily recognisable in relatively late apoptotic phagosomes (Fig. 1C). This programming by the cell involves gene activation and the synthesis of a rather specific DNA degradation endonuclease enzyme which characteristically cleaves the DNA in the intranucleosomal regions into fragments that are multiples of about 200 base pairs in length (180 to be precise). The consequence of the action of this enzyme is that DNA fragments which are multiples from discrete 1.2.3....n times 200 base pair lengths. When the DNA is extracted from cells dying via apoptosis and run on gel electrophoresis, a series of bands are generated. This so-called DNA ladder is very characteristic of apoptosis. Although the generality of DNA ladders in apoptotic cells is currently being questioned. Fragmentation into 50 k base fragments may be a more universal characteristic. However, in order to

---

a typical crescent shape commonly seen in apoptotic nuclei. (C) shows another phagosome containing a fragment of an apoptotic cell with several fragments of the nucleus with condensed chromatin and many mitochondria which even at this relatively late stage, still show intact internal structures. At the top of this picture are two Paneth cell granules. This phagosome is probably incorporated into the cytoplasm of a Paneth cell. (D) shows two apoptotic fragments at a late stage in their life cycle since the internal structures are now in the process of degradation. I am grateful to Dr. T. Allen for these photomicrographs.

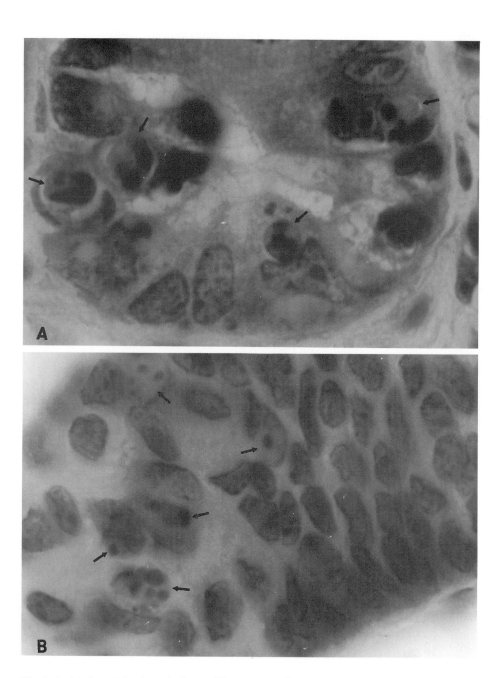

Fig. 2. Apoptotic cell death at the base of the crypt in a haematoxylin-stained section. The lower regions of the crypt is illustrated with several cells undergoing apoptosis (arrows). Fragments can be seen at the very base of the crypt and above the large apoptotic body arrowed in the centre of the field.

obtain a DNA ladder, large numbers of roughly synchronous dying cells are required in order to be able to extract sufficient DNA. This cannot be achieved with tissues like the intestine. Hence, here the identification of apoptosis relies solely on morphological criteria. In the past, dying cells in a tissue like intestine were often described as pycnotic nuclei as a consequence of the condensation of the chromatin material and the fragments that were generated were referred to as the consequence of karyorrhexis.

In twenty years of studying the destructive effects of radiation and a wide variety of cytotoxic drugs [9–11] all the cell death observed has been consistent with the process of apoptosis. A low level of spontaneous cell death can be observed in the small intestinal crypts of unirradiated animals (see Refs. [12,13]) which has been linked to the normal homeostatic mechanisms that govern stem cell numbers [4,14,16]. Both the radiation-induced and the spontaneous apoptosis are found to be predominantly associated with the stem cell position in small intestinal crypts.

Techniques have relatively recently been developed that are based on the ability to detect the broken ends of DNA strands. The principles that are involved include the use of polymerase enzymes and DNA bases that are tagged with molecules that can be recognised by appropriate antibody and immuno-histochemical techniques. A variety of names have been applied to the approach, but probably the most appropriate here is *in situ* end labelling (ISEL). Such ISEL techniques have been successfully used to identify apoptotic cells with their broken DNA in various tissues, however, these techniques have not been applied successfully to the gastrointestinal tract. Use of the techniques tend to result in considerable non-specific staining of the cells throughout the epithelium with particularly strong staining of the cells on the villus. Although this has been reported in the literature as indicating that villus cells are undergoing apoptosis [15], these villus cells with a few possible rare exceptions [25], do not exhibit any of the morphological features of apoptosis. Conversely, apoptotic cells in the crypts either occurring spontaneously or induced by radiation often tend to be unlabelled using these approaches. It is likely that by appropriate modification of the procedures, these techniques can be made to be sensitive and specific for apoptosis in the gut, but this has yet to be achieved.

An alternative mode of death for cells is necrosis. This occurs in tumours, for example subject to ischaemia and also in tissues as a consequence of thermal injury and a good example of this is in the testis where subtle changes in temperature result in bursts of cells dying by apoptosis or necrosis depending largely on their position within the spermatogenic cell hierarchy [17]. The features of necrosis, that distinguish it from apoptosis are that it involves an initial swelling of the cell and hence the cytoplasm becomes paler. A rapid degradation of the cytoplasmic organelles with the mitochondria quickly losing their characteristic features and a condensation of chromatin material scattered in irregular patches throughout the entire nucleus. The presence of necrotic cells invariably triggers an inflammatory response in the tissue which is never seen in apoptosis.

In the small intestine, over a period of 15 years, using a wide variety of cytotoxic agents and a range of doses the cell death produced has all been much more characteristic of apoptosis than necrosis. Because of the way in which these studies are performed, we cannot rule out completely the possibility that some occasional cells that we call apoptotic are in fact dying through necrosis.

Apoptosis is believed to be a programmed form of cell death controlled in part by a series of specific genes. Recent work has suggested that p53 is a gene that is involved in the recognition and identification of damage within a cell [18] and the subsequent changes that either allow time for the repair of the damage or the initiation of apoptosis. bcl-2 is a gene that is believed to suppress apoptosis in cells and hence allow them to undergo the other processes for which they are programmed — proliferation and/or differentiation [19]. The oncogene c-myc has also been implicated in controlling the balance between proliferation and apoptosis [20] in relation to variable concentrations of growth factors such that in the presence of high growth factor concentration and the activation of myc, proliferation is favoured. In low growth factor concentrations the activation of myc, may result in apoptosis. The interaction between such genes and the occurrence of yet other genes is a current area of rapidly developing research interest.

If we consider the occurrence of apoptosis in both normal and irradiated intestines of mice, there are a number of important characteristic points. The first of these is that in normal healthy unirradiated mice, there is a constant low level expression of apoptosis. This spontaneous cell death occurs at a frequency of about 0.1–0.2 apoptotic events per crypt section. In other words, one apoptotic event in every 5–10 crypt sections. Although this is a low yield, when expressed on the basis of the percentage of proliferating crypt cells dying at any moment in time it is more significant (about 0.5–1.0% of all crypt cells). However, this apoptotic death is characteristically restricted to the lower regions of the crypt and more specifically to about the 4th position, i.e., the stem cell region. Since in any one crypt section there are only two cells at the 4th position, this death could represent a cell death frequency of between 10–20% for the cells at the 4th position. The full significance of this frequency is of course dependent on the length of time that it takes a cell to go through the full sequence of events that characterise apoptosis. This has not been precisely determined, but in the crypt it looks as if the half-life for apoptosis is about 5 h. Thus over a period of about 10 h, most cells would have gone through the complete sequence. The duration of apoptosis may be roughly comparable to the duration of DNA synthesis and these apoptotic indices therefore have a similar significance for the stem cells as the labelling index determined with tritiated thymidine. The biological significance of this spontaneous cell death remains unclear, but two obvious explanations come to mind. Firstly, these dying cells could represent the removal of cells that are produced excess to requirements by the stem cells. If stem cells normally undergo asymmetric divisions producing a stem cell and a transit cell at each division, but occasionally divide symmetrically producing two stem cells, apoptosis may be the mechanism by which these extra healthy stem cells are then removed. This process is in some ways similar to the apoptosis that characterises certain stages of development in embryos when large numbers of healthy cells are removed by apoptosis to allow the restructuring of tissues. The second explanation for the levels of spontaneous apoptosis is that these cells are a reflection of the low levels of spontaneous DNA damage induced by environmental factors or errors incurred during the process of DNA replication. As we will discuss later, there may be protective advantages in removing such cells with minor damage rather than attempting to repair the damage. For reasons discussed later, the former explanation seems the most likely.

The second important point in relation to radiation induced apoptosis is that following exposure, the appearance of new apoptotic cells is extremely rapid. Elevation in the numbers of apoptoses per crypt begins to be observed at about 1.5 h after irradiation and reaches peak levels between 3 and 6 h after irradiation [12]. Following low doses of radiation (less than 1 Gy) the levels of apoptosis decline rapidly thereafter reaching control levels at times beyond 24 h. Following higher doses, although a clear early peak at 3–6 h is observed, the reattainment of control levels can take some considerable time with oscillating levels of apoptosis in the intervening period. The third important observation is that following exposure to radiation, the early peak in apoptosis that is observed at 3–6 h is characteristically distributed around the 4th position from the bottom of the crypt, i.e., this early peak is a phenomenon that appears to be associated with the stem cell population. If the full positional distribution of apoptosis is determined, most of the cell death occurs below the 10th position and the distribution is quite unlike the distribution of proliferative cells which is relatively low at the 4th position and persists well up to the 20th positions. So the apoptotic death is not a process associated with the rapidly cycling cells of the crypt but associated with the more slowly cycling crypt base cells. The fourth and final significant point about the radiation induced apoptosis concerns its dose response relationship. Analysis of the yield of apoptosis at the time of the early peak, i.e., between 3 and 6 h after irradiation, shows that the yield increases progressively with increasing dose, up to about 1 Gy. Thereafter, it either plateaus or assumes a very shallow dose response relationship. At the time of the plateau, the yield is equivalent to about 4 apoptotic events per crypt section. Taking into account the fact that the apoptotic cells tend to be centripetally positioned in relation to the centrifugally positioned column of cell nuclei, this figure is equivalent to a total of about 6 cells per crypt being killed by a dose of 1 Gy or approximately 40% of the cells at cell position 4. Although higher doses of radiation clearly cause DNA damage and reproductively kill cells, these damaged cells do not initiate apoptosis readily. They may undergo apoptosis at some time subsequent to the early peak, they may repair the damage and continue to function normally, or they may persist as differentiated, but non-proliferative cells (prematurely aged). The surprising feature of the dose response relationship is the very high sensitivity of some of the cells in the stem cell region. This sensitivity is such that 1 rad (0.01 Gy) elevates the apoptotic yield and 0.05 Gy can be very readily detected. This makes these cells amongst the most radiosensitive cells in the mammalian body [12]. They have a sensitivity as high as the most sensitive spermatogonia and oocytes and higher than the peripheral lymphocytes which have always been thought of as being very sensitive. These three types of experiment, temporal, spatial and dose-dependent are summarised in Fig. 3.

A final feature of this apoptotic response in the small intestine is that the occurrence of even small elevated levels of apoptosis are apparently effectively detected by the surrounding neighbouring cells which respond by changing their proliferative characteristics [21,22]. This implies a tightly controlled regulatory process linking apoptosis and proliferation. A variety of experiments have indicated that the levels of mitosis, the cell cycle parameters as determined by % labelled mitosis techniques, the labelling pattern in the crypt base and even probably the stem cell self-maintenance probability are changed very rapidly following the induction of low levels of apoptosis. Thus although these cells delete themselves very readily after low levels of damage, the system compensates for this by responding in terms of proliferation to replace the lost cell. In this way the hypersensitive stem cell compartment becomes re-established after irradiation [23]. The sensitivity of these 6 cells at the stem cell region is such that damage anywhere in the DNA appears to precipitate the apoptotic process. This implies an extremely efficient DNA self-screening programme and an absence or prohibition of DNA repair processes which themselves may cause errors. Thus apoptosis may be an efficient protective mechanism for removing potentially harmful damaged stem cells, but it operates in conjunction with an extremely efficient system for recognising apoptosis and replacing the dying cells by cell division in other more resistant stem cells that are capable of undergoing repair of DNA damage. However, these processes nevertheless carry a minimal risk of transferring damage back to the early stem cells or to the stem cell compartment as a whole.

Studies involving eighteen different cytotoxic agents at different doses and studied at different times have indicated that the cells that are targeted by

Opposite: Fig. 3. Summary of three different types of experiments investigating apoptotic cell death in small intestinal crypts. The upper panel shows the temporal response for two different doses of radiation. Peak values are observed between 3 and 6 h after irradiation. The centre panel shows the spatial distribution of apoptotic bodies at any time between 3 and 6 h post-irradiation (bar diagram). Peak levels of apoptosis are seen in the third and fourth cell positions with high levels also observed at the fifth and sixth position. Relatively little apoptosis is seen at the tenth position which represents the peak of proliferative activity (dashed line). The lower panel shows the dose response relationship at 3–6 h post-irradiation. NB both scales are logarithmic. The control levels of spontaneous apoptosis are shown by the lower dashed line, a significant elevation in the levels of apoptosis can be observed following a dose of 0.02 Gy, the yield increases progressively with increasing dose up to about 1 Gy when it appears to saturate. This level of saturation is equivalent to about 4 cells/crypt section or about 6 cells in total/crypt.

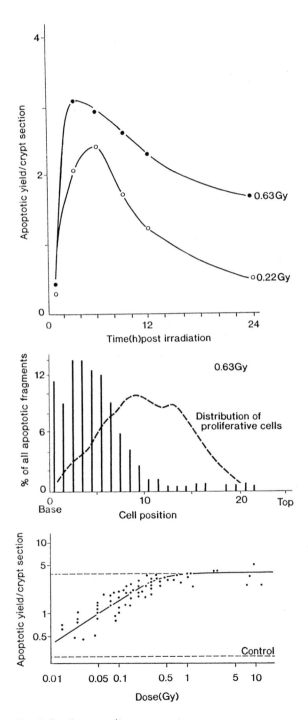

Fig. 3 Caption opposite.

different agents can have different positions within the crypt [9–11]. One group of agents including radiation appears to target the cells at around the 4th position, i.e., the stem cells. A second group tend to target cells at positions 6–8 in the crypt and these are clearly affecting cells early in the dividing transit part of the lineage, yet other agents target cells between cell positions 8 and 11 and these are clearly affecting cells in the middle of the transit population. What these experiments show quite clearly is that all cells in the crypt possess the necessary genetic programmes to activate apoptosis, but under normal circumstances this is suppressed (by genes such as bcl-2 and possibly myc when associated with high levels of growth factors) and that different drugs and cytotoxic agents can release cells from this suppression of apoptosis and allow them to initiate the process.

Measurements of the levels of apoptosis in small intestinal crypts have been used to investigate the effects of dose rate and linear energy transfer (LET). These studies have shown that the incidence of apoptotic cells induced by low doses of gamma rays was independent of the dose rate within the range 0.0027 and 4.5 Gy/min and the relative biological effectiveness (RBE) values for 14 MeV and 600 MeV neutrons was 4.0 and 2.7 respectively. The data for the dose response relationships which generally have the shape illustrated in the lower panel of Fig. 3 can be interpreted to provide survival curves for the cells sensitive to apoptotic death. The earlier studies such as illustrated in Fig. 3 and subsequent studies [26] provide survival curves for gamma rays with D_0 values for apoptosis (reciprocal of the slope) of about 0.24 Gy. The survival curve for 14 MeV neutrons has a D_0 value of 0.06 and that for 600 MeV neutrons, 0.09 Gy. The approach has also been used to quantitate the amount of cell killing induced by different doses of intracellular radiation delivered by the decay of tritium from tritiated thymidine incorporated into the DNA [27]. The dose response curve here has a shape similar to the lower panel in Fig. 3.

Less information has been obtained on radiation-induced apoptosis in the colon. However, the studies that have been performed clearly indicate that apoptosis is initiated following irradiation. The results show two clear differences from the response in the small intestine. Firstly, the apoptosis is concentrated in the mid-crypt region and not at the crypt base where the stem cells are believed to be located (at least in the mid colon). Secondly, there are indications that the dose response relationship is not saturated following doses of about 1 Gy, but continues to increase until about 6 Gy. Again the full temporal relationships have not been established in the colon, but the time of the peak yield appears to be similar to that in the small intestine. This differential positional response in the colon compared with the small intestine has also been observed following treatment with 4 different mutagenic and carcinogenic chemicals [5,16]. These chemicals target cells at the 4th position in the small intestine, but on average cells at cell position 10 in the large bowel. These observations have been interpreted to suggest that apoptosis may be an important protective mechanism in the small bowel in the stem cell population. The cells recognise the existence of DNA damage and respond by committing suicide, thus effectively removing the damage. This process does not seem to operate or is defective in the colon and thus cells with DNA damage have the potential to persist either carrying low levels of damage that are undetected, or damage that has been repaired, or damage that has been misrepaired. As a consequence of this the cells have a greater risk of sustaining perpetual genetic errors that might ultimately lead to cancers and this has been proposed as one additional explanation for the high levels of cancer incidence in the large bowel compared to the negligible levels of cancer incidence in the small bowel (in humans the incidence ratio is approximately 100:1).

The gene p53 has been suspected of being involved in the detection of DNA damage, i.e., the surveillance process and also in the initiation of apoptosis, and it is interesting in this respect that p53 expression rises rapidly in the small intestine 3 h after exposure to radiation, i.e., at a time concomitant with the rise in apoptosis and that this p53 expression is specifically located in the lower regions of the crypt (Ref. [24] and Fig. 4). In contrast, in the large bowel, p53 expression also rises following irradiation at 3 h, but here, the positive cells are distributed throughout the entire crypt. In mice which have had the p53 gene knocked out and then delivered a dose of 8 Gy, no apoptotic figures were found in either the small intestine or the large intestine 4.5 h after the exposure. These observations provide indications of a positive link between DNA damage induction, p53 expression, and apoptosis.

bcl-2 is a gene that has been linked with suppression of apoptosis and hence survival and proliferation of cells. Preliminary studies show that under normal circumstances bcl-2 expression is negligible or low in the small intestine of both untreated and irradiated animals and is high in both untreated and irradiated large intestine. These data correlate well with the above hypothesis.

Cells in a tissue can clearly die in a variety of ways in much the same fashion as humans can die in a variety of ways. As with current medical ethics, the question of how one defines human death, when precisely death occurs and which markers are most appropriate, similar questions and considerations apply to the identification of death of cells in a tissue. Clearly certain metabolic poisons, heat, and chemicals such as those used in fixatives, e.g., formalin or alcohol, can kill a cell instantly and the morphological consequence of this death may not be evident on a histological preparation or could manifest themselves as necrosis. Other agents or lower levels of injury may damage the cell in such a way that the self-deletion apoptotic sequence could be initiated and the morphological consequences of this can be recognised as apoptosis in sectioned material. Yet other possibilities are that the damage is such that apoptosis is not triggered, but the reproductive potential of the cell is impaired. The cell may be completely reproductively sterilised but it may persist as a cellular entity in the tissue. It may be capable of struggling through one or a few cell divisions which represents a reduction in its proliferative potential prior to exposure to the damaging agent. If we consider the stem cell compartment, such impairment of reproductive potential may result in a stem cell effectively becoming a dividing transit cell with limited potential, or indeed

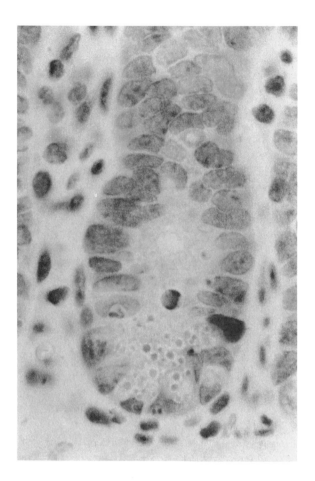

Fig. 4. Section through a small intestinal crypt 3–4 h after irradiation, stained with an affinity purified polyclonal antibody to p53 gene product. A single positive cell can be seen on the right hand side of the crypt at about cell position 4 immediately above the Paneth cells. A clear apoptotic cell can be seen in the centre of the field. Other apoptotic fragments are recognisable in the section. The function of the single p53 positive cell at the stem cell position remains to be elucidated as does the significance of the fact that the apoptotic cell is p53 negative. I am grateful to Anita Merritt for the section from which this photograph was taken. (See also colour plate on p. xiv.)

becoming a differentiated functional cell, a process that we may refer to as premature differentiation or maturation. There are indications that all these possibilities do in fact occur following a dose of radiation. The loss of reproductive potential is normally studied by looking at the number of cells that retain a fully functional reproductive capacity. Such approaches form the basis of the clonal regeneration assays that are available in many tissues including the intestine and these will be discussed in greater detail in Chapter 3.

3. CHANGES IN PROLIFERATION

Over the years there have been many independent studies, of varying precision and detail, that have indicated fairly clearly that after a dose of radiation, the cell cycle time of the majority of the cells in the crypt is reduced by approximately 20%. Depending on the data considered the average cycle time of cells in the crypt ranges between about 10–14 h in unirradiated animals (see Fig. 5 in Chapter 1). Following irradiation with moderate doses the cycle time for the average cells in the crypt may be reduced to 8–10 h. One of the more detailed analyses was performed by Lesher in 1967 [28] where a whole series of percent labelled mitosis curves were generated at various times after a dose of approximately 3 Gy. Here the cycle time was reduced from 13.1 h to 10.4 h, 24 h after irradiation. This type of cell cycle shortening is mainly attributable to reductions in the length of G_1 although other phases of the cycle may also be perturbed (see Fig. 5). Our own data on BDF1 mice indicate a 33% reduction in the average cycle time from 13.4 h to 9.0 h on the 3rd day after irradiation (8 Gy) [29]. Animals exposed to continuous or repeated daily exposures to radiation also show a reduction in the average cycle time.

Several of these studies showed that the cycle time for the cells at the base of the crypt in the small intestine is much more dramatically altered, for example it is reduced by 60% from 25.5 h to 10.1 h on day 3 after a dose of 8 Gy [29] and similarly, under conditions of continuous irradiation the cycle time at the crypt base was reduced by nearly 40% to between 9–10 h while the average for the mid-crypt cells were only reduced in their cycle time by 14% [31]. Other studies have indicated that damage caused by irradiation initiates rapid changes in the cell cycle even after the very small doses which result in 1 or 2 apoptotic cells per crypt [21,22,30]. The experiments here have involved studies looking at the recruitment of clonogenic cells into rapid cycle where they can be killed by metaphase arrest agents, changes in the number of cells in mitosis and changes in the number of mitotic figures that are radioactively labelled and changes in the migration of the leading edge of the labelling index versus cell position distributions which have been interpreted as indicating that the stem cell self-maintenance probability has been raised from 0.5 to a higher figure closer to 1.0 very rapidly after irradiation. Many of these studies have involved small doses (0.5 Gy) or doses of tritiated thymidine (slightly larger than conventional cell kinetic doses, i.e. 100 μCi or 3.7 MBq) which result in small increases in the levels of apoptosis. These rapid changes in various proliferation indices can only occur of course in cells that are not killed via apoptosis or cells that are not completely reproductively sterilised. These cell kinetic changes can only occur once the cells have overcome another well known effect of radiation which is to block the progression of cells through G_2. Such a block results in a fall in mitotic activity and this process is commonly known as mitotic delay or G_2 arrest. The rapid recruitment of cells into cycle discussed above and the mitotic delay phenomenon can be reconciled by the fact that the assays for rapid recruitment generally either involve times longer than the G_2

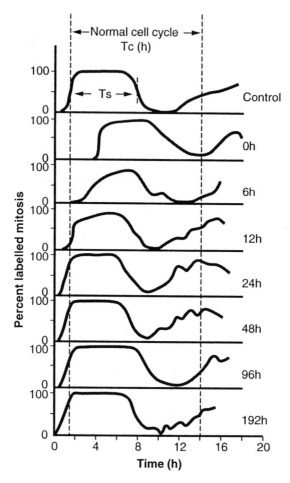

Fig. 5. A resumé of an extensive series of experiments performed and reported by Lesher in 1967 [28]. The experiments involved performing percent labelled mitoses experiments which were initiated by an injection of tritiated thymidine at various times (shown on the right) after 3 Gy of irradiation. Samples were taken at various times thereafter and analysed for the percent of mitotic figures that are radioactively marked in autoradiographs. The technique allows the duration of the cell cycle to be estimated (as shown by the vertical dotted lines for the control experiment at the top of the graph). It also allows the individual phases of the cell cycle to be identified (the duration of S, T_s, as shown for the control graph). The data show dramatically the effects of irradiation on cell cycle activity. The graph initiated at 0 h illustrates clearly, the G_2 arrest phenomenon. The graph at 24 h illustrates clearly the significant shortening in the cell cycle time. At 8 days post-irradiation (lowest panel), the shape of the curve is approximately identical to that in the control. At 4 days the S-phase still appears to be perturbed.

arrest phenomenon (for example, 12 h) or they involve an analysis of the movement of cells into the S-phase of the cycle as opposed to the movement of cells into M. This reconciliation is shown by the data of Lesher in 1967 where PLM analyses indicated a shortening of the cell cycle time shortly after irradiation, but the first wave in mitotic activity was delayed by several hours due to the G_2 arrest phenomenon (see Fig. 5). The conventional dogma concerning G_2 arrest suggests that the cells are delayed for about 1 h for each Gy of radiation delivered. This statement is based on studies with fibroblast cells in culture. For the bulk of the cells in the crypt this is also broadly the case. However, cells towards the base of the crypt appear to be more sensitive and are delayed for between 2–3 h for each Gy of radiation [32]. For 1 Gy the mitotic delay was estimated to be 2.8 h for cell positions 1–5 and 1.0 h for cell positions 16–20 and for 2.5 Gy the respective values were 5.5 h and 2.0 h.

There are many experiments that have been performed looking at the distribution of mitotic cells and DNA synthesizing cells (labelling index) at each cell position in the crypt at various times after a dose of radiation. The principles of the scoring procedure are shown in Fig. 6. Such experiments have been formed by us in BDF1 mice and have been performed extensively in rats (Sprague–Dawley) by Becciolini and his group (see Chapter 5). Similar studies have been performed by many other workers in the field including some of the pioneers of cell kinetics and radiobiology (e.g., see Ref. [31]). When the distributions of labelled cells in mice are considered, the general features of the response are as follows: there is a progressive fall in the average labelling index over a period of about 15 h. However, following a medium sized dose such as 8 Gy the average labelling index never falls below about 34% of the control value at any time which suggests that many cells continue to enter DNA synthesis and replicate their DNA. Cells also continue to emigrate from the crypt during the post-irradiation period. This cell migration process can be shown to be remarkably radioresistant and continues after doses of 12 Gy at near normal rates for at least the first two days [33–35]. Clearly with the occurrence of cell death, blockage in mitosis, damage to reproductive potential, combined with continued near normal emigration from crypt to villus the crypt population rapidly declines in size and this is probably the main explanation for the fall in the average labelling index. Between 15 h and 60–72 h post-irradiation, the crypt increases in size and the average labelling index increases progressively with time reaching control levels at around 40 h. Since the labelling index continues to increase with time there is a considerable overshoot in both labelling and mitosis between about 40–60 h. After about 72 h there is a regression in the average labelling index back towards the control levels. The overshoot however, is followed by some oscillations which is a phenomenon commonly observed in injured tissues. The changes in labelling index with time after a dose of 8 Gy are summarised in Figs. 7–9 [36].

The changes in the average labelling index have been reported by us and others, however, these cell positional frequency distributions provide further more detailed information. In particular, it can be seen that the regenerative process in terms of cell proliferation begins in the lower positions of the crypt when a clear burst of proliferative activity as measured by labelling index occurs at the crypt base between 3 and 12 h. This wave of DNA synthesis is followed by 2 successive waves for the crypt base population (Fig. 9). Very

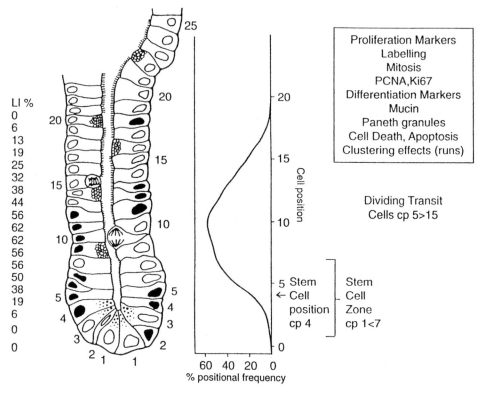

Fig. 6. Diagram illustrating the principles of the cell positional scoring techniques that have been used extensively in our studies and early pioneering work [31], and the group of Becciolini in Florence (see Chapter 5). A typical longitudinal section of a crypt is shown, the cells are numbered starting at the bottom of the crypt and various parameters (as shown in the box) can be determined on a cell positional basis. The numbers on the left represent an actual set of labelling index data for unirradiated animals and the graph illustrating this is shown in the middle of the diagram. Such cell positional data are usually expressed with frequency on the vertical scale and position on the horizontal scale and from such distributions, individual positions within the crypt can be analysed and characterised.

similar trends are observed when the mitotic frequency plots are considered. These and some of the other preceding observations suggest that the regenerative process following a radiation injury begins near the crypt base in the small intestine, i.e., in the stem cell compartment. Mathematical modelling studies have suggested that the early patterns of regeneration in the crypt can be explained solely on the basis of regulatory processes operating on the stem cells of the crypt [37].

In terms of the cellular populations and the proliferative rate of the cells in the crypt following irradiation injury the following general statements can be made. The first effects to be observed are acute cell death. The maximum yield of cell death occurs very early within about 3–6 h. This is at a time when p53

Postirradiation labelling indexes in crypts

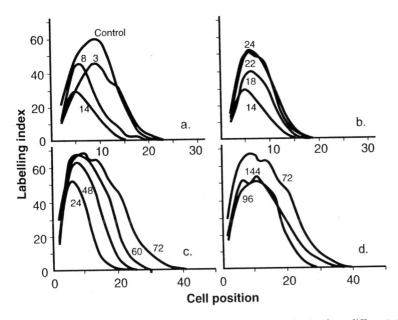

Fig. 7. Representative labelling index frequency plots obtained at different times (shown as numbers on the graph) following a dose of 8 Gy. Each line is the smoothed average for a minimum of 4 mice per time point. In this experiment, altogether 35 time points were investigated, the lines shown here are representative examples. All the time points are summarised in Fig. 8 (from Ref. [36]).

expression is raised and when there are some indications of an induced proliferative response in some of the non-killed cells. This rapid proliferative response has to accommodate the fact that progression through G_2 is a radio-sensitive process and this G_2 arrest is particularly pronounced in the stem cell population. Yet, other cells in the crypt have their reproductive potential impaired and may not go through their full programme of cell division. If they do not complete their full proliferative potential they may migrate onto the villus where they may be capable of performing some of the normal functions of intestinal epithelial cells. This process we have called 'Premature Differentiation or Maturation'. Some of the cells whose reproductive potential is impaired may have been potential clonogenic cells or regenerative cells. The consequence of these various forms of injury (death, delay in cycle progression, premature maturation, reduced proliferative potential) combined with the continued migration of cells from the crypt to the villus means that the crypt shrinks rapidly in size. If this process happens in too many crypts (i.e., if the dose of radiation is sufficiently large), eventually there will be a deficiency of cells for the villus and the integrity of the epithelial barrier is impaired. Generally, this impairment of the integrity of the mucosa does not manifest

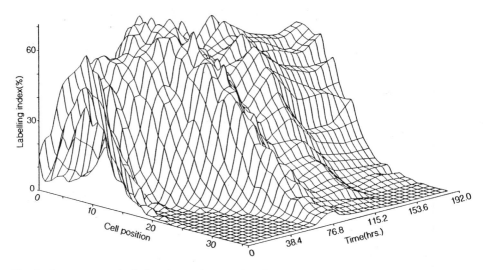

Fig. 8. A summary of all the time points analysed using tritiated thymidine labelling as a proliferation marker at various times following a dose of 8 Gy. This 3-dimensional plot shows labelling index on the vertical scale, cell position in the crypt and time after irradiation. The initial shrinkage in the labelling index distributions seen in Fig. 7 at early times can be seen. There is a gradual expansion and increase in the proliferative compartment with a significant overshoot at around 72 h and a gradual regression back to control levels at 192 h (data from Ref. [36]).

itself until times in excess of about 3 days which is the time that it takes for cells to move from the base of the villus to its tip, i.e., the villus transit time. The fact that even after high doses the integrity of the mucosa can be maintained for 3 days indicates that a large proportion of the crypt cells are capable of surviving the dose of radiation in the sense that they can emigrate and contribute to the mucosal integrity.

While the processes described above lead to a depletion in the overall cellularity of the crypt over a period of about two days, regeneration of the crypt will be initiated by any surviving clonogenic cells. The number of clonogenic cells per crypt is between about 6 and 30 depending on the level of injury that has been induced (see Fig. 15, Chapter 1 and also Chapter 3). If a single clonogenic cell survives, the crypt will be regenerated over a period of 2–3 days. Generally speaking, by the third day, the regenerating crypt is somewhat larger in terms of physical dimensions and cellularity than a controlled crypt. If no clonogenic cells survive, the crypt will generally shrink away over a period of two days. The differentiated Paneth cells at the base of the crypt tend to be much more radioresistant as would be expected for differentiated cells and may persist for some period of time marking the location of the dead crypt. Regeneration from clonogenic cells located in the lower regions of the crypt begins very soon after irradiation as demonstrated by the changes in labelling and mitotic activity at the crypt base (Fig. 9).

Radiobiological response of small intestine

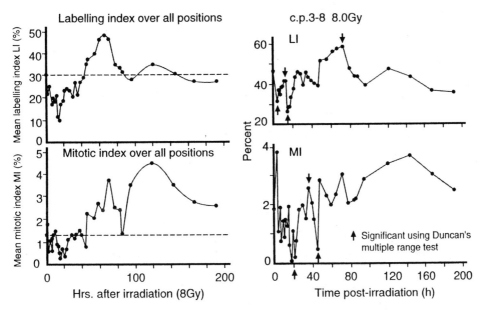

Fig. 9. The data shown in Figs. 7 and 8 can be summarised as the average labelling index value for each individual frequency distribution plot. Such data for labelling and mitotic activity for the crypt as a whole are shown in the two left hand panels. The dashed line shows the control values. The reduction in proliferation at early times, the regenerative phase and the overshoot phase can be clearly seen. Broadly speaking, the mitotic activity changes mimic those seen with labelling. The frequency distribution plots can be analysed to investigate specific regions in the crypt as illustrated in Fig. 6. It is difficult to define a single precise stem cell position in such an experiment because the size and shape of the crypt is varying throughout the time course. However, the data shown on the two right hand panels give the labelling and mitotic data for the lower regions of the crypt which are believed to contain the small intestinal stem cells. Statistically significant peaks and troughs in proliferation can be observed, the earliest of which represents the initial steps in crypt regeneration (taken from Ref. [1]).

If the mucosal integrity is jeopardised, what this means in simple terms is that the surface covering ends up with holes in it, i.e., there is 'naked' connective tissue. This means that the animal is no longer protected from the environment, the water balance and the electrolyte balance are affected, loss of fluids and blood into the lumen of the gut can occur and bacterial contamination can move the other way. The consequences of such damage are generally expressed as the *gastrointestinal radiation syndrome* which is characterised by anorexia, vomiting, diarrhoea, loss of electrolytes, septicaemia and ultimately death if the symptoms are sufficiently severe. These symptoms generally begin to express themselves on around the third day and with severe levels of damage, mice will succumb to the gastrointestinal radiation syndrome and die over the period 3–7 days.

While these negative effects of radiation are proceeding, regeneration phenomena are also taking place providing the dose of radiation was not supralethal in terms of the clonogenic cells. These regenerative processes start early after irradiation at the bottom of the crypt, are characterised by rapid cell cycles and the re-establishment of the cellular compartment of the crypt within a period of 48–72 h. The occurrence of the gastrointestinal radiation syndrome and the ultimate survival of the animal depends on the competitive actions of crypt depopulation and crypt regeneration and the absolute number of surviving clonogenic cells (see Fig. 14, Chapter 1). If enough clonogenic cells survive, sufficient crypts will be regenerated to maintain the integrity of the mucosal barrier. The regenerative capacity of the clonogenic cells is truly remarkable and is illustrated by the response following a dose of about 12 Gy. This is a dose that is approximately equivalent to the LD_{50} dose for mice, i.e., a dose at which half the animals will succumb within a period of 6–7 days and half will survive. This dose results in a depopulation of the crypts by about 80%. Thus in these animals, about 1 surviving clonogenic cell in every 5th crypt is compatible with the survival of half the animals. This means that in those animals that survive an epithelium is re-established and the integrity maintained by 1 surviving clonogenic cell in every 5th crypt.

These observations can be viewed in the light of what has become known as the first law of radiobiology, mainly the statements made by Bergonie and Tribondeau in 1906. They stated that the sensitivity of cells to irradiation is in direct proportion to their reproductive activity and inversely proportional to their degree of differentiation. As a generalised statement this clearly applies to the intestine. The intestine is characterised by rapid proliferation and, therefore, would be expected to be radiosensitive and indeed it is. However, the statement of Bergonie and Tribondeau needs to be modified to take into account the concept of cellular hierarchies. In fact in the small intestinal crypt, the most rapidly proliferating cells do not seem to be the most sensitive. The mid-crypt cells have a cycle time of about 12 h and many of these cells seem to be capable of maintaining some cell cycle activity and certainly differentiating to villus cells. In contrast, cells near the base of the crypt, the stem cells, have a longer cell cycle time of around 24 h and are much more radiosensitive. Some of these cells exhibit all the characteristics of a radiosensitive population. However, the radiosensitivity of the stem cells (stem cells in their broadest sense including the clonogenic compartment) must be quite heterogeneous. Some cells within the stem cell compartment are in fact exquisitely sensitive and die very easily after small doses and this can be seen by the occurrence of apoptotic cells. However, only about 6 cells in the crypt can be killed in this way. These very sensitive cells must be largely unable to repair DNA damage and must have very efficient mechanisms for detecting the occurrence of damage. However, the stem cell compartment must also contain more resistant cells which are capable of repairing damage (which accounts for their resistance) and under normal circumstances, these more resistant cells can repopulate the sensitive compartment. These more resistant cells comprise much of the potential clonogenic compartment. Crypts cannot be destroyed until all the potential stem cells have been reproductively sterilised. Under normal circumstances and low doses of radiation, the crypt may contain another 6 of these more resistant cells, but if the damage is more severe, it is capable of calling upon a greater number of potential clonogenic cells (up to 30). Thus the crypts may contain up to 4–6 actual, very sensitive, stem cells, about 6 more resistant clonogenic cells and up to about 30 other potential resistant clonogenic cells which are called into action after high levels of injury (see Chapter 3).

The changes in histological appearance of the crypts and villi can be seen in paraffin sections cut through the tissue and at appropriate times, the reduction in the villus height and in crypt cellularity is clearly evident. The foci of regeneration can be easily recognised because of the intense staining (chromophilic nature) of the healthy rapidly proliferating, regenerating epithelium (see Fig. 13, Chapter 1 and Fig. 1, Chapter 3). The changes in villus appearance after irradiation have also be documented using the scanning electron microscope [38], when the villi become abnormal shaped, squat, and eventually flat. These studies also reported changes in the stroma that supported the epithelium [39]. The stromal changes that are involved include a loss of the considerable degree of organisation observed in the sub-epithelial or pericryptal regions and damage to the basal lamina. There are also changes in the deep stromal regions with cells becoming more irregular shaped with cytoplasmic inclusions and sometimes vesicles, the ground substance also showed some disorientation of its ordered nature. Changes were observed in the arterioles with damage to the lining of the vessels, there are also some less well defined changes in the muscle layers and small changes in the nervous tissue. These studies led to attempts to formulate a numerical index of damage to the tissue taking into account all the various morphological changes that were observed [40]. Studies have also been performed on the effects of radiation on the endothelial cells in the mesenteric arterioles [41] After high doses of radiation (45 Gy) there was a significant depletion of cells over a protracted period of time. Even after these high doses there is some evidence of a gradual repopulation of cells from some very radioresistant surviving cells.

Thus, although the predominant and most sensitive element of the gastrointestinal tissue is the epithelial mucosa, changes also occur in the connective tissue and in particular, the vascular elements (see Fig. 2, Chapter 1 and Chapter 7). These changes will affect the overall response of the tissue and also its functional competence. However, higher doses of radiation are generally required to produce some of the observed effects.

References

1. Potten, C.S. (1990) A comprehensive study of the radiobiological response of the murine (BDF1) small intestine. Int. J. Radiat. Biol. 58, 925–974.
2. Kerr, J.F.R., Wyllie, A.H. and Currie, A.R. (1972) Apoptosis: a basic biological phenomenon with wide-ranging implication in tissue kinetics. Br. J. Cancer, 26, 239–257.
3. Potten, C.S. (1983) Stem cells in gastrointestinal mucosa. In: E.M. Skolnick and A.J. Levine (Eds.), Tumor Viruses and Differentiation. Alan R. Liss Inc., New York, pp. 381–398.
4. Potten, C.S. (1992) The significance of spontaneous and induced apoptosis in the gastrointestinal tract of mice. Cancer Metastasis Rev. 11, 179–195.
5. Li, Y.Q., Fan, C., O'Connor, P.J., Winton, D. and Potten, C.S. (1992) Target cells for the cytotoxic effects of carcinogens in the murine small bowel. Carcinogenesis 13, 361–368.
6. Harmon, B.V., Takano, Y.S., Winterford, C.M. and Potten, C.S. (1992) Vincristine induces cell death by apoptosis in intestinal crypts of mice and in human Burkitt's lymphoma. Cell Prolif. 25, 523–536.
7. Thakkar, N.S. and Potten, C.S. (1992) Abrogation of adriamycin toxicity *in vivo* by cycloheximide. Biochem. Pharmacol. 43, 1683–1691.
8. Kerr, J.F.R., Searle, J., Harmon, B.V. and Bishop, C.J. (1987) Apoptosis. In: C.S. Potten (Ed.), Perspectives on Mammalian Cell Death. Oxford Scientific Publications, Oxford, pp. 93–108.
9. Ijiri, K. and Potten, C.S. (1983) Response of intestinal cells of differing topographical and hierarchical status to ten cytotoxic drugs and five sources of radiation. Br. J. Cancer 47, 175–185.
10. Ijiri, K. and Potten, C.S. (1987a) Further studies on the response of intestinal crypt cells of different hierarchical status to cytotoxic drugs. Br. J. Cancer 55, 113–123.
11. Ijiri, K. and Potten, C.S. (1987b) Cell death in cell hierarchies in adult mammalian tissues. In: C.S. Potten (Ed.), Perspectives on Mammalian Cell Death. Oxford University Press, pp. 326–356.
12. Potten, C.S. (1977) Extreme sensitivity of some intestinal crypt cells to κ and γ irradiation. Nature 269, 518–521.
13. Potten, C.S., Al-Barwari, S.E., Hume, W.J. and Searle, J. (1977) Circadian rhythms of presumptive stem cells in three different epithelia of the mouse. Cell Tissue Kinet. 10, 557–568.
14. Potten, C.S., Merritt, A.J., Hickman, J., Hall, P. and Faranda, A. (1994) The characterisation of radiation-induced apoptosis in the small intestine and its biological implications. Int. J. Radiat. Biol. 65, 71–78.
15. Gavrieli, Y., Sherman, Y. and Ben-Sasson, S.A. (1992) Identification of programmed cell death *in situ* via specific labelling of nuclear DNA fragmentation. J. Cell. Biol. 119, 493–501.
16. Potten, C.S., Li, Y.Q., O'Connor, P.J. and Winton, D.G. (1992) Target cells for the cytotoxic effects of carcinogens in the murine large bowel and a possible explanation for the differential cancer incidence in the intestine. Carcinogenesis 13, 2305–2312.
17. Allan, D.J., Harmon, B.V. and Kerr, J.F.R. (1987) Cell death in spermatogenesis. In: C.S. Potten (Ed.), Perspectives on Mammalian Cell Death. Oxford Scientific Publications, Oxford, pp. 229–258.

18. Lane, D.P. (1992) News and views: p53 guardian of the genome. Nature 358, 15–16.

19. Vaux, D.L., Cory, S. and Adams, J.M. (1988) *Bcl*-2 gene promotes haemopoietic cell survival and co-operates with *c-myc* to immortalise pre-B cells. Nature 335, 440–442.

20. Evan, G.I. and Littlewood, T.D. (1993) The role of *c-myc* in cell growth. Curr. Opin. Genet. Devel. 3, 44–49.

21. Potten, C.S. (1991a) Regeneration in epithelial proliferation units as exemplified in the small intestine. CIBA Foundation Publ. 160, John Wiley, Chichester, pp. 64–76.

22. Potten, C.S. (1991b) The role of stem cells in the regeneration of intestinal crypts after cytotoxic exposure. In: B.E. Butterworth, T.J. Slaga, W. Farland and M. McClain (Eds.), Chemically Induced Cell Proliferation. Implications for Risk Assessment. John Wiley, New York, pp. 155–171.

23. Ijiri, K. and Potten, C.S. (1984) The re-establishment of hypersensitive cells in the crypts of irradiated mouse intestine. Int. J. Radiat. Biol. 46, 609–624.

24. Merritt, A.J., Potten, C.S., Hickman, J.A., Kemp, C., Ballmain, A., Hall, P. and Lane, D. (1994) The role of p53 paper in spontaneous and radiation-induced intestinal cell apoptosis in normal and p53 deficient mice. Cancer Res. 54, 614–617.

25. Potten, C.S. and Allen, T.D. (1977) Ultrastructure of cell loss of intestinal mucosa. J. Ultrastruct. Res. 60, 272–277.

26. Hendry, J.H. and Potten, C.S. (1982) Intestinal cell radiosensitivity: a comparison for cell death assayed by apoptosis or by a loss of clonogenicity. Int. J. Radiat. Biol. 42, 621–628.

27. Ijiri, K. (1988) Cell death induced in mouse intestine by tritiated thymidine and gamma rays. Proc. 3rd Japan–US Workshop on Tritium Radiobiology and Health Physics, Nov. 8–10, pp. 217–222.

28. Lesher, S. (1967) Compensatory reaction in intestinal crypt cells after 300 Roentgens of cobalt^{60} gamma-irradiation. Radiat. Res. 32, 510–519.

29. Potten, C.S. (1986) Cell cycles in cell hierarchies. Int. J. Radiat. Biol. 49, 257–278.

30. Potten, C.S., Chadwick, C., Ijiri, K., Tsubouchi, S. and Hanson, W.R. (1984) The recruitability and cell cycle status of intestinal stem cell. Int. J. Cell Cloning 2, 126–140.

31. Cairnie, A.B. (1967) Cell proliferation studies in the intestinal epithelium of the rat: response to continuous irradiation. Radiat. Res. 32, 240–264.

32. Chwalinski, S. and Potten, C.S. (1986) Radiation induced mitotic delay: duration, dose and cell position dependence in the crypts of the small intestine in the mouse. Int. J. Radiat. Biol. 49, 809–819.

33. Kaur, P. and Potten, C.S. (1986a) Circadian variation in migration in small intestinal epithelium. Cell Tissue Kinet. 19, 591–600.

34. Kaur, P. and Potten, C.S. (1986b) Cell migration velocities in the crypts after cytotoxic insult are not dependent on mitotic activity. Cell Tissue Kinet. 19, 601–610.

35. Kaur, P. and Potten, C.S. (1986c) Effects of puromycin, cycloheximide and noradrenalin on cell migration within the crypts and on the villi of the small intestine. A model to explain cell movement in both regions. Cell Tissue Kinet. 19, 611–626.

36. Potten, C.S., Owen, G. and Roberts, S.A. (1990) The temporal and spatial changes in proliferation within the irradiated small intestinal crypts. Int. J. Radiat. Biol. 57, 185–199.

37. Paulus, U., Potten, C.S. and Loeffler, M. (1992) A model of the cellular regeneration

in the intestinal crypt after perturbation based solely on local stem cell regulation. Cell Prolif. 25, 559–578.

38. Carr, K.E., Hamlet, R., Nias, A.H.W. and Watt, C. (1983) Damage to the surface of the small intestinal villus: an objective scale of assessment of the effects of single and fractionated doses. Br. J. Radiol. 56, 467–475.

39. Carr, H.E., Hamlet, R., Nias, A.H.W., Boyle, F.C. and Fife, M.G. (1985) Stromal damage in the mouse small intestine after Co^{60} gamma irradiation. Scanning Electron Microscopy IV, 1615–1621.

40. Carr, K.E., McCullough, J.S., Nunn, S., Hume, S.P. and Nelson, A.C. (1991) Neutron and X-ray effects on small intestine summarised by using a mathematical model or paradigm. Proc. Roy. Soc. Lond. B. Biol. Sci. 243, 187–194.

41. Hirst, D.G., Denekamp, J. and Hobson, B.0 (1980) Proliferation studies of the endothelial and smooth muscle cells of the mouse mesentery after irradiation. Cell Tissue Kinet. 13, 91–104.

C.S. Potten and J.H. Hendry (Eds.), *Radiation and Gut*

CHAPTER 5

Radiation Effects on Proliferation and Differentiation in the Rat Small Intestine

A. Becciolini[1], M. Balzi[1] and C.S. Potten[2]

[1]*Laboratory of Radiation Biology, Department of Clinical Physiopathology, University of Florence, Viale Pieraccini 6, 50134 Florence, Italy*
[2]*CRC Department of Epithelial Cell Biology, Paterson Institute for Cancer Research, Christie Hospital NHS Trust, Wilmslow Road, Manchester M20 9BX, UK*

1. INTRODUCTION

The mechanisms involved in the interaction of ionising radiation with biological systems can be studied at various levels from the molecular, to microbiological, to cells in culture. However, more specific approaches are needed for complex systems to understand the damage induction and damage repair processes within cells, tissues, organs and within the entire organism. Studies on animals are very informative, but do not necessarily allow a direct extrapolation to the human situation, however, in spite of this such systems do allow the damage induction and repair processes involved in acute responses and late injury to be studied.

The intestinal epithelium is a good model to study the effects of physical and chemical cytotoxic agents, because

(a) the tissue has a high proliferative activity and a rapid turnover which means that damage is manifest within a short time of exposure,

(b) the proliferative compartment is distinct from the differentiated compartment and is easily identified,

(c) differentiation occurs according to cell position on the crypt/villus axis and is characterised by the synthesis of particular molecules such as brush border enzymes, and

(d) different differentiation pathways exist, all of which are believed to be derived from a common stem cell (see Chapter 1 for further details).

A knowledge of the processes involved in the intestine following exposure to cytotoxic agents such as irradiation are important in humans because the intestine is one of the common limiting tissues in radiotherapy and chemotherapy of cancer patients. Regions of normal healthy intestine are commonly included in the radiation field and the entire intestine is exposed when systemic cytotoxic drugs are used. Radiation can be regarded as a good 'model' cytotoxic agent to study the consequences of such injury, in part because doses can be measured accurately. The effects of radiation on human intestine are well documented and are summarised in Chapter 8. Irradiation of part of the intestinal epithelium is common in the treatment of patients with abdominal and pelvic tumours (for the most part gynaecological tumours) and this results in the malabsorption syndrome [1–3]. Differential absorption of different elements in the diet can be observed depending on whether the molecules are absorbed through active or passive transport mechanisms. Such studies are based on the analysis of individual molecules in blood samples taken during treatment and after the administration of test meals of specific composition, the results being compared with data obtained before therapy. Amongst the various molecules studied, proteins and amino acids showed little variation during treatment whereas statistically significant reductions were observed in fatty acid, vitamin and carbohydrate absorption [1–3]. Disaccharides showed the greatest reduction, these molecules requiring preventive hydrolysis by disaccharidases in the brush border. The biggest effects in most cases were observed half way through the treatment following 25–30 Gy. For doses between 45 and 55 Gy, carbohydrates particularly, showed an additional reduction in absorption towards the end of the treatment.

The gastrointestinal radiation syndrome typically involves diarrhoea and water and electrolyte loss. By analysing plasma, blood and total body water volume during the active phase there was no significant variation during, or at the end of the treatment or exposure period which demonstrates the existence of compensatory mechanisms to prevent dehydration [4]. Similar studies have shown that there is no modification in the pancreatic enzyme activities as measured in the contents of the duodenum [5]. These studies reinforce the view that cell structure, organisation, proliferation and differentiation are all important in determining the severity of the reaction to cytotoxic agents.

1.1 The structure of the intestinal epithelium

The structure of the intestinal epithelium is summarised in Chapter 1. Here we wish to emphasis the importance of section orientation for a proper analysis of proliferation, differentiation, cell death, etc., in relation to the crypt/villus axis. Chapter 1 also describes the technical approach of measuring cell proliferation, differentiation and death on a cell positional basis which using appropriate software and microcomputers, can be analysed to generate frequency plots for the various differentiated cell types along the crypt/villus axis. Using appropriate normalisation procedures, it is possible to compare such frequency plots with one another. Examples of such plots are shown in Fig. 1, which confirm that in the small intestine, the proportion of labelled cells (S phase cells) at the bottom of the crypt is low and that the incidence of differentiated

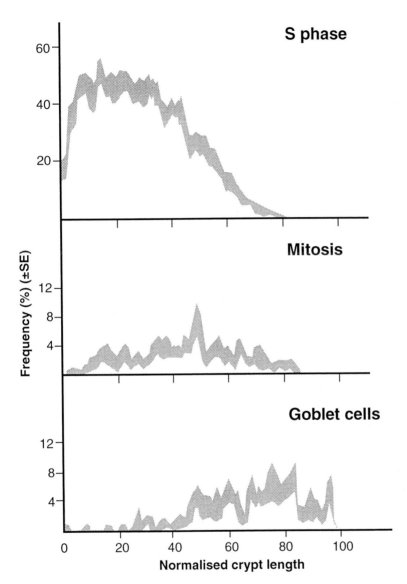

Fig. 1. Frequency distributions of S-phase cells, mitoses and goblet cells in different positions of the crypt, for control rats sacrificed at the same time of day. Total height of the crypt has been normalised to 100%. The curves represent the standard error limits on the mean. (Modified from Ref. [45]).

goblet cells increases gradually with increasing cell position. Such frequency plots are consistent with the existence of differentiated Paneth cells at the crypt base and goblet cell differentiation in the later phases of the dividing transit populations [6] and with the existence of more slowly cycling (or quiescent, G_0) pluripotent stem cells in the lower positions of the crypt. The proportion of S phase cells in the rat is about 50% in the mid crypt region and the proportion of S phase cells reaches 0 about three-quarters of the distance up the crypt as shown in Fig. 1. The frequency plot for mitosis is slightly displaced to the right since mitosis follows S phase in the cell cycle and the cells are migrating up the crypt as they pass through the cycle, hence mitotic figures are seen as far as 85% up the crypt length compared to 75% for the S phase cells.

In the rat, goblet cells are rarely observed in the lower 25% of the crypt. The highest levels (between 6 and 8%) are seen in the region between 50 and 85% of the crypt length (Fig. 1). The figures in the rat appear to be lower than corresponding numbers in the mouse [6]. In both species, the frequency of goblet cells falls towards the very top of the crypt for reasons that remain somewhat obscure. The data in general suggest the existence of some differentiated cells (Paneth cells) at the very base together with some proliferative cells with a longer cell cycle or quiescence. On the whole, differentiation occurs in the upper 25% of the crypt in relation to goblet cells and chief cells. This pattern is also typical of the synthesis of characteristic enzymes which are localised in the external protein layers associated with the microvillus membrane. These enzymes are involved with the terminal digestive processes (membrane digestion) which result in the hydrolysis of monosaccharide and amino acid dimers and trimers.

1.2 Digestion and absorption in the small intestine

Digestion and absorption of the simple molecular constituents resulting from the hydrolysis of macromolecules are the main functions of the gastrointestinal epithelium. The epithelial cells are not only a lining, but they actively participate in absorption through active or passive transport mechanisms or through pinocytosis. Several years ago, an additional process was reported which was also observed in the epithelium of proximal tubules of the kidney namely membrane digestion [7–8]. This process of terminal digestion involves the dimer and trimer forms of amino acids and monosaccharides and their hydrolysis and subsequent absorption by specific carriers located in the membranes. The scheme which was proposed by Ugolev [9,10] is summarised in Fig. 2.

The brush border enzymes are glycoproteins with high molecular weights (about 200 kD) and they form approximately 10% of the brush border membrane proteins. They are synthesized in the cytosol, glycosylated in the Golgi apparatus, and then transferred to the membrane. The synthesis is first observed in the cells located in the upper part of the crypt ie, in the region of decycling (loss of proliferative activity) and terminal differentiation. These brush border enzymes which are active in the outer layers of the membrane tend to be lost into the lumen through pancreatic protease action and are replaced by newly synthesized enzymes [11].

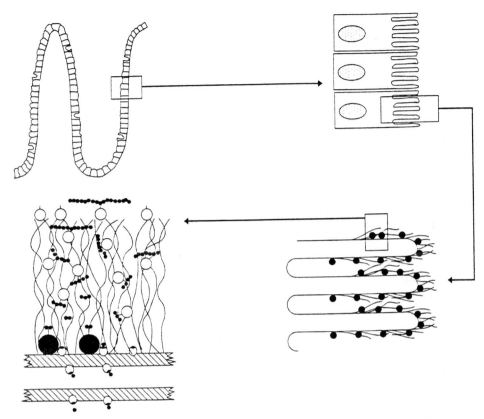

Fig. 2. Schematic representation of the membrane digestion process. A part of the epithelium is enlarged and analysed at the brush border level where the macromolecules of food are progressively hydrolysed to dimeric forms. The white circles represent enzymes in the lumen entangled in the fuzzy coat. Black circles represent brush border enzymes associated with carriers to the outer layer of the cell membrane. (Modified and expanded from Ref. [9]).

1.3 Polysaccharide digestion and absorption

The different disaccharidase enzymes are structurally similar to each other, but they differ in their specificity for hydrolysis of different molecular bonds. Maltase, invertase, isomaltase, trehalase and lactase each hydrolyse the corresponding disaccharides to produce glucose, fructose, or galactose and it is the absorption of the monosaccharides that it is the rate limiting step because the hydrolysis is rapid.

The distribution of brush border enzyme activities along the gastrointestinal tract is not uniform. Activity is absent in the stomach, increases gradually from the duodenum to the jejunum and mid-ileum and then decreases to very low levels in the terminal ileum (Fig. 3). Activity is absent in the large bowel.

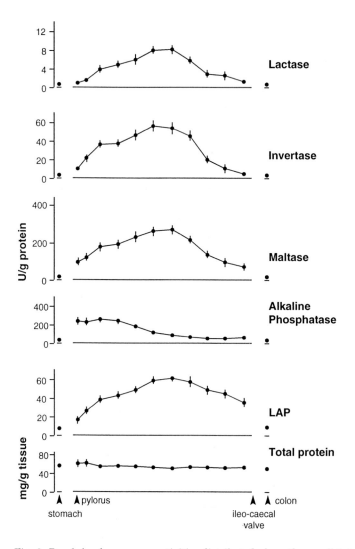

Fig. 3. Brush border enzyme activities distributed along the small intestine, lactase, invertase, maltase, alkaline phosphatase and leucineaminopeptidase. The mean values ± SE of control rats sacrificed at the same time of the day are reported. The values in the stomach and colon are also presented. (Unpublished data).

Trehalase and alkaline phosphatase are present at high levels in the duodenum and jejunum and then decrease rapidly in the ileum. Individually, the levels of the enzymes vary considerably. Maltase is the most abundant and trehalase and lactase are present at low levels. In mammals, the enzyme activities vary with age; lactase activity being very high in suckling rats and the other enzymes being very low. After weaning, the lactase is reduced 10-fold and maltase and invertase and other disaccharidases increase considerably. In the adult and old rat, lactase levels decrease further and in man some elderly subjects exhibit hypolactasia and therefore have an intolerance to milk. These brush border enzymes are affected by diet and in some individuals enzyme deficiencies may develop. Numerous pathological situations have been linked to malabsorption of carbohydrates and one of the causes may be brush border enzyme deficiencies due, for example, to anatomical changes as in the case of coeliac disease, tropical sprue, or gastroenteritis. In situations where the mucosa is apparently normal, and there is still malabsorption, this could be due to congenital defects in the synthesis of specific enzymes [12–14]. Some congenital enzyme deficiencies may result in severe intolerance to specific carbohydrates. Lactase deficiency is the commonest one in man and it differs in its frequency in various ethnic groups [13]. Here the deficiency lies in the regulatory genes which control the synthesis of the enzymes and not in an inactive variant of the molecules [14]. Another example of malabsorption of disaccharides can be seen in the intestinal intolerance in some infants before and during weaning. The deficiency again may be congenital and lactose which is not hydrolysed by the enzyme is then metabolised by intestinal bacteria which can result in the production of lactic acid, aldeids, etc., which irritate the bowel and can result in diarrhoea [15]. Once the lactose is removed from the diet, the situation returns to normal.

1.4 Digestion and absorption of proteins and amino acids

The digestion and absorption of proteins occur through mechanisms that are similar to those for polysaccharides. However, in general there is a greater number of processes involved along the length of the intestine and malabsorption conditions usually are not observed. Endoluminal digestion of proteins which follows the protease action initiated in the stomach is performed by pancreatic enzymes to produce oligomer forms. Digestion continues by further splitting of the molecules by brush border hydrolases. Some of these enzymes act on the longer oligopeptide molecules and these are located in the brush border with dipeptidases. Only dipeptidases are observed in the cytosol [16]. As with the disaccharidases, amino peptidases are synthesised in the rough endoplasmic reticulum then glycosylated in the Golgi apparatus and incorporated into the plasma membrane where they are anchored by small hydrophobic peptide sequences [17]. In both rats and humans, the absorption of amino acids from dipeptides is more rapid than can be demonstrated in equivalent solutions of free amino acids. Some dipeptides are absorbed intact and hydrolysed by the cytosolic peptidases. Such mechanisms reduce the frequency of malabsorption of protein hydrolysis products.

1.5 Distribution of other molecules along the small intestine

Lysosomal enzyme activity such as beta-glucuronidase, beta-acid galactosidase, and acid phosphatase, shows an even distribution along the small intestine,

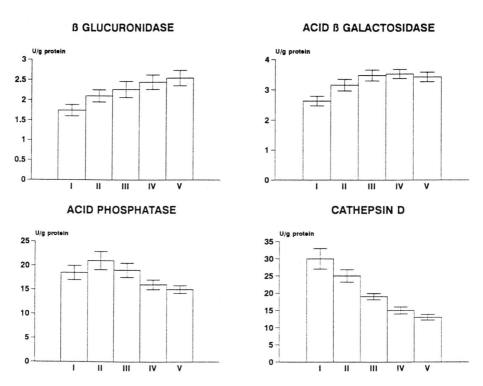

Fig. 4. Lysosomal enzyme distribution (β glucuronidase, β acid galactosidase, acid phosphatase and cathepsin D) in the 5 regions of the small intestine of control animals. The mean values ± SE of control rats sacrificed at the same time of the day are presented. (Data from Ref. [65]).

with only a small increase from the duodenum to the terminal ileum. Cathepsin D in contrast shows its highest activity in the duodenum with decreasing activity in the ileum (Fig. 4). Protein and DNA contents show an even distribution along the small intestine.

1.6 Bioperiodic dependence

The metabolism, function and activity of organisms often shows cyclic functions that have highly variable periods which can last from fractions of seconds (for example those seen in neural membranes and muscular cells) to as long as seasons or even decades. Such bioperiodic oscillations have been observed in many physiological functions, however, it is only recently that the clinical use of these periodic functions has been studied. One such biorhythm is the circadian cycle (the cycle of approximately 24 h) which is very common in mammals and is related to the light/dark, day/night cycle and the related variations in the levels of activity, feeding etc. The precise mechanisms involved in these rhythms and the anatomical structures involved in receiving the stimuli and regulating the rhythms are largely unknown, but the current view is that it is a multi-oscillatory system and that the supra-chiasmatic nuclei and the epiphysis plays a role. These rhythms influence experimental results and the design of experiments and must be taken into account in the interpretation of data. Both proliferative and differentiative activity (e.g., enzyme and metabolic activities) can vary with the time of day. Studies of circadian rhythm in proliferative activity are important when considering cytotoxic agents that might have differential sensitivities for cells at various stages of the cell cycle. For an agent that has some specificity for a particular stage of the cell cycle it would be important to consider the time of administration of such cytotoxic agents in relation to the time of day. This might become important in the treatment of cancer where the appropriate administration of cytotoxic agents could minimise the damage to normal healthy tissue. Animal studies are useful for determining whether agents which affect proliferation or differentiation may act differently depending on the time of day they are administered. Once the variations in rhythmic cycles of sensitivity to a damaging agent are known, the timing of the administration of such an agent becomes important [18]. The data published using animals to investigate these questions are sometimes conflicting, probably because of variations in such factors as the housing conditions and because the amplitude of the rhythm is sometimes small.

1.7 Bioperiodic phenomena in the small intestine

Bioperiodic rhythms exist in the small intestine, but there is a lack of consistency between the various reports. For example some reports suggest high proliferative activity during the night [19,20], or during the day [21,22]. These rhythms in proliferation can be reversed by altering the light/dark cycle [23] or changing the feeding programme [22]. Some reports state that the maximum number of cells that line the epithelial crypt occurs when the proliferation is lowest [24,25]. It has been suggested by some that the abrasive activity of food in the lumen of the gut removes cells from the villus which may provide a signal to stimulate proliferation in the crypt [25].

1.8 Brush border enzyme activities

One parameter which certainly shows a circadian dependence is the level of brush border enzymes and the levels of these enzymes can be influenced by the feeding regime. In both rats and mice, fed ad libitum and kept in a 24 h light/dark cycle with the lights on from 0630 h to 1830 h, the highest activity in enzymes is observed soon after midnight [26,27], with small changes in the phases according to which enzyme is analysed. The lowest activity is observed in the afternoon. These observations are consistent with the fact that in these nocturnal animals, the highest motor and metabolic activity occurs during the night. If food is available only for a few hours per day and not ad libitum, the highest levels of enzyme activity are observed during the feeding period [28,29] provided a period of adaptation is allowed. When food is withheld, the maltase and leucinaminopeptidase cycle (LAP) remains normal for at least 2 days after which the oscillations decrease and disappear by the 5th day. When the animals are re-fed, the LAP cycle returns immediately while the normal disaccharidase cycle requires 2 days for its reappearance. Animals placed in continuous light or continuous dark have the same cycles when feeding is allowed *ad libitum*. For the group kept in continuous light, biorhythms are only observed in the animals that received timed feedings [30]. From these studies it is possible to conclude that the light/dark cycle and the period of feeding influence each other and that the control of the circadian cycle for various enzymes is achieved by different mechanisms. Circadian rhythms, for example of invertase, are not present in the rat foetus and they appear after birth only when the animals have been weaned and begin to eat mostly in the period of darkness [31].

1.9 Enzyme activity and age

Experiments have been performed to investigate the effects of the age of the rat on damage induced by radiation taking into the account the circadian rhythm. Two-month-old rats were used and compared with 18-month-old animals, both kept in rigidly controlled conditions in terms of the light/dark cycle (lights on at 0630 h and off at 1830 h). In control animals sacrificed at 0900 or 2100 h, there was no statistically significant differences in the number of crypt cells or in the entire crypt-villus system when young animals were compared to old ones. Nor were there any differences between the respective groups sacrificed at different times of day. However, the mitotic index in the old rats was lower by 40% compared to the young animals (p < 0.01), but there was no significant difference in the mitotic index at different times of day [32].

There was no difference in brush border enzyme activity between the young and old animals. There were circadian oscillations when the 0900 and 2100 h groups were compared, with similar trends for maltase, invertase, trehalase, LAP and alkaline phosphatase. These differences are statistically significant (p < 0.01). For the lysosomal enzymes, beta-glucuronidase, beta-acid galactosidase and acid phosphatase, the activity is higher at 2100 than at 0900 h, but the differences are not statistically significant. There was no evidence of differences in the protein content of the small intestinal homogenate of animals of different ages or of animals sacrificed at different times of day [32].

1.10 Polyamines in the small intestine

Polyamines which are derived via ornithine catabolism play a very complex biological role which involves many reactions in different metabolic pathways. Their polycationic nature allows the stabilisation of nucleic acids and they thus influence proliferation and differentiation [33,34]. If polyamine synthesis is

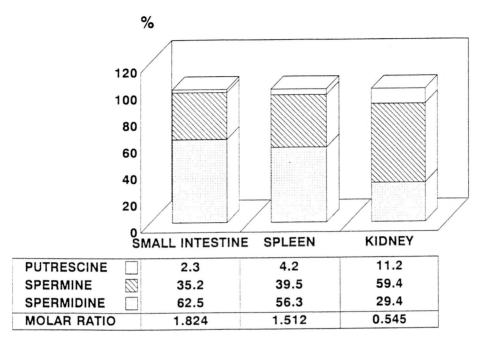

		SMALL INTESTINE	SPLEEN	KIDNEY
PUTRESCINE	☐	2.3	4.2	11.2
SPERMINE	▨	35.2	39.5	59.4
SPERMIDINE	☐	62.5	56.3	29.4
MOLAR RATIO		1.824	1.512	0.545

Fig. 5. Levels of polyamines (putrescine, spermine, spermidine) in the small intestine, spleen and kidney of control animals sacrificed at the same time of day. The values are expressed as a percentage of the total polyamine content.

stopped, cells are blocked in G_1 [35]. The polyamine content in tissue homogenates differs according to the mitotic activity. Spermidine is the polyamine that has the highest concentration in tissues with the highest proliferative activity such as small intestine and spleen, whilst spermine is higher in the less proliferative tissues. Putrescine concentrations are very low. In the kidney there are high levels of spermine and relatively high levels of putrescine, probably due to the specific function of the kidneys (Fig. 5). Putrescine is present in high quantities in urine. The ratio of spermidine to spermine can be used as a distinctive parameter related to the proliferative activity. This ratio has levels higher than one in tissues with a rapid turnover and lower than one in slow or non-proliferative tissues [36].

In rats maintained as described above, the circadian rhythm in polyamines has been investigated. In the small intestine, putrescine and spermidine levels remain constant through the day whereas spermine shows low concentrations at midnight with concentrations increasing progressively until about 1830 h ($p < 0.01$) [37]. It should be noted that tritiated thymidine uptake levels in the small intestine measured an hour after injection did not show any significant difference throughout the day [37]. The relationship between tissue polyamine concentration and proliferative activity could be used to characterise tumour growth [38–40].

2. RADIATION EFFECTS

The classical description of the sequence of events which takes place in the gastrointestinal epithelium after irradiation was presented by Quastler in 1956 [41]. These changes have been summarised in Chapters 3, 4 and 6. Briefly, they involve the following effects:

2.1 Cellular damage

A block in the cell cycle of proliferating cells. Besides the death of a certain number of cells, this results in a mitotic delay if the cell injury is reparable or in a reproductive death if it is not. Any sub-lethally damaged regenerative cells may survive, repair their damage and by division restore the epithelium to its normal conditions.

2.2 Tissue damage

The epithelium suffers a loss of cell production, the differentiated cells continue to be extruded from the apex of the villus, while production from the crypt is decreased. This results in a reduction in the height of the villus which will appear collapsed and an alteration can be seen in the shape of the epithelial cells as they attempt to cover the greatest possible surface area.

2.3 Organ damage

With the continued loss of epithelial cells exceeding the production of new cells, there will be regions where the epithelium is lost completely.

2.4 Damage to the organism

As a consequence of the denuded epithelium, the animal may die due to infection caused by bacteria, toxic effects as a consequence of the loss of the intestinal barrier, damage caused to the mucosa by proteolytic enzymes, hypovolemic shock due to the loss of water and electrolytes caused by the ensuing diarrhoea, which in extreme cases will contain blood. At sub-lethal doses, intracellular repair mechanisms will operate and repopulation and regeneration of the epithelium will occur rapidly. If this takes place too slowly, or the damage is so extensive that it cannot be compensated for by regeneration, death will occur within 3–8 days.

Specific changes that can be detected include:

Body weight changes
In rats irradiated with doses from 3–12 Gy, there is a dose dependent reduction which starts the first days after exposure. The degree and duration of the fall in body weight depends on the dose [44]. After a dose of 3 Gy, the

Body weight

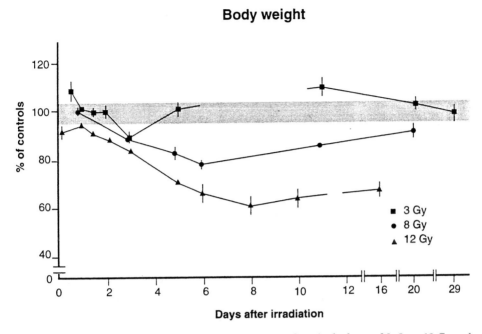

Fig. 6. Variations of body weights in groups of rats exposed to single doses of 3, 8, or 12 Gy and sacrificed at different times after irradiation, expressed as a percentage of controls. (Mean values ± SE). The SE of the control rats is represented by the band at 100%. (Modified from Ref. [42]).

minimum in weight is reached 2 days after irradiation and represents a loss of 15%. The values return to normal after 5 days (Fig. 6). At higher doses including studies where the abdomen only is irradiated, there is a major and progressive reduction in body weight up to 6–8 days with a gradual return to control levels. After 12 Gy the decrease is more dramatic, but there is a trend to return to normal levels in rats surviving the intestinal radiation syndrome. There were no significant differences between different groups irradiated at different times of day.

2.5 Modification in the weight of the small intestine

After 3 Gy, there is a rapid reduction in the weight of the small intestine with a minimum reached between 24 and 36 h and a gradual return to normal values at 72 h followed by an overshoot at 5 days which is maintained for more than 11 days (Fig. 7). For animals irradiated at different times of the day, there was a sharper initial reduction when irradiation was delivered at midnight and a greater overshoot after 5 days when compared with rats irradiated at 0600 h. Following 8 Gy abdominal irradiation, the initial reduction is more dramatic and the duration and overshoot are more evident and longer lasting. In rats surviving 12 Gy the decrease is much more marked and the return to normal and the overshoot appear at later intervals in the small intestine [42] (Fig. 7).

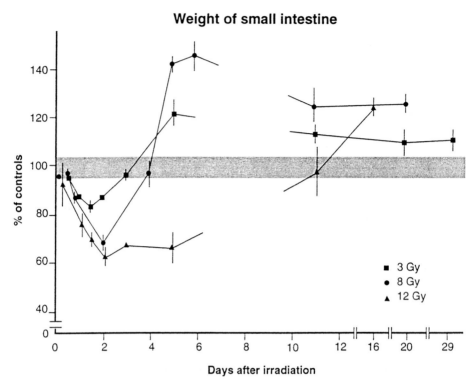

Fig. 7. Variation in the weight of the small intestine from rats exposed to single doses of 3, 8, or 12 Gy and sacrificed at different times after irradiation expressed as a percentage of controls. (Mean values ± SE). The SE of the control rats is represented by the band at 100%. (Modified from Ref. [42]).

2.6 Radiation injury, qualitative morphologic modifications

The qualitative morphologic modifications are quite similar in the proximal and distal jejunum and the terminal ileum. The temporal sequence of injury to the proliferative cells in the crypt have been studied with different doses administered to the entire body, to the abdomen only and also to sections of exteriorised intestine. Even extremely low doses have been studied to evaluate the cytotoxic effects on cells at particular positions within the crypt of the mouse [43].

Morphological damage caused by radiation

The changes that occur in the crypts following a dose, for example, of 6 Gy to the abdomen show a range of characteristic temporal alterations which can be summarised as follows [44,45].

1. Within 30 min — only minor changes are noted, a few swollen nuclei and a reduction in the number of mitoses.
2. After 1 h — mitoses are rare and in the lower part of the crypt, there are indications of swelling of the nucleus and evidence of very rare chromophilic nuclear fragments (apoptotic bodies).
3. After 2 h — apoptotic bodies increase in number and some cells at the crypt base have larger swollen nuclei. The literature abounds with reports of pycnosis, karyolysis and karyorrhexis. Many of these earlier reports are undoubtedly reporting the occurrence of apoptosis. Mitosis is still very rare at this time.
4. After 4 h — mitotic figures are still absent, very numerous apoptotic figures occur in the lower regions of the crypt.
5. After 6 h many apoptotic fragments are present and occasional mitotic figures can be seen. The apoptotic cells appear to fragment into more bodies, each of which is smaller, than is seen in the mouse (see Chapter 4); see also Fig. 8.
6. After 8 h — the nuclei in the crypt appear enlarged and misaligned, there are fewer cells altogether and the altered cells occur at higher positions in the crypt. Apoptotic bodies are less frequent, but clearly present in a variable fashion from animal to animal.
7. After 12 h — the apoptotic bodies are very common. There are altered enlarged cells in the lower two-thirds of the crypt with increased distance between the nuclei. In the lower portions of the crypt there are now rare mitotic figures.
8. After 16 h — cells with an altered morphology occupy the entire crypt and even the base of the villus. The chromophilic fragments become rare with mitosis becoming more numerous particularly at the base of the crypt.
9. After 24 h — the cells damaged by radiation continue to migrate along the villus. Normal enterocytes are observed only at the higher positions on the villus.
10. After 36–40 h — both the crypts and the villus are reduced in height and are covered by radiation damaged cells with swollen nuclei.
11. After 44–48 h — cellular damage is very clear on both the villus and in the crypt, however, in the crypt there are now numerous cells in mitosis.
12. After 60 h — the villus is similarly abnormal, but in the lower portion of the crypts there are cells with a normal morphology reappearing and many mitotic figures.
13. At later times, there is a continued return towards normality and from 108 h onwards, the morphological characteristics are comparable to those in control animals with the exception that there is an increase in the number of cells in the crypts compared to controls, i.e., an overshoot.

Beginning at the 16th hour after irradiation, there is a progressive increase in an inflammatory infiltrate in the stroma. This infiltrate increases and reaches its highest levels 48 and 60 h after irradiation and returns to normality when the epithelium returns to normal.

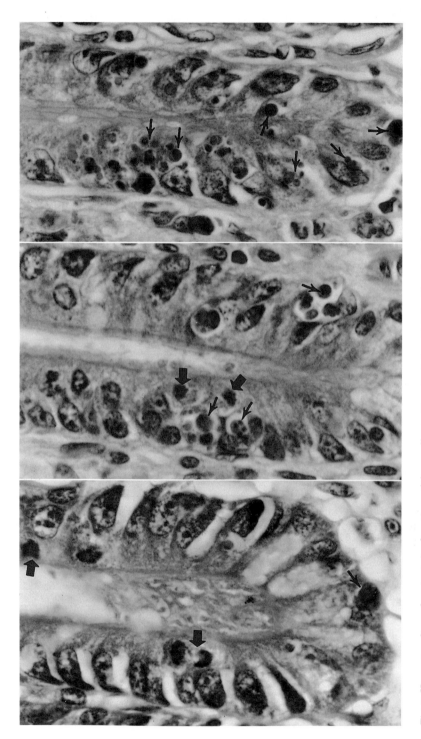

Fig. 8. Haematoxylin and eosin stained sections of the small intestine of rats irradiated with a single dose of γ rays showing mitotic cells (large arrows) and apoptotic fragments of cells (small arrows). Left hand panel, control unirradiated rats showing a spontaneous apoptotic cell. Middle panel, 6 h after 1 Gy, and right hand panel 6 h after 8 Gy. Many small apoptotic fragments are seen in the right hand panel. (See also colour plate on p. xv.)

At lower doses, the temporal sequence of events is similar, particularly during the first 24 to 36 h. There will be fewer dead cells and a shorter block in proliferative activity and a more rapid return to normality. With higher doses the number of surviving cells is decreased. The damage to the epithelium generally is more serious and it returns to control levels at a slower rate. At supra-lethal doses (greater than 12 Gy), the repopulation cannot compensate for the damage and the denudation of the epithelium and the animal dies [46].

It is interesting to note that especially after higher doses, the repopulation is not homogeneous, but has a focal distribution, both within different crypts in the same sections and within different regions of the same animal and in different animals sacrificed at the same time. The reasons for these variations remain obscure at present.

Ultrastructural changes

Within 30 min of 6 Gy ultrastructural modifications are apparent in the lower part of the crypts [44]. Lysosome-like dense bodies, apoptotic bodies and amorphous dense material in the smooth membranes all are apparent. These changes become progressively more severe and both the nucleus and the cytoplasm of the crypt cells are altered. The chromatin concentrates as dense clumps close to the nuclear membrane, while the inner part of the nucleus becomes more transparent. These changes are consistent with the process of apoptosis and a number of dense bodies appears in the cytoplasm of cells consistent with phagocytosed apoptotic fragments. Some cells appear to be extruded directly into the lumen of the crypt. Between 1 and 12 h after exposure, there is a remarkable increase in the number of free ribosomes, particularly in the cells at the transition between the crypt and villus. The changes in the crypt cells gradually disappear with time and also move to appear at higher positions in the crypt and in the lower regions of the villus. Between 24 and 32 h after irradiation, only severely altered cells are seen. In the lower part of the villus, the cells show an increase in free ribosomes and a swelling of the mitochondria. There is also a slight reduction in the height of the microvilli. With time, this reduction is more evident and involves most of the cells on the villus. Between 36 and 48 h, the villus is covered with cells of a grossly altered morphology, lacking apical microvilli, having a very clear cytoplasm, a swollen appearance and some fragmentation of the organelles. Other cells appear smaller with dense cytoplasm and packed organelles, and these may be extruded into the lumen. While these changes can be detected on the villus, between 36 and 48 h after irradiation, the cells in the crypts are progressively returning to a more normal appearance. At 5 days after irradiation, some cells on the villus still show numerous ribosomes and at later intervals, the villus morphology is normal.

Quantitative morphological modifications

In a steady-state situation, such as exists in the normal intestinal epithelium, any impairment in the process of cell replacement will result in alterations in the tissue. One of the most obvious of these is the shortening of the villus. The proliferative cells in the crypt are the most sensitive cells, while the differentiated cells are quite radioresistant. Because cells are constantly moving from the crypt to the villus, damage in the crypt becomes manifest on the villus at later times [44,47,48]. A large number of studies have been undertaken to study and quantitate the morphological changes in the rat intestine following various doses of radiation [32,44–46,49–54]. The changing number of epithelial cells along one side of the crypt in sections following a dose of 8 Gy delivered at midnight, 0600, midday or 1800 h are shown in Table 1. The number of cells is expressed as a percent of the control value in rats sacrificed at the same time of the day. Irradiation at all the times of day produced very similar general changes with a reduction in the cellularity reaching a minimum value at 48 h. Following this, repopulation re-establishes the cellularity and this regeneration occurred earlier in the group irradiated at midday. Between 72 and 96 h, the control values were re-established and following this, there was an overshoot in numbers. The overshoot was less marked in the group irradiated at 0600 h. The overshoot persisted for at least 20 days after exposure. Only crypts with a relatively normal organisation were analysed (i.e., degenerating crypts were excluded).

TABLE 1

Variations in the number (mean ± SE) of epithelial cells along the side of the crypts in animals irradiated with 8 Gy to the abdomen at different times of the light/dark cycle and sacrificed at different intervals after exposure. The values are expressed as percent of the control values for animals sacrificed at the same time of the day (unpublished data).

Time of sacrifice after irradiation	Time of irradiation			
	24.00	6.00	12.00	18.00
6 h	90±2	74±2	76±3	83±2
12 h	71±5	70±2	71±2	65±4
20 h	63±2	53±1	64±1	57±1
36 h	50±2	52±2	50±2	54±4
48 h	49±1	51±2	43±0.3	50±3
72 h	55±2	68±9	82±5	54±9
96 h	115±2	104±5	98±7	117±3
126 h	119±3	103±3	112±3	120±3
150 h	122±1	110±2	118±2	120±3
11 days	111±2	99±6	119±1	119±2
20 days	109±5	105±1	114±1	109±3

TABLE 2

Variations of the labelling index in the crypts of the small intestine of animals irradiated, with 8 Gy to the abdomen, at different times of the light/dark cycle and sacrificed at different intervals after exposure. The values are expressed as percent of the control values for animals sacrificed at the same time of the day (unpublished data).

Time of sacrifice after irradiation	Time of irradiation			
	24.00	6.00	12.00	18.00
6 h	33±4	34±7	24±5	37±5
12 h	26±2	34±9	11±4	43±11
20 h	44±5	44±3	53±5	52±5
36 h	50±14	57±8	91±11	73±14
48 h	89±10	110±14	74±6	135±12
72 h	165±3	157±11	154±21	196±10
96 h	145±28	150±12	135±5	101±5
126 h	144±12	110±11	105±5	121±15
150 h	142±20	113±3	118±7	124±2
11 days	125±5	105±3	83±21	97±7
20 days	97±6	97±3	95±13	90±0

The changes in proliferative activity are described in Table 2 as a percent of the control values. A marked block of proliferation can be seen at 6 h with the lowest values being obtained at 12 h. There was then a progressive increase so that values close to control were reached at 48 h. This recovery to control values appeared to occur earlier in the groups of rats irradiated at 0600 and 1800 h. There was then a significant overshoot in proliferative activity at 72 h where values between 150 and 200% of controls were obtained. There was a tendency to return to control levels, but only after 11–20 days. Thus proliferation values returned to normal at a time when the cellularity was still elevated.

Following exposure to 3 Gy, similar patterns of behaviour were observed [55]. At 12 h the number of cells was between 70 and 80% of controls reaching its lowest level at 20 h. The return to control occurred at 48 h for the groups irradiated at midday and 1800 h and occurred later in the other irradiation groups. There was a significant overshoot at 72 h (p < 0.01) and control values were re-established between 5 and 11 days after irradiation, with the groups irradiated at 0600 h returning to normal at the earlier time. The proliferation in these 3 Gy irradiated animals was very low at 12 h (20–50% of control), but quickly increased and at 36 h is significantly higher than controls in all groups. The highest levels of proliferation were seen at 48 h which was followed by a progressive reduction back to control levels at 5 days for the groups irradiated at midday and 1800 h or at 20 days in the other groups. These studies following both 3 and 8 Gy indicate that irradiation at different times of the day does produce some differences in the response showing that there are radiosensitivity differences amongst the cells of the small intestinal crypt that are related to the circadian rhythms.

2.7 The frequency of labelled cells at each cell position along the side of the crypt

If animals are injected with tritiated thymidine and sacrificed one hour later and autoradiographs prepared, the distribution of labelled cells at each cell position along the side of the crypt is a useful way to study the structure and function of the proliferative compartment as has been described in Chapter 1 and 4. In order for this to be effective, the orientation of the section has to be precise to obtain longitudinal sections through the crypt-villus structure. This allows the base of the crypt and the crypt-villus junction to be recognised. The effects of radiation were predominantly observed as changes in the cells of the crypt, since the differentiated cells on the villus are relatively radioresistant and changes in the differentiated compartment are only observed at appropriate intervals after exposure to radiation. The timing of these changes was dependent on the turnover time of the cells in the crypt. Using appropriate software, data on proliferative indices can be obtained for the cells at each position along the crypt-villus axis and these data can be normalised to take into account variations in the length of the crypt. In this way, changes between groups of animals can be compared [56]. A number of experiments have been performed in rats. For animals sacrificed at different times of the light/dark period, changes in the S-phase distribution differing according to the time of sacrifice were observed. The general shape of the curves was similar, but a gradual modification was observed as one moves from groups of rats sacrificed at 0600 h to groups sacrificed at 1800 h. In the latter, the S-phase frequency was lower in the cell positions near the bottom of the crypt while there was an increase in the upper regions of the crypt where differentiation occurs. At intermediate times, the differences were not significant and the curves appeared similar. Studies on the frequency of mitotic cells showed similar distributions. Mitoses were present at very low frequencies near the base of the crypt and there was a progressive increase with maximal levels in the central regions of the crypt (about 4–5%). In the upper half of the crypt, the mitotic frequency decreased and in the upper 85% of the total crypt length, no mitotic cells were observed. There are no clear differences in the mitotic distributions at different times of the day. In relation to the S phase distribution, mitotic figures tended to reach higher cell positions as is shown in Fig. 1 [56].

Labelled cell (S phase) distribution after irradiation
The labelled cell distribution has been analysed following different doses of irradiation. At early times (a few hours) after irradiation, a marked reduction was observed throughout the crypt, but particularly in the lower half of the crypt where the highest frequencies was observed in unirradiated conditions [57,58]. Twelve hours after 8 Gy to the abdomen, there were only a few S phase cells localised in the lower half of the crypt, whereas at 20 h, the frequency was

8Gy

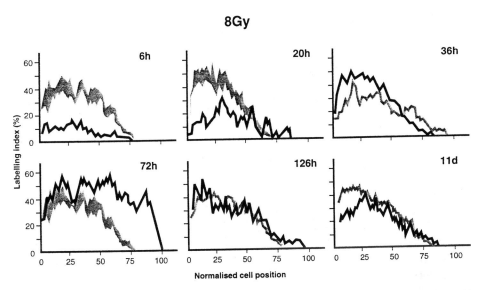

Fig. 9. S phase cell distributions in the crypts of groups of animals treated with a single dose of 8 Gy at the same time of the day and sacrificed at different intervals after irradiation. The curves represent the mean values (treated) and the limits of the SE for controls sacrificed at the same time of the day. (Data taken from Refs. [57,58]).

beginning to return towards normality, but was still significantly reduced compared to controls (see Fig. 9). This return to normality became more evident at successive time intervals and by 72 hours, the labelling index could reach 50% in the middle regions of the crypt and there was a considerable expansion in the proliferative compartment to higher cell positions (Fig. 9). The distributions returned towards normality between days 5 and 11. There were no particular differences observed in these labelled cell distributions when groups of animals were irradiated at the same dose at different times of the day, except for a more marked initial reduction in those animals exposed at noon [57,58].

These results are useful in helping to understand the behaviour of the brush border enzymes during the post-irradiation period. In fact, brush border enzymes increased at a time when the frequency of S-phase cells was greatly reduced and the enzyme levels were close to zero during the recovery phase for proliferation. Specifically, during the period of 4–7 days after irradiation when there was an expansion in the proliferative compartment and a return to near normal cell morphology, the brush border enzymes were decreased in activity and only returned to normal levels at later times.

2.8 Changes in the number of goblet cells

Groups of animals sacrificed at different times of day showed no important differences in the goblet cell index in the crypts. The average values ranged between 2.6±0.2% and 3.1±0.2% [59]. Only goblet cells with positive mucus staining and an associated nucleus in the crypt section were counted. The behaviour of goblet cells after exposure to a single dose of radiation is characterised by 3 phases.

(a) Initially, there was a marked increase in the number of goblet cells,

(b) this was followed by a reduction to very low levels, and

(c) a phase where the numbers gradually returned to normal.

A statistically significant increase in the number of goblet cells was observed within a few hours after irradiation. This was due partly to a reduction in the epithelial cell numbers, but also to a real increase in goblet cell numbers. For example, after a dose of 8 Gy delivered to animals exposed at different times of the day, the number of goblet cells at 12 and 20 h after irradiation reached values ranging between 120% of controls (for the group exposed at 0600 h) and 160% (for the group exposed at midnight) with the goblet cell index ranging between 200 and 270% [59]. During the period 48 to 72 h after exposure (the acute phase of irradiation injury), the goblet cell index was reduced to about 20% of the control values in all groups. Thereafter, there was a progressive increase, but the values only reached control levels 20 days after irradiation for the groups irradiated at 0600 and 1800 h.

3. MALABSORPTION FOLLOWING IRRADIATION

Irradiation of the abdomen causes malabsorption of carbohydrates, lipids and vitamins mainly and to a lesser extent, amino acids and proteins. This malfunction is related to 3 components of absorbtion, (1) passive absorbtion, (2) active transport and (3) membrane digestion. Pinocytotic activity is impaired by cell oedema. Studies into the changes in brush border enzyme activity give some insight into the mechanisms involved in malabsorption.

3.1 Brush border enzyme activity

Within a few hours of exposure to ionising radiation, brush border enzyme activity was significantly increased (specifically the di- and trisaccharidases and the di- and tripeptidases). The threshold for these effects was about 2 Gy and if higher doses were given, the time dependent changes could be investigated [49,50]. The increase in enzyme activity began at about 2 h after exposure and continued to be elevated until about 36–40 hours after which significantly lower values were observed than in controls with minimum values reached 60–72 h after irradiation [44,46,49,50,60]. The higher the dose, the greater was the initial increase in enzyme activity and the lower the value found during the acute injury phase. Also the higher the dose, the longer it took for control levels to be reattained. There were no significant changes amongst the different enzymes and sham irradiated animals showed patterns of enzyme activity similar to controls. Circadian rhythms influence these results and hence animal housing and timing have to be carefully controlled. During the radiation-induced intestinal syndrome, processes that interfere with the normal physiological rhythms such as digestion, absorption, and cellular proliferation all have an influence. A lack of appetite, the presence of morphologically evident mucosal damage, changes in the intestinal content (either in fluid, molecular composition or molecular concentrations), and changes in the intestinal flora all change the physiological environment for digestion and absorption. Figure 10 shows the time course for the changes in maltase activity (1–4 α glycosidase) in the third of five regions of the small intestine that were studied. The second to third regions were the area in which the enzyme activity was highest. The effects of two different doses (3 and 8 Gy) administered at four different times of the light/dark cycle were studied [51,54,61–66]. The results when these doses were administered at either midnight or midday ie, near to the time of the circadian maximum and minimum for enzyme activity are reported in Fig. 10A,B. Significant changes can be noted with the passage of time relative to the control value at time zero. The importance of the circadian oscillation in brush border enzyme is evident in Fig. 11A,B where the same data as shown in Fig. 10A,B are presented as a percentage change relative to the control value for rats sacrificed at the same time of day.

The early rise in enzyme activity and its subsequent fall was clearly evident. At both 3 and 8 Gy, the peak in activity occurs at 20 h and the minimum values are obtained at about 72 h. If the animals are irradiated at the time of the minimum in the circadian rhythm of maltase activity, the changes induced by radiation were of a lower magnitude. Following the higher dose of radiation, the minimum value obtained at 72 h represents less than 20% of the control values and the return to control levels takes about twice as long as after the lower dose (11 days compared to about 5 days). The animals irradiated at midday did not return to control levels within the period of study (30 days).

Similar results were observed for the other disaccharidases such as invertase and threalase [51,54]. This was also especially true for alkaline phosphatase in the first 2 segments of the small intestine, where the principle component of the phosphatase is a brush border enzyme. The same behaviour as seen for maltase was observed for leucine-aminopeptidase [64].

Figure 12 shows the same general trend as was seen for maltase when lactase activity was studied (βD galactosidase). However, this enzyme because of its particular characteristic of being induced by components in the diet, shows some important differences. Notably, these are: a more marked reduction in activity and a slower return to normal levels as exemplified by the 3 Gy groups irradiated at midday which returned to control levels at 11 days compared to those irradiated at midnight which take 45 days to reach control levels which is longer than was seen for maltase-activity. Following a higher dose (8 Gy) lactase activity disappeared completely at 72 h and only started to reappear in some situations after about 6 days.

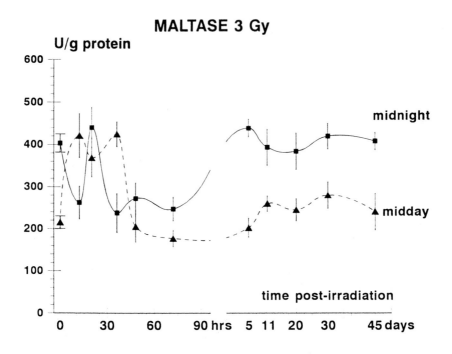

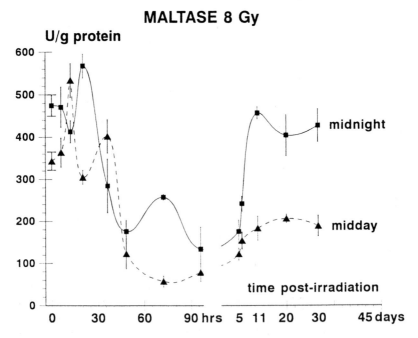

Fig. 10. Variations in maltase activity in the third segment of the small intestine of rats irradiated at 2 different times of the day (midday, dotted line, and midnight, solid line) and sacrificed at different times after exposure. The activity is expressed as units per gram of protein; (mean values ± SE). Top panel: results after a 3 Gy dose; bottom panel: those after 8 Gy are shown.

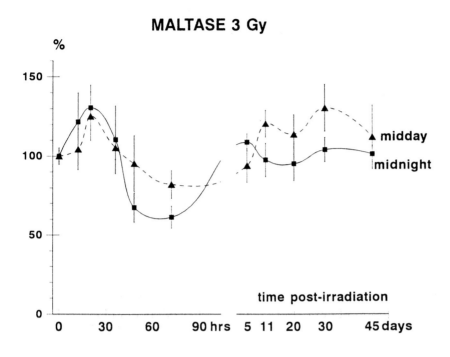

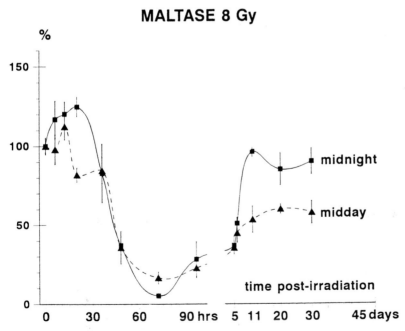

Fig. 11. Variations in maltase activity in the small intestine of rats. The same data as shown in Fig. 10, in terms of a percentage of control values (see Fig. 10 for further details).

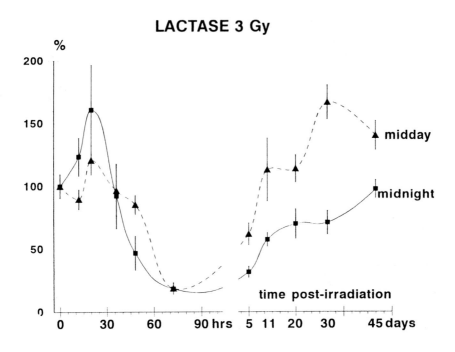

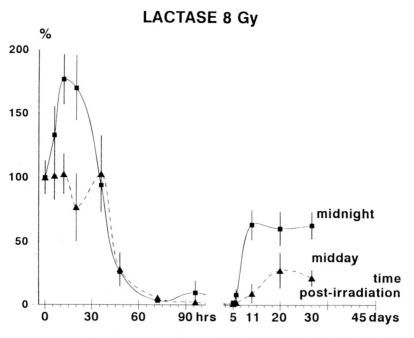

Fig. 12. Variations in lactase activity in the small intestine of rats irradiated with 3 and 8 Gy administered at two different times of day. The activity is expressed as a percentage of the relevant controls (see Fig. 10).

The results of irradiation on brush border enzyme activity can be summarised as follows. There is:

1. An increase in activity over the first 36 h.

2. A highly significant reduction in activity between 48 and 72 h.

3. A general tendency to return to control levels over a period of about 11 days.

These changes began to appear after a dose of about 2 Gy [45,49,50]. There were changes following sublethal doses that were dependent on the time of day at which radiation was administered. If irradiation was given at midnight, when the enzyme activity was maximal, the early increase in enzyme activity was more dramatic. In animals irradiated when the enzyme activity was decreasing (for example 0600 h), there was little early change in enzyme activity. Exposure at midday (when the enzyme activity is close to its minimal value) resulted in a very small early increase whereas irradiation at 1800 h (when the enzyme activity is increasing) resulted in a very significant early increase. These effects are all more pronounced with higher doses of irradiation. The time that it took for the brush border enzymes to return to control values was inversely proportional to dose. After a dose of 8 Gy, there were variations in enzyme levels at different times of the day in the animals sacrificed between 120 and 150 h after irradiation, although these fluctuations were smaller than the circadian fluctuations observed in controls and were not obviously related to the control circadian rhythm [58,63]. After even higher doses (for example 12 Gy), the restoration of enzyme activity took longer and at even higher doses, intestinal death ensued [46,50].

Striking differences were noted in the times that were required for the enzyme activity to return to normal values depending on the time of day at which the irradiation was given. For example, following 8 Gy delivered at the time of maximal enzyme activity, the return to control levels was observed earlier than in a comparable group, irradiated at the time of minimal enzyme activity expression. The full details of the experiments investigating the changes in maltase activity are summarised in Figs. 10 and 11. Five separate segments of the small intestine were investigated following a dose of 8 Gy and irradiations were delivered at midnight, 0600 h, midday and 1800 h. Animals were sacrificed at various times after irradiation for the determination of enzyme levels. The circadian variation in the total maltase activity in the entire small intestine of unirradiated animals is shown in the top left hand panel in Fig. 13. Similar variations were seen in all five separate regions of the small intestine. Evidence of circadian rhythms can be clearly seen. The levels of activity in the five different regions can vary considerably. Six hours after irradiation, there was still some evidence of a rhythm, but some changes relative to the control could be seen. At this and the following times, the overall levels of activity increased (as discussed earlier), with the increase being more pronounced when the radiation was given at the time of high enzyme activity. By 48 h, the levels of enzyme activity were significantly reduced in all regions and at six days after irradiation, the beginnings of a circadian rhythm were

8 Gy Maltase

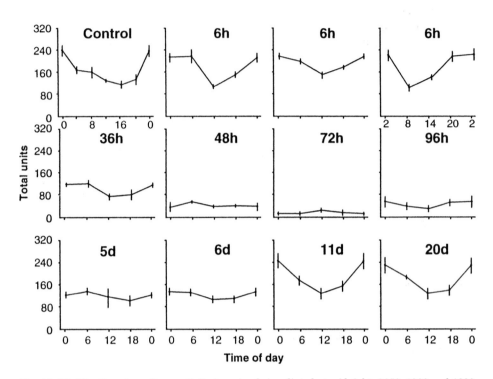

Fig. 13. Modifications in maltase activity in animals irradiated at midnight, 0600, 1200 and 1800 h with 8 Gy and sacrificed at different times after exposure. These chronograms illustrate the presence of the circadian oscillations in enzyme activity in irradiated animals. (Control data are presented in the top left panel). (Data from Refs. [54,62]).

again appearing. By 11 days, the biorhythm was clearly present. By 20 days after irradiation, the curves are similar to the controls. At lower doses the effects are less pronounced with evidence of a circadian rhythm still being present at 72 h. The return to normal levels of enzyme activity and normal circadian rhythms occurs at five days after 3 Gy.

Figure 14 summarises the effects of 3 and 8 Gy given at 4 different times during the circadian rhythm. Here, the results have been normalised as a percent of the corresponding control values. There was an early increase in activity which is significant in some cases and not in others, and a progressive decline to essentially zero values at 72 h particularly at the higher dose. Control values were reached after about 5 days after the lower dose, and between 11 and 20 or more days, after the high dose. Rather similar changes have been observed for the other disaccharidases, alkaline phosphatase and leucineami-nopeptidase.

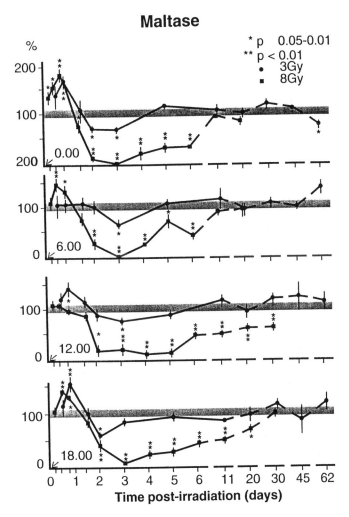

Fig. 14. Variation in maltase activity in rats irradiated with 3 (closed circles) and 8 Gy (closed squares) administered at midnight, 0600, 1200 and 1800 h respectively. The mean values ± SE in the second segment of the small intestine are presented. The results are expressed as a percentage of control values. The standard errors of the control values are represented by the horizontal band. The levels of statistical significance are represented with one asterisk if p < 0.05 or with two asterisks if p < 0.01. (Unpublished data).

3.2 Changes in lysosomal enzyme activity

The various biochemical alterations in the intestinal epithelium depend on a variety of factors. Firstly, epithelial cells damaged by irradiation and inflammatory cells (granulocytes, plasma cells, macrophages, etc.) which are localised in the stroma, increase in number with the seriousness of the injury. β-acid galactosidase (at a pH of 2.9), acid phosphatase, β-glucuronidase, have been

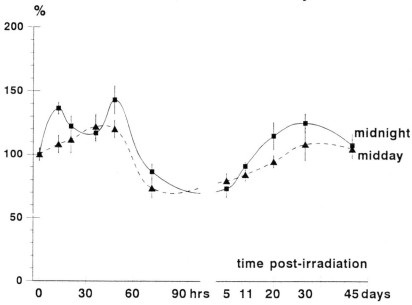

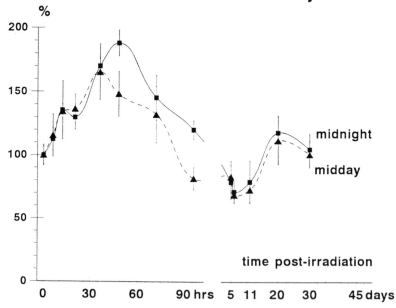

Fig. 15. Variations in acid β galactosidase activity in the third segment of the small intestine of rats irradiated at midday (dotted line) and midnight (solid line) with 3 Gy (top panel) and 8 Gy (bottom panel). (mean values ± SE). The results are expressed as a percentage of control values.

assayed in various experiments. These enzyme activities lack a circadian variation, but the values do increase from the duodenum to the terminal ileum and after irradiation, they all show similar changes. After all doses between 3 and 20 Gy, there was a progressive increase in enzyme activity in the first hours after irradiation [45,46,65]. The maximum levels of enzyme activity were found at 48 h. During the process of tissue regeneration, the activity was reduced compared with controls, the control levels were reached about 11 days after irradiation. As an example, Fig. 15 shows the changes in β-galactosidase after 3 and 8 Gy in animals irradiated at midnight and midday. The curves are very similar in both cases, with only minor changes depending on the time of day of irradiation. The lower levels of morphologic injury induced by 3 Gy accounts for the smaller changes of enzyme activity; irradiation at midnight seems to cause a more severe damage (increase of enzyme activity). The increase in enzyme activity seen immediately after irradiation, could be linked to the autolytic processes that result from the occurrence of damaged epithelial cells. Inflammatory cells are particularly abundant between 36 and 72 h after 8 Gy. As the morphology returned to normal, inflammatory cells became progressively less frequent and the lysosomal enzyme activities became lower.

3.3 Protein content

Protein levels in the homogenates of the small intestine do not show circadian rhythms, but slightly higher protein levels were found at midday. After irradiation there was a progressive reduction in protein levels with a minimum at 48 h, as shown in Fig. 16. There was then a time dependent increase in protein levels which after 8 Gy reached control values between 5 and 11 days after irradiation. Following 3 Gy, control levels were re-established after about 72 h. There was thus a dose dependence for the time that it took to return to the control levels. On the whole, the irradiation caused more effect, when administered at midnight, but the overshoot at later times tended to be greater when the irradiation was given at midday.

3.4 DNA levels

The level of DNA extracted in homogenates of intestinal tissue did not show any circadian rhythm although slightly higher levels were found in the animals sacrificed at midday. A dose of 3 Gy caused a significant reduction that began about 12 h after irradiation, was greatest in the group irradiated at midnight, but control levels were regained at 48 and 72 h. Tritiated thymidine uptake (1 h pulse labelling) was maximum in the latter part of the dark period, (i.e., the early hours of the morning). After 3 Gy, there was a complete block of thymidine uptake at 12 h, an increased uptake at 20 h and a significantly higher level than in controls at 36 h [37]. Maximum uptake was obtained at 48 h and significantly higher levels were still present at 72 h after irradiation. Following this the thymidine uptake levels returned to normal [37].

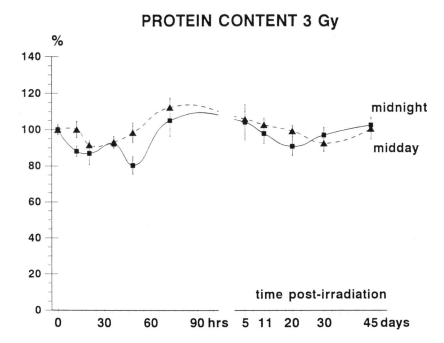

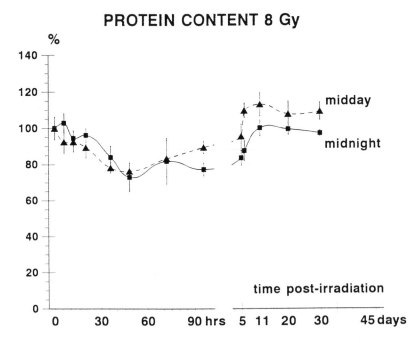

Fig. 16. Variations in protein content in homogenates of the third segment of the small intestine in rats irradiated at midday (dotted line) and midnight (solid line). The results after 3 Gy (top panel) and 8 Gy (bottom panel) are shown as a percentage of control values.

4. THE EFFECTS OF IONISING RADIATION ON GUT POLYAMINES

The behaviour of polyamines has been analysed following a dose of 3 Gy delivered at four different times of day (0.00, 6.00, 12.00 and 18.00 h). Between 12 and 20 h after irradiation, polyamine levels decreased in a highly significant way (Fig. 17). Putrescine levels, the polyamine that has the lowest concentration, reached values slightly lower than 40% of controls and returned to control values at 72 h. This was followed by a second reduction in levels with control values being re-established at about 30 days. Rats exposed at 1800 h showed a more marked initial reduction whereas those exposed at midnight and 0600 h showed a longer lasting reduction.

Similar changes were observed for spermidine, but the effects were much less marked. Control levels were re-established by 36 h. The changes in the level of spermine were similar to those for spermidine. Also shown in Fig. 17 are the changes in tritiated thymidine uptake which show a similar general trend, but with more pronounced variations. At 12 h, the levels of labelled cells were nearly zero, and in contrast were greatly elevated during the repopulation phase. The similarity in the shape of the thymidine curve is worth noting since this confirms that these polyamines are related to the proliferative activity

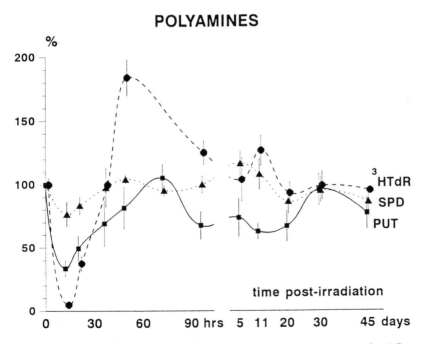

Fig. 17. Variations in polyamine concentration in the entire small intestine after 3 Gy are presented for animals sacrificed at different intervals after irradiation (mean values ± SE). Putrescine (solid line, PUT), spermidine (dotted line, SPD) and ³H thymidine uptake (dotted line ³HTdR) expressed as a percentage of controls.

changes induced by injury of this rapidly proliferating tissue. This was further confirmed by the assays of polyamine content in spleen and kidney [36,67]. In fact, the response in the spleen was very similar to that of the small intestine with a slower return to normal levels because of the slower turnover of this tissue. In the kidney, where proliferative activity was very low, there was little change in polyamine concentrations. Thus, polyamines are useful biochemical markers of radiation injury and could be used to identify the block in mitotic activity, the repopulation phase and the time of the return to normal morphologic and functional conditions.

5. PERFUSION STUDIES

Supralethal doses (more than 10 Gy) cause clear functional and metabolic alterations in the intestine. Malabsorption of many compounds was evident, particularly sugars, sodium, etc. [68–70]. Some of these modifications were evident even after sublethal doses. The changes that were observed in enzyme activities of the brush border suggest that there may also be impairment at the functional level of the process of membrane digestion. In order to study this, perfusion techniques have been used in unirradiated animals and following a dose of 20 Gy [70]. The absorption of carbohydrates has been investigated using *in vitro* preparations such as everted sacs. Although such techniques provide information on the mechanisms and kinetics of absorption, they do not relate directly to conditions *in vivo* since the intestine is severed from its blood supply. In order to overcome this, the intestinal absorption of tracers with loading amounts of glucose and sucrose under *in vivo* conditions have been studied [71]. This approach has been used to study the absorption of sodium ions during the course of the gastrointestinal radiation syndrome [69]. Using ^{14}C labelled glucose, it could be seen that radioactivity appeared in the blood of the portal vein 30–60 s after injection of the tracer into the intestinal lumen and the level remained constant during the 6 min of the experiment. At the end of this period about 70% of the tracer dose and about 10% of the loading dose (50 mg) of glucose were absorbed. The 30% of remaining radioactivity spread into the neighbouring intestinal segments. Chromatography of intestinal homogenates and of the plasma revealed that about 80% of the radioactivity was attributable to glucose at the end of the experiment and about 20% attributable to lactic acid [70]. Using different substrate levels, it could be shown that the reaction followed saturation kinetics. Absorption of sucrose occurred at a somewhat slower rate than for glucose, but displayed a similar apparent Michaelis constant. The mean percentage of the tracer dose of glucose infused into the duodenum, jejunum and colon of 6 animals with the standard errors of their means were respectively 15.8±0.86, 19.2±1.3, and 10.3±1.2. The corresponding values for sucrose were 6.4±1.35, 7.95±0.83 and 3.59±0.75. These results illustrate the different absorption capabilities along the length of the intestine.

In rats analysed at different times after 20 Gy whole body irradiation it was shown that at 20 h there was a statistically significant increase in the absorption

TABLE 3

Absorption rate (mean ± SE) of different amounts of glucose and sucrose injected into the duodenum of control and irradiated rats (20 Gy) sacrificed 20 and 72 hours after irradiation. The number of rats in each group is shown in parentheses. (Data published in part, Ref. [70]).

Molecule	Time after irradiation 20 Gy	Absorption rate mg/min (mean ± SE)			
		Tracer	8 mg	20 mg	50 mg
Glucose in H_2O	Control	0.3±0.1 (6)	0.6±0.03 (2)	0.9±0.3 (3)	0.9±0.2 (3)
	20 h	0.4±0.1 (4)	0.7±0.1 (2)	1.5±0.3 (3)	1.7±0.2 (3)
	72 h	0.1±0.03 (6)	0.2±0.02 (2)	0.4±0.07 (3)	0.5±1.1 (3)
Sucrose in H_2O	Control	0.1±0.05 (6)	0.3±0.03 (2)	0.5±0.08 (3)	0.6±0.2 (3)
	20 h	0.1±0.03 (5)	0.4±0.1 (2)	0.5±0.07 (3)	0.6±0.08 (2)
	72 h	0.03±0.005 (6)	0.07±0.02 (2)	0.1±0.02 (3)	0.2±0.04 (3)

of glucose with respect to the controls, while at the same time, the absorption of sucrose was unchanged. At 72 h, the absorption of glucose and sucrose was reduced at all the doses that have been studied (see Table 3). The kinetic constants for absorption of glucose from the duodenum of normal and irradiated rats were v_{max} ($\mu mol \cdot min^{-1}$), 6.0, 12.0, and 3.0 respectively in the controls and at 20 and 72 h after irradiation. The Km values ($\mu mols$) were 28, 50 and 50 respectively for glucose. The same parameters for sucrose were v_{max} 2.3, 2.3 and 1, Km 37, 30.5 and 75.

Using different loading conditions, it could be shown that at 20 h after irradiation, the active transport of glucose was already impaired although the maximum velocity was increased. At 72 h, when the epithelium was grossly altered, the absorption was notably reduced, but the small intestine still appeared to be able to supply, at least in part, the glucose needed by the organism. The disaccharide, sucrose, must be hydrolysed by invertase before it can be absorbed. At 20 h after irradiation, there was no increase in sucrose absorption with respect to controls in spite of a statistically significant increase in invertase activity (Fig. 18). This can be explained by the hypothesis that the enzyme activities represent newly synthesised molecules produced perhaps during the early differentiation process that remain inside the cell and do not transfer into the brush border membrane. This may complicate functional studies associated with the activity of these molecules. At 72 h, the brush

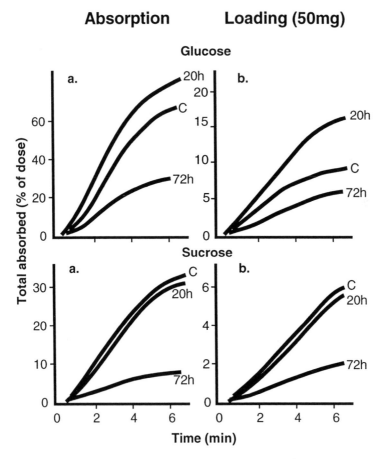

Fig. 18. Absorption of glucose for tracer and loading amounts of glucose (50 mg) in control rats and for 20 and 72 h after 20 Gy (panels A and B). Absorption of sucrose for tracer and loading amounts (50 mg) in control rats, and 20 and 72 h after 20 Gy (panels C and D). (Modified from Ref. [70]).

border enzyme activity was very low which explains why the reduced concentration of glucose after loading with sucrose occurred.

6. FRACTIONATED IRRADIATION

There is a need to assess the tolerance of normal healthy tissues to the types of radiation procedures that are adopted in radiotherapy using appropriate types of radiation sources and at appropriate schedules. The schedules most commonly used involve fractionation of the dose which is based on the knowledge that cell and tissue repair processes can occur during the interval between fractions. From the cellular level this usually means repair of sublethal cellular injury and from the tissue aspect, it involves the regeneration or repopulation of the tissue via stimulated cell proliferation [72–75]. A particular feature of dose–effect curves is that after an initial shoulder region, the higher the dose per fraction, the lower is the cell surviving fraction. The higher the injury the more difficult it is for cells to repair the damage and the longer it takes for the tissue to be repopulated. Fractionation in radiotherapy allows high total doses to be delivered, the dose limitation being, the tolerable level of damage to healthy tissues. The gut is often included in an irradiation field when tumours of the abdomen are treated and with its high sensitivity the study of this tissue during fractionation is of particular interest (see also Chapter 6).

Numerous studies have been conducted on laboratory animals and many fractionation schedules have been used with different doses per fraction. The interval of time between doses is of great importance since it is during this time that repair of sublethal damage occurs. In terms of analysing the results, the general practice has been to consider the time at the end of irradiation as the starting point for analysis. A number of experiments have been performed in rats over a number of years by our group in Florence where the experimental conditions (radiation source, light-dark cycle, strain, age, sex, diet, etc.) have

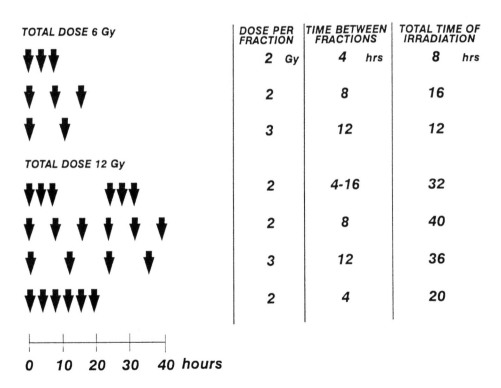

	DOSE PER FRACTION	TIME BETWEEN FRACTIONS	TOTAL TIME OF IRRADIATION
TOTAL DOSE 6 Gy	2 Gy	4 hrs	8 hrs
	2	8	16
	3	12	12
TOTAL DOSE 12 Gy	2	4-16	32
	2	8	40
	3	12	36
	2	4	20

0 10 20 30 40 hours

Fig. 19. Scheme for a series of experiments carried out at the Radiation Biology Laboratory in Florence to evaluate the effects of different schedules of fractionation to study the modifications in the small intestine of Wistar rats. ^{60}Co γ rays, dose rate 70–100 cGy/min, abdomen-only irradiated.

all been carefully controlled and are identical to those used in single dose studies. The experiments on rats involved irradiation of the whole abdomen with the first fraction administered in the afternoon. Total doses of 6 and 12 Gy were studied and the fractionation regimes are described in Fig. 19. The results obtained following 2 Gy per day and 2 Gy × 6 4 h apart are not reported since the former produced only small changes and the second was lethal. Two 6 Gy fractions delivered at intervals between 6 h and 5 days resulted in lethality in many animals when the interval between fractions was less than 24 h [76]. In order to facilitate comparison of the results, the data are expressed as a percent of controls of animals the same age, sacrificed at the same time of day to take into account circadian variations.

6.1 Body weight

All fractionation regimes resulted in a clear reduction in body weight beginning on the second day after the end of radiation treatment. The reduction was particularly marked when 2 doses of 6 Gy were administered at intervals between 6 h and 5 days. If the interval between the 2 doses was less than 48 h, the effects on body weight were greater than was seen after a single 12 Gy dose (42). In the rats surviving such 2 fraction exposure, the body weight returned to normal earlier than after single dose irradiation. When the interval between fractions was greater than 2 days, the fall in body weight was less and the return to normal was earlier. When the total dose of 12 Gy was administered as multiple daily fractions, no changes were noted within a period of 3 days. Thereafter, a fall in body weight was observed which was greater than that seen after a single dose of 8 or 12 Gy. In the fractionation protocol where 2 Gy was given 3 times, 4 h apart, followed 16 h later by another course of 3 doses 4 h apart (abbreviated here to (2 Gy × 3) × 2), the changes in body weight were similar to that observed after a single dose of 8 Gy. The weights returned to control levels 19 days after the end of irradiation. Other multiple fractionation schemes showed behaviour similar to that seen after a single dose of 6 Gy, except for 2 Gy × 6, with an 8-h interval, which showed a smaller reduction and a later return to normality in terms of body weight [42].

6.2 Small intestine weight

A marked decrease in the weight of the small intestine was observed in all fractionation experiments [42]. Two doses of 6 Gy administered within 48 h caused a particularly marked decrease greater than that seen after a single dose of 12 Gy. For longer intervals between fractions, the reduction was lower and the return to normality was quicker. Multiple fractionation produced an initial decrease similar to that seen after a single dose of 12 Gy, the general pattern of response was similar to that seen after a single dose of 8 Gy. Two Gy every 8 h produced an earlier return to normality than was seen with the other multiple fractionation regimes.

6.3 Qualitative modifications in morphology after 3 Gy fractions

When 2 fractions of 3 Gy were delivered, the changes seen at early times (1–4 h after the last dose) were similar to those observed after a single dose of 3 Gy. The changes included swelling of cells, the appearance of pycnotic nuclei and fragmentation of the nuclei. At 12 h, apoptotic bodies were present at lower numbers than early times, but mitoses were still largely absent. Goblet cells were very numerous and the cytoplasm was filled with mucopolysaccharide. At 36 h, the entire crypt villus structure was changed, mitosis and labelled cells were very numerous. Inflammatory cells were evident in the stroma. By 72 h, cells of altered morphology were only present on the villi and at later times, the epithelium looked normal [77].

After fractionation involving 4 fractions of 3 Gy, alterations in cellular morphology were observed 1 and 4 h after the last fraction (37 and 40 h respectively from the beginning of the fractionation regime) in the crypts and over two thirds of the villus length. Few apoptotic bodies were present and mitoses were rare, whereas goblet cells were numerous and filled with secretory material. Numerous inflammatory cells were evident in the stroma [77]. Twenty-four and 36 h after the last fraction, the most severe alterations were evident. Repopulation took place over later times and in a heterogeneous fashion with some crypts regenerating and others showing severe morphological changes. Five days after irradiation, altered cells were apparent on the upper parts of the villi and by 11 days, the epithelium had returned to normality.

6.4 Quantitative morphological changes

The total number of epithelial cells in the vertical column along the crypt side and the labelling index showed changes after multiple fractionation of 6 and 12 Gy (Figs. 20 and 21). The changes seen after 3 Gy single dose and 3 Gy delivered twice were somewhat similar with the mitotic index in the former reduced to about 30% of the controls and in the latter to zero. After a single dose, the number of cells increased progressively and reached control values after 36 h. Following 2 doses of 3 Gy, the effect of the second dose became evident as a delay in the return to normality [77]. The labelling index following a single dose of 3 Gy results in a significant overshoot at 48 h (about 150% of control). A similar overshoot was seen in the dose-fractionation groups. By about 5 days, both irradiation groups returned to normal.

The progression of damage during irradiation was well demonstrated in the multiple fractionation regime of 3 Gy delivered 4 times. Here the number of epithelial cells was greatly reduced to about 50% of control and it remained at this level until about 36 h. This was followed by an increase and a modest but significant overshoot from about 3 to 20 days (Fig. 20). The repopulation processes that occurred during the course of treatment could be seen in the labelling index data. One hour after the end of fractionation, the labelling index

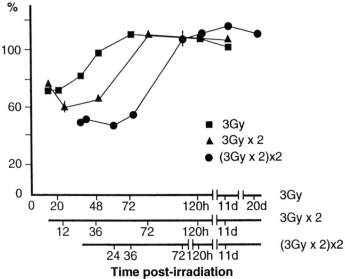

Fig. 20. Number of epithelial cells along the side of crypts in the jejunum of rats irradiated with 3 Gy single dose, 3 Gy × 2 and 3 Gy × 4 sacrificed at different times after exposure (mean values ± SE). The results are expressed as a percent of controls sacrificed at the same time of day. (Modified from Refs. [55,66,77]).

was more than twice that seen after other doses (Fig. 21). At 24 h, the LI was significantly higher with respect to controls and reached its maximum value at 3 days which is the time when the epithelial cells of the crypt have a normal morphology. Following this, the labelling index returned to normal values, however, there was an overshoot in crypt cell numbers. Hence the number of S-phase cells was higher than in controls. The mitotic index data were more variable as a consequence of the lower levels of mitosis in relation to S-phase cells, however, the general features seen with labelling index were also observed with mitotic index. The mitotic delay seen one hour after the end of irradiation could be observed after these fractionation treatments [77].

The number of goblet cells and goblet cell index at the end of the multiple fractionation treatments were 2–3 times higher than seen in controls (Fig. 22). Following 2 doses of 3 Gy at 36 h the goblet cell index was similar to controls. It fell to its lowest value (about 50% of controls) at 72 h and at 5 days after the last fraction, control values were restored. After 4 fractions of 3 Gy, the lowest levels (about 15% of controls) were observed at 72 h. The values returned to normal after 11 days which was many days after the return of normal morphology [59]. The increase in the number of goblet cells seen soon after a single dose could be a consequence of early differentiation induction whereas the delay in appearance of goblet cells when the radiation doses had undergone repair and

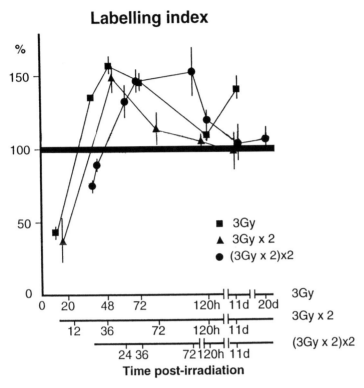

Fig. 21. Variations in the labelling indices in the same experiments as reported in Fig. 20. (Modified from Refs. [55,66,77]).

recovery, could be explained by a temporary defect in differentiation and a preference for proliferation.

6.5 Other multiple fractionation protocols

The results for a variety of different fractionation regimes showed similar responses (3×2 Gy every 4 h, 3×2 Gy every 4 h followed by a delay of 16 h and then a second course of 3×2 Gy every 4 h). The following protocols were also investigated; 2 Gy every 8 h until a total dose of 6 or 12 Gy has accumulated. In the case of 12 Gy, irradiations were initiated at midday or midnight [78]. There were no significant differences between these various fractionation regimes in qualitative and quantitative response except for slightly more initial injury when the first fraction was started at midnight [79]. In this group, repair and repopulation took place slightly earlier than in the group which was irradiated at midday. Quantitatively the number of crypt cells was significantly lower than controls (about 50%) until at least 36 h after the last fraction (Fig. 23). When fractions were given every 8 h to a total of 12 Gy, the total cell number was higher and there was a delayed overshoot when compared with

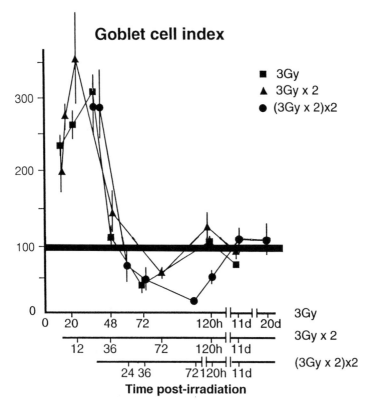

Fig. 22. Variations in Goblet Cell Index in the same experiment as reported in Fig. 20. (Modified from Ref. [59]).

the other fractionation regimes [79,80]. There was a certain amount of variability amongst the animals in each group, particularly during the regeneration phase. Six doses of 2 Gy delivered every 8 h showed a lower reduction in the labelling index which confirmed the fact that there is better tolerance of this fractionation regime. Four hours after the last fraction, the values were similar to controls in comparison with 4 fractions of 3 Gy, where control values were reached at 24 h. Control values were reached even later in the groups which received (2 Gy × 3) × 2 (Fig. 24). The overshoot in labelling index following 6 fractions of 2 Gy 8 h apart was considerably lower than for the other fractionation regimes where the overshoot reached values of 135–145% of controls at 72 h after the last fraction. Control values in all cases were reached between 5 and 11 days after the last dose, but considerable variability from animal to animal was noticed. The mitotic index data generally followed the same pattern.

The goblet cell index showed similar changes to those reported earlier, but slightly higher values were observed at 1 and 4 h after irradiation [59]. Six fractions of 2 Gy every 8 h did not result in an initial increase in the number

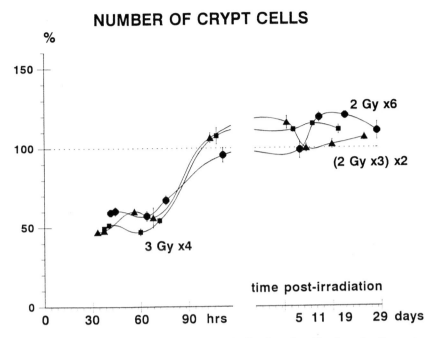

Fig. 23. Variations in the number of epithelial cells along the side of crypts after various multiple fractionation schedules (2 Gy × 3) × 2 (closed triangles), 3 Gy × 4 (closed squares) and 2 Gy × 6 (asterisk) using a total dose of 12 Gy. The results are expressed as a percent of control values (mean values ± SE). (Modified from Refs. [66,77,78]).

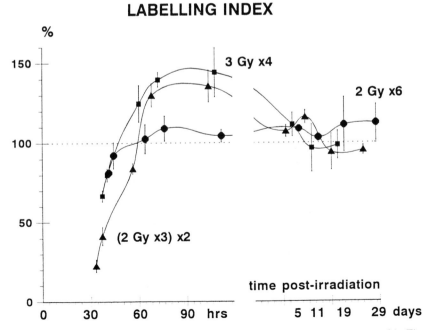

Fig. 24. Variations in the Labelling Indices in the same experiments as reported in Fig. 23.

and index of goblet cells. Here, the length of the fractionation treatment was 40 h and the first intervals of sacrifice were later than with the other fractionation regimes and occurred during the phase of a decrease in goblet cell number. Thus during this phase the values obtained were similar to those of controls. These observations were in agreement with other studies using fractionation regimes and showed an earlier return to control values for all regimes in comparison with a single dose of 8 Gy and this confirmed the tolerance of the small intestine to fractionated regimes.

6.6 S-phase distribution

Following multi-fraction treatment there was a statistically significant reduction of labelled cells at all cell positions along the crypt axis at the first time interval studied which confirmed the changes that were observed in the overall labelling index. The results for various fractionation regimes are shown in Figs. 25, 26 and 27. Following 2 doses of 3 Gy 12 h apart, there was a general suppression in the distribution of labelled cells 1 h after the last treatment, 13 h after the beginning. One hour after the last of 4 fractions 12 h apart (33 h after exposure), there was a suppression of labelling in the lower part of the crypt, but normal levels in the upper part. Four to 24 h after irradiation, there was an increase in the labelled cell frequency that was observed after both 6 and 12 Gy total dose [81]. A comparison of the labelling index frequency plot 36 h after the end of treatment (Fig. 26) showed an increase in proliferative activity in all cases. This was particularly pronounced in the upper regions of the crypt for the fractionation regimes. By 5 days after the end of the treatment, control patterns for labelling index distribution were observed in all groups except for a partial expansion in the proliferative compartment in the 3 Gy × 4 fractionation group (Fig. 27) [81].

6.7 Other multiple fractionation regimes

Three fractions of 2 Gy resulted in similar changes in the labelling index as reported above. The fractionation regime with a 16-h split (2 Gy × 3) × 2 showed a larger early decrease in labelling index up to 24 h after the end of irradiation, thereafter, a similar response was observed.

An analysis was performed on groups of rats killed at 4 times of the day, 11 days after fractionation. These showed that the S-phase distributions were similar to those of controls killed at the same time of day, even though there was an expansion of the proliferative compartment [78]. It was only after 19 and 29 days, that the frequency of labelled cells was similar to controls. After 6 fractions of 2 Gy, the initial reduction in S-phase cells was lower and the return to normal earlier than for other fractions [79].

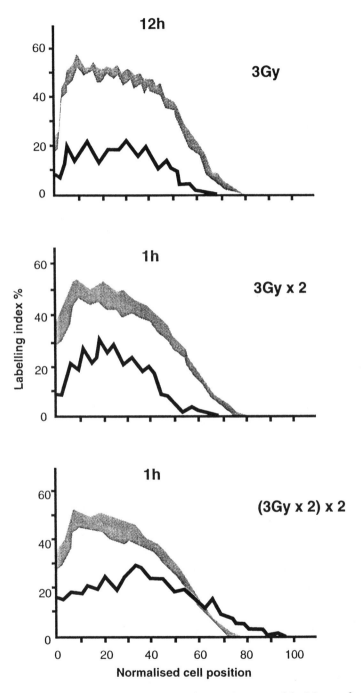

Fig. 25. Normalised labelled cell distributions in crypts of the jejunum from rats irradiated with 3 Gy, 3 Gy × 2 and 3 Gy × 4 and sacrificed respectively 12 and 1 h after exposure. The limits of the SE are shown for the controls and the mean value for the irradiated group. The error limits shown for the controls are typical throughout. (Modified in part from Ref. [81]).

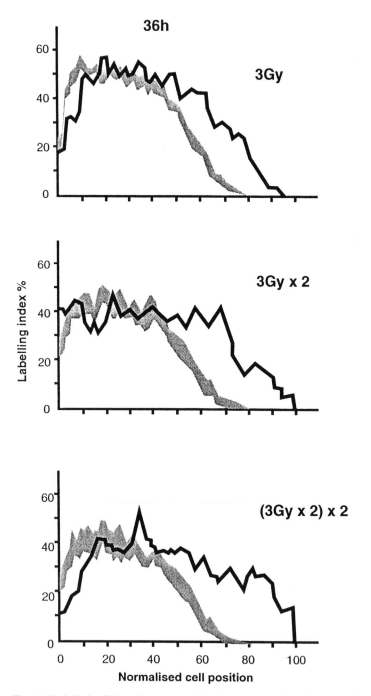

Fig. 26. Labelled cell distributions at 36 h after the end of irradiation in the same experiments as presented in Fig. 25. (Modified in part from Ref. [81]).

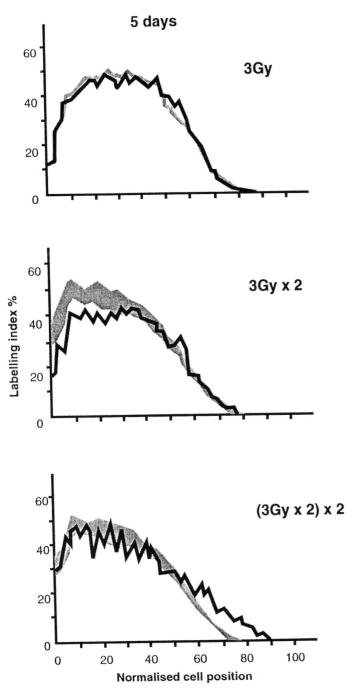

Fig. 27. Labelled cell distributions at 5 days after the end of irradiation in the same experiments as present in Fig. 25. (Modified in part from Ref. [81]).

6.7 Biochemical changes after fractionation

Brush border enzyme activity

The changes in brush border enzyme activities following fractionation were similar to those observed after single exposures when the length of treatment was taken into account. The initial increase, the reduction and the return to normal levels occurred after all fractionation regimes. In the case of 2 fractions of 6 Gy, the later exposure occurred during the acute phase of the radiation damage induced by the first dose that is between 24 and 72 h and the early increase in brush border enzyme activity was absent, but there was an earlier return to control levels [76]. The increase in brush border enzyme activities after 2 doses of 3 Gy was statistically significant one hour after the end of treatment. The levels of disaccharidases and leucine-aminopeptidase (LAP) increased progressively until a maximum was observed at 12 h. For maltase and LAP, values similar to control were subsequently observed which was followed by minimum levels of about 70% of control at 36–72 h after irradiation. This was then followed by a return to control values [82]. Following a regime of 4 doses of 3 Gy, the disaccharidase and dipeptidase activities were slightly higher than controls at 1 and 4 h after the end of irradiation. Thereafter they decreased rapidly to very low levels (10–20% of controls) between 24 and 72 h, which represents the minimum. By 5 days, maltase, invertase, trehalase and LAP all returned to normal values which are reached by 29 days after irradiation. Lactase activity was generally lower than the other brush border enzymes.

Figures 28 and 29 summarise the results obtained for 3 Gy alone, 2 doses of 3 Gy and 4 doses of 3 Gy. For maltase and lactase activity in the second of the 5 segments into which the small intestine was cut, the enzyme activity showed a progressive reduction with the lowest levels occurring during the acute phase of injury. After 4 doses of 3 Gy, the reduction tended to be more evident than for the other irradiation schedules and returned to normal conditions at a slower rate. Following the fractionation regime of 2 Gy 3 times with an interval of 16 h between two such schedules, there was an increase in brush border enzyme activity at one hour and 4 h after irradiation. Following this, the activities of the enzymes decreased to levels lower than seen after any other fractionation regime and returned to control values after 11 days. Following 6 fractions of 2 Gy, the changes were more modest and generally in the acute phase of injury the values were higher than seen for the other fractionation regimes. When these results were compared with the effects after a single dose of 8 Gy, the fractionation regimes resulted in a longer period of elevated enzyme activity, a lower minimal value and an earlier return to control levels.

Lysosomal enzyme activities

Following two doses of 3 Gy, lysosomal enzyme activities showed an increase above the values seen for 3 Gy alone at the earliest time intervals. The highest levels were reached at 36 h after irradiation and returned to control values after 5 days [83]. Figure 30 shows the changes in β glucuronidase activity in

MALTASE

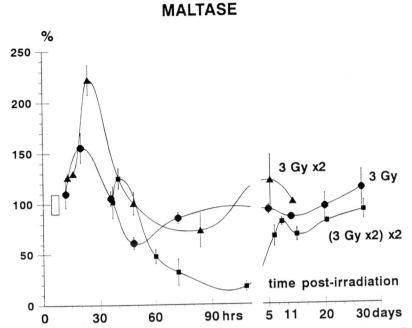

Fig. 28. Variations in maltase activity in the second segment of the small intestine of rats irradiated respectively with 3 Gy, 3 Gy × 2 and 3 Gy × 4. The values are expressed as a percent of control values (mean values ± SE).

LACTASE

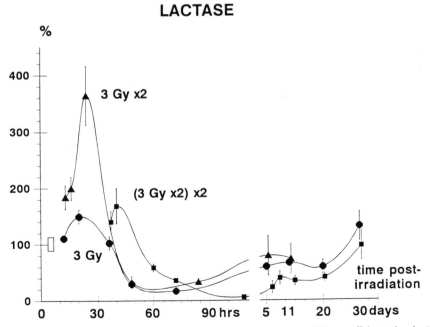

Fig. 29. Variations in lactase activity in the second segment of the small intestine in the same experiments as presented in Fig. 28.

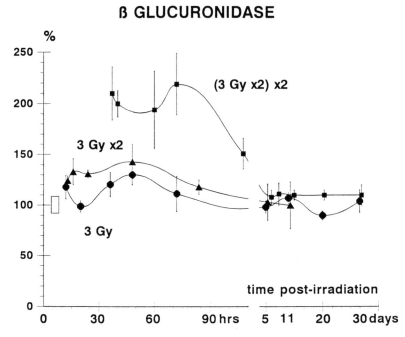

Fig. 30. Variations in β glucuronidase activity in the second segment of the small intestine in the same experiments as presented in Fig. 28.

the second of the 5 segments of the intestine that were analysed. The other segments of the small intestine showed similar changes, but with less marked variations. Following 4 doses of 3 Gy, there was a very marked increase soon after irradiation that persists until at least 36 h after irradiation. The enzyme activity begins to return to normal between 3 and 5 days post-irradiation [83]. Acid phosphatase and cathepsin D activities showed similar behaviour with statistically significant increases at the early times and an earlier return to normal values. The other fractionation regimes analysed showed a similar pattern of response.

7. GENERAL CONCLUSIONS

The usefulness of the small intestine as a model for the evaluation of the effects of radiation is evident. The cellular organisation allows analysis of the structure of the crypt and of the mechanisms which regulate proliferation, programmed cell death and differentiation. The latter is characterised by the synthesis of specific functional proteins, the brush border enzymes, that occur in the cells in the upper part of the crypt close to the junction with the villus. The strong circadian dependence in brush border enzyme activities necessitated studies into their variation together with those of cell kinetic parameters during the light/dark cycle. The activities of brush border enzymes are regulated by factors such as motor activity and food intake which are greatest at night in rats. Indications that the circadian variations are tied to specific functional activities is provided by the lack of a circadian dependence of lysosomal enzyme activity and protein content. Proliferative activity also showed some circadian variation in the small intestine, but at a much lower level than that seen for the brush border enzyme activity.

The high level of proliferation and the rapid turnover of the small intestine necessitates a continuous production of new cells to compensate for those extruded continuously at the apex of the villi. Proliferation activity tends to be highest in the early hours of the morning and lowest in the mid afternoon. Because of these strong circadian variations, animals have to be housed in rigidly controlled light/dark conditions and the times of irradiation have to be particularly defined. The aims of our work over the years have been the following:

(a) to evaluate irradiation damage and repair and recovery mechanisms after different doses ranging from 2 to 20 Gy administered as a single acute dose;

(b) to evaluate the effects of fractionation by using different total doses, different doses per fraction and different time intervals between fractions.

In all of our experiments, groups of rats were sacrificed at several different times after exposure between 1 h and 20–45 days. For all our studies, female Wistar rats, 10–12 weeks of age were used. These animals were kept in an artificial light/dark cycle of 12 h (with lights on at 0630 h) for at least 3 weeks, with the same diet always being available *ad libitum*. The radiation source was a telecobalt unit with a dose rate of 70–100 cGy/min. The whole abdomen was exposed except for the 3 Gy study where the animals were irradiated to their entire body. The studies primarily concerned the small intestine which was divided into 3 zones — proximal, distal jejunum, and terminal ileum. In fact the small intestine was cut into 5 different segments, but the results demonstrated that the radiation response in terms of morphological changes, cell kinetic and biochemical changes, were very similar in the different areas [49,50, 76]. By analysing a large number of different parameters, one can get a comprehensive view of the response of this rapidly proliferating tissue to an insult such as radiation. Qualitative and quantitative morphological analysis of the distribution of S-phase cells along the side of the crypt confirms the structure and function of the proliferative compartment and its changes during different phases of intestinal radiation damage. Studies into the lysosomal enzyme activity can help understand epithelial cell death and the inflammatory response in the stroma during the acute phase of injury and during repopulation. Studies into parameters such as polyamine content and total thymidine incorporation have been used to confirm the other more morphological analyses. Analyses into the brush border enzyme activity enable one to understand the functional damage to the tissue that results in malabsorption problems. The behaviour of a variety of enzymes (disaccharases, dipeptidases, non-specific alkaline phosphatase) are similar and are related to the differentiation processes that occur at the top of the crypt. Brush border enzyme activities increase within a few hours after exposure to both acute and fractionated doses and this increase persists for up to 36 h. It has been suggested that this represents an induced differentiation process, since it occurs during a phase of significant reduction in proliferative activity (labelling index). This reduction in the percentage of S-phase cells is contemporaneous with a significant increase in the goblet cell number and its index which seems to confirm the hypothesis of an early induced differentiation. Such early differentiation phenomena induced by ionising radiation have been observed in various mammalian cells [84,85]. This induction of differentiation by radiation in a tissue with a high proliferative activity is confirmed by studies on the kidney. In this organ, the epithelial cells of the proximal tubules represent a brush border similar to that in the small intestine. Here, disaccharidases, dipeptidases and alkaline phosphatase and other molecules are localised. The function of the brush border enzymes is membrane digestion of dimeric and trimeric forms of monosaccharides and amino acids and their subsequent absorption as monomers into the blood system [86–88]. In this way, kidney is involved in the re-absorption process of many molecules that would otherwise be lost in the urine. The kidney is characterised by a very low mitotic activity, with a labelling index ranging from 0.08–0.2% at different times of the light/dark cycle [89]. There is not a statistically significant variation throughout the light/dark cycle in the kidney [90,91] and irradiation of the kidney produces no statistically significant modification of the brush border enzyme activities when doses of 6 and 8 Gy were administered to the abdomen [92,93]. Maltase and alkaline phosphatase do show an increase within 20 h after exposure with 8 Gy, but to a much less marked extent when compared with the small intestine. Even in old rats exposed to 8 Gy, the brush border enzymes of the kidney do not show any significant variations in activity in relation to the controls within 5 days of irradiation [94]. During these same intervals lysosomal enzymes (β glucuronidase, β acid galactosidase, acid phosphatase and cathepsin D) show some small variations [93,94]. In the small intestine, during the acute phase of damage with sublethal radiation doses, the number of epithelial cells is reduced and there is an increase (after the initial decline) in the number of S-phase cells and mitotic activity spreads into the upper regions of the crypt where under normal circumstances, differentiation occurs.

Analysis of histological sections during the acute phase of damage shows very significant morphological changes in the villi with abundant inflammatory cells in the stroma and low levels of brush border enzymes and goblet cells at a time when there are maximum lysosomal activities. Between 3 and 5 days after exposure, the proliferative activity is still elevated, but the distribution of the S-phase cells is shrinking back to normal patterns. During this time, the morphological appearance of the epithelium returns to normal, both from a qualitative and quantitative point of view. Lysosomal enzyme activities return to normal, but the goblet cell index and brush border enzyme activities remain at a low level for several days. The re-establishment of normal differentiation patterns is slow to return to normal. These observations seem to suggest that the return to normal function, i.e., enzyme activity, is delayed during the repopulation phase after irradiation, although the cell numbers may return to normal, or even be higher than normal values. These cells are almost exclusively chief cells exhibiting none of these differentiation functions. The reduction in enzyme activity is particularly evident for lactase and during this period, it is likely that malabsorption of disaccharides and dipeptides and other molecules from the diet is occurring. It is only after about 11 days, that these things return to normal.

Only modest variations in proliferative activity are seen throughout the day. When rats were irradiated with the same sublethal dose at different times of the light/dark cycle, differences in the morphological and cell kinetic properties were not particularly evident. However, some differences were observed. Exposure at midnight produces an earlier repair and recovery with respect to animals irradiated at midday. The evolution of intestinal injury following fractionated radiation follows a pre-described schedule determined by proliferation, differentiation and the overall turnover time. This is true if the total duration of treatment is less than about 40 h. If it is longer than this, then the delivery of some of the doses of irradiation occurs during the acute response phase for the first few radiation exposures and as a consequence, some of the changes are not observed, e.g., the early increase in enzyme activity.

A dose of 12 Gy fractionated into 2, 4 or 6 fractions results in significantly less changes in the intestinal epithelium compared with a single dose of 12 Gy. This is approximately a 30% lethal dose for the rats. By comparing different multiple fractionation regimes with the same total dose administered to the abdomen over similar total times, some interesting results can be observed, even if the general response is similar. The $(2 \text{ Gy} \times 3) \times 2$ with a 16-h split results in the largest changes, whereas 2 Gy in 6 fractions results in the greatest tolerance. In the former case, the split of 16 h appears to be insufficient to repair the damage induced by the first course of 3 fractions every 4 h. In the latter case, because of the longer time during irradiation, the first few hours after the treatment does not show an increase in brush border enzyme activities and the results are similar to controls.

Overall, the results show that the small intestine is an important and valid model for the evaluation of the effects of cytotoxic chemicals and physical agents on a tissue with a high proliferative activity. Studies into the various parameters involved in the cellular organisation and function of the tissue has led to a better understanding of proliferation and differentiation processes. Such studies also provide information on repair and repopulation phenomena after treatment with perturbing agents. Such studies enable one to determine the real tolerance of the tissue and to predict new or different treatment schedules with cytotoxic agents.

Acknowledgements

The studies are supported by the CNR, Accordo Bilaterale n. 9300211CT04 and 9402354. The authors are very grateful to Drs. Sauro Porciani, Valentino Giaché, Aldo Lanini and all others that have worked at the Radiation Biology Laboratory for their help with the experimental work and to Ann Kaye for her patient help with the manuscript.

References

1. De Giuli, G., Dalla Palma, L. and De Domincis, R. (1967) Prophylaxis and treatment of intestinal damage due to radiation. Proc. XIth Int. Cong. of Radiology. Rome, September, 1965. Int. Cong. Series 105, Excerpta Medica, Amsterdam, pp. 1609–1616.
2. Dalla Palma, L. (1968) Intestinal malabsorption in patients undergoing abdominal radiation therapy. In: M.F. Sullivan (Ed.), Gastrointestinal Radiation Injury, Excerpta Medica, Amsterdam, pp. 261–275.
3. Cionini, L., Becciolini, A., Dalla Palma, L. and De Giuli, G. (1971) Intestinal absorption of radioiodine labelled human serum albumin, mono-iodotyrosine and di-iodotyrosine following abdominal radiation therapy. Acta Radiol. 10, 342–352.
4. Cionini, L., Becciolini, A. and Giannardi, G. (1976) Water (electrolyte) balance after abdominal therapeutic treatment. Strahlentherapie 172, 78–82.
5. Becciolini, A., Cionini, L., Cappellini, M. and Atzeni, G. (1979) Biliary and pancreatic secretions in abdominal irradiation. Acta Radiol. Ther. Phys. Biol. 18, 145–154.
6. Paulus, U., Loeffler, M., Zeidler, J., Owen, G. and Potten, C.S. (1993) The differentiation and lineage development of goblet cells in the murine small intestinal crypt: experimental and modelling studies. J. Cell Sci. 106, 473–484.
7. Borgstrom, B., Dahlquist, A., Lundh, G. and Siovall, S. (1957) Studies of intestinal digestion and absorption in the human. J. Clin. Invest. 36, 1521–1536.
8. Crane, R.K. (1966) Enzymes and malabsorption: a concept of brush border membrane disease. Gastroenterology 50, 254–262.
9. Ugolev, A.M. (1968) Physiology and Pathology of Membrane Digestion. Plenum Press.
10. Ugolev, A.M. and De-Laey, P. (1973) Membrane digestion. A concept of enzyme hydrolysis on cell membranes. Biochim. Biophys. Acta 300, 105–128.
11. Alpers, D.H. and Tedesco, F.J. (1975) The possible role of pancreatic proteases in the turnover of intestinal brush border proteins. Biochim. Biophys. Acta 401, 28–40.
12. Gray, G.M. (1981) Carbohydrate absorption and malabsorption on physiology of the gastrointestinal tract. In: L.R. Johnson (Ed.), Physiology of the Gastrointestinal Tract. Raven Press, New York, pp. 1063–1072.
13. Simoons, F.J. (1978) Geographic hypothesis and lactose malabsorption: a weighing of the evidence. Am. J. Dig. Dis. 23, 963–980.
14. Gray, G.M., Conklin, K.A. and Townley, R.R.W. (1976) Sucrase-isomaltase deficiency. Absence of an inactive enzyme variant. New Engl. J. Med. 294, 750–753.
15. Hammerli, M.P., Kistler, H.J., Amman, R., Marthaler, T., Semenza, G., Auricchio,

S. and Prader, A. (1965) Acquired milk intolerance in the adult caused by lactose malabsorption due to a selective deficiency of intestinal lactase activity. Am. J. Med. 38, 7–18.

16. Hegarty, J.E., Fairclough, P.D., Moriarty, K.J., Kelli, M.J. and Clark, M.L. (1982) Effects of concentration on *in vivo* absorption of a peptide-containing protein hydrolysate. Gut 23, 304–309.

17. Quaroni, A., Kirsh, K. and Weiser, M.M. (1979) Synthesis of membrane glycoproteins in rat small intestinal cells. Redistribution of L (1, 5, 6-3H) glucose labelled membrane glycoproteins among Golgi, lateral, basal and microvillus membrane. Biochem. J. 182, 213–221.

18. Halberg, F (1969) Chronobiology. Am. Rev. Physiol. 31, 675–725.

19. Sigdestad, C.P., Bauman, J. and Lesher, S. (1969) Diurnal fluctuation in the number of cells in mitosis and DNA synthesis in the jejunum of the mouse. Exp. Cell Res. 58, 159–162.

20. Klein, R.R. (1980) Analysis of intestinal cell proliferation after guanethidine-induced sympathectomy. III Effects of chemical sympathectomy on circadian variation in mitotic activity. Cell Tissue Kinet. 13, 153–162.

21. Al-Dewachi, H.S., Wright, N.A., Appleton, D.A. and Watson, A.J. (1976) Studies on the mechanism of diurnal variation of proliferative indices in the small bowel mucosa of the rat. Cell Tissue Kinet. 9: 459–467.

22. Scheving, L.E., Tsai, T.H. and Scheving, L.A. (1983) Chronobiology of intestinal tract of the mouse. Am. J. Anat. 163, 433–438.

23. Sigdestad, C.P. and Lesher, S. (1971) Photo-reversal of the circadian rhythm in the proliferative activity of the mouse small intestine. J. Cell Physiol. 78, 121–125.

24. Al-Nafussi, A.I. and Wright, N.A. (1982) Circadian rhythm in the rate of cellular proliferation and in the size of the functional compartment of mouse jejunal epithelium. Virchows Arch. (Cell Pathol.) 40, 71–79.

25. Stevenson, N.R., Day, S.E. and Sitren, H. (1979) Circadian rhythmicity in rat intestinal villus length and cell number. Int. J. Chronobiol. 6, 1–12.

26. Saito, M., Murakami, E. and Suda, M. (1976) Circadian rhythms in disaccharidases of rat small intestine and its relations to food intake. Biochim. Biophys. Acta, 421, 177–179.

27. Becciolini, A., Romano, S., Porciani, S., Buricchi, L., Benucci, A. and Casati, V. (1977) Circadian rhythms of some enzymes in the small intestine of rat. Chronobiologia 4, 100.

28. Stevenson, N.R. and Fierstein, J.S. (1976) Circadian rhythms of intestinal sucrase and glucose transport: cured by time of feeding. Am. J. Physiol. 230, 731–735.

29. Furuya, S., Sitren, H.S., Zeigen, S., Offord, C.E. and Stevenson, N.R. (1979) Alteration in the circadian rhythmicity of rat small intestinal function. J. Nutr. 109, 1962–1969.

30. Saito, M., Murakami, E., Nishida, T., Fuyisawa, Y. and Suda, M. (1976) Circadian rhythms in digestive enzymes in the small intestine of rats. III. Effects of fasting and refeeding. J. Biochem. 80, 563–568.

31. Henning, S.J. and Guerin, Q.M. (1983) Role of nocturnal feeding in the development of the diurnal rhythm of jejunal sucrase activity. Proc. Soc. Exp. Biol. Med. 172, 232–237.

32. Becciolini, A., Benucci, A., Nardino, A., Giannardi, G. and Balzi, M. (1983) Enzyme activities in ageing small intestine and modifications after irradiation. Strahlentherapie 159, 41–50.

33. Porter, C.W. and Bergeron, R.J. (1983) Spermidine requirement for cell prolifera-
     tion in eukaryotic cells: structural specificity and quantitation. Science 219, 1083–
     1085.
34. Marton, L.J. and Morris, D. (1987) Molecular and cellular function of the polyami-
     nes. In: P.P. McCann, A.E. Pegg and A. Sioerdsma (Eds.), Inhibition of Polyamine
     Metabolism. Academic Press, Orlando, pp. 79–105.
35. Luk, G.D., Marton, L.J. and Baylin, S.B. (1980) Ornithine decarboxylase is impor-
     tant in intestinal mucosa maturation and recovery from injury in rats. Science 210,
     195–198.
36. Becciolini, A., Porciani, S. and Lanini, A. (1993) Polyamines. In: A. Ballesta, G.C.
     Torre, E. Bombardieri, M. Gion and R. Molina (Eds.), Updating on Tumor Markers
     in Tissue and in Biological Fluids: Basic Aspects and Clinical Applications. Min-
     erva Medica Torino, pp. 413–434.
37. Becciolini, A., Porciani, S., Lanini, A. and Attanasio, M. (1989) Polyamines in the
     small intestine of rats after whole body irradiation. Int. J. Radiat. Biol. 56, 67–73.
38. Becciolini, A., Porciani, S., Lanini, A., Balzi, M., Cionini, L. and Bandettini, L.
     (1991) Polyamine levels in healthy and tumor tissues of patients with colon
     adenocarcinoma. Dis. Col. Rect. 34, 167–173.
39. Becciolini, A., Porciani, S., Lanini, A., Cionini, L. and Santoni, R. (1992) Urinary
     polyamines in patients with advanced or recurrent cervical cancer during and after
     radiotherapy. Acta Oncol., 31, 327–331.
40. Becciolini, A., Porciani, S., Balzi, M., Lanini, A., Scubla, E., Pacini, P., Benucci, A.
     and Distante, V. (1992) Cell kinetics and biochemical parameters in breast cancer.
     Int. J. Biol. Markers 7, 16–20.
41. Quastler, H. (1956) The nature of intestinal radiation death. Radiat. Res. 4,
     303–320.
42. Becciolini, A., Porciani, S., Nardino, A., Giache, V. and Lanini, A. (1982) Unconven-
     tional dose administration: modifications of body and small intestine weights.
     Strahlentherapie 158, 183–189.
43. Potten, C.S. (1977) Extreme sensitivity of some intestinal crypt cells to x and γ
     irradiation. Nature 269, 518–521.
44. Becciolini, A., Arganini, L., Tedde, G., Vannelli, G. and Cariaggi, P. (1976) Bio-
     chemical and morphological changes in the epithelial cells of the small intestine
     after irradiation. Int. J. Radiat. Oncol. Biol. Phys. 1, 915–925.
45. Becciolini, A. (1987) Relative radiosensitivity of the stomach and small and large
     intestine. In: J.T. Lett and K.J. Altman (Eds.), Relative Radiosensitivities of
     Human Organ Systems. Advances in Radiation Biology Vol. 12. Academic Press,
     New York, pp. 83–126.
46. Becciolini, A., Gerber, G.B., Buracchi, A. and Deroo, J. (1977) Intestinal enzyme
     distribution after supralethal irradiation. Strahlentherapie 153, 484–488.
47. Quastler, H. (1963) Effects of irradiation on intestinal mucosal cell population.
     Fed. Proc. 22, 1330–1335.
48. Cairnie, A.B., Lamerton, L.F. and Steel, G.G. (1965) Cell proliferation studies in
     the intestinal epithelium of the rat. Determination of the kinetics parameters. Exp.
     Cell. Res. 39, 528–538.
49. Becciolini, A., Ravina, A., Arganini, L., Castagnoli, P. and De Giuli, G. (1972) Effect
     of ionising radiations on the enzymes of the intestinal mucosa of rats at different
     time intervals after abdominal irradiation. Radiat. Res. 49, 213–225.
50. Becciolini, A., Cariaggi, P., Arganini, L., Castagnoli, P and De Giuli, G. (1974)

Effect of 200, 650 and 1200 R on the intestinal disaccharases and dipeptidases. Acta Radiol. 13, 142–152.

51. Becciolini, A., Benucci, A., Casati, V., Nardino, A., Porciani, S. and Rizzi, M. (1979) Post-irradiation enzyme activities of the rat small intestine: effects on circadian fluctuation. Strahlentherapie 155, 869–874.

52. Becciolini, A., Cremonini, D., Balzi, M., Fabbrica, D. and Cinotti, S. (1982) Irradiation at different times of the day: morphology and kinetic of the small intestine. Acta Radiol. Oncol. 21, 169–175.

53. Casati, V., Benucci, A., Nardino, A., Rizzi, M., Giannardi, G., Pelà, G. and Becciolini, A. (1981) Influenza dell'età sulle attività enzimatiche delle intestino tenue di ammiferi irradiati. Aggiornamenti di Radiobiogia, A. Becciolini (Ed.), Uncimi Pierucci, Firenze, pp. 257–258.

54. Becciolini, A., Giache , V., Scubla, E. and D'Abbondio, D. (1987) Circadian phenomena and irradiation: modifications of enzyme activity in the small intestine after sublethal exposure. Acta Oncol. 26, 477–481.

55. Becciolini, A., Balzi, M., Fabbrica, D. and Potten, C.S. (1995) Cell kinetics in rat small intestine after irradiation with sublethal dose at different times of the day. Submitted to Int. J. Rad. Biol.

56. Becciolini, A., Balzi, M., Cremonini, D., Cinotti, S. and Fabbrica, D. (1983) Behaviour of the proliferative compartment of the small intestine at different times of the day. Acta Radiol. Oncol. 22, 201–207.

57. Becciolini, A., Balzi, M., Cremonini, D. and Fabbrica, D. (1983) S-phase cell distribution in the small intestine irradiated at different times of the day: I — Acute irradiation injury. Acta Radiol. Oncol. 22, 305–313.

58. Becciolini, A., Balzi, M., Cremonini, D. and Fabbrica, D. (1983) S-phase cell distribution in the small intestine irradiated at different times of the day: II — Recovery phase. Acta Radiol. Oncol. 22, 337–344.

59. Becciolini, A., Fabbrica, D., Cremonini, D and Balzi, M. (1985) Quantitative changes in the goblet cells of the rat small intestine after irradiation. Acta Radiol. Oncol. 24, 291–299.

60. Becciolini, A. and Ravina, A. (1970) Effect of ionising radiations on intestinal disaccharidase rats. Br. J. Radiol. 43, 150–151.

61. Becciolini, A., Romano, S., Porciani, S., Buricchi, L., Benucci, A. and Casati, V. (1981) Circadian rhythms of some enzymes in the small intestine of rat. Proc. XIII Int. Conf. Soc. Chronobiol., F. Halberg, L.E. Scheving, E.W. Powel, D.K. Hayes (Eds.) Il Ponte, Milano, pp. 11–18.

62. Becciolini, A., Bini, R., Lanini, A., Giache, V., Porciani, S and Drighi, E. (1981) Modification of circadian dependence of intestinal maltase after irradiation. Int. J. Chronobiol. 7, 207.

63. Becciolini, A., Lanini, A., Giache, V., Balzi, M. and Bini, R. (1982) Modifications of the brush border enzymes of the small intestine after irradiation at different times of the day. Acta Radiol. Oncol. 21, 273–279.

64. Becciolini, A., Benucci, A., Porciani, S., Nardino, A. and Lanini, A. (1982) Dipeptidase activity in the small intestine after irradiation at different times of the day. Strahlentherapie 158, 368–374.

65. Becciolini, A., Giache, V., Lanini, A., Cremonini, D. and Drighi, E. (1982) Modifications of small intestine lysosomal enzymes after irradiation at different times of the day. Acta Radiol. Oncol. 21, 61–66.

66. Becciolini, A. (1991) Radiosensitivity of the small and large intestine. In: R.

Dulbecco (Ed.), Encyclopedia of Human Biology. Academic Press, New York, 6, pp. 469–480.

67. Becciolini, A., Porciani, S., Lanini, A. and Balzi, M. (1987) Polyamine content as a marker of radiation injury in the rat spleen. Int. J. Radiat. Biol. 52, 676–774.
68. Altman, K.I. and Gerber, G.B. (1970) Radiation Biochemistry. Academic Press, New York.
69. Gits, J. and Gerber, G.B. (1973) Electrolyte loss, the main cause of death from the gastrointestinal syndrome. Radiat. Res. 55, 18–28.
70. Becciolini, A., Gerber, G.B. and Deroo, J. (1977) *In vivo* absorption of carbohydrates in rats with gastrointestinal radiation syndrome. Acta Radiol. Ther. Phys. Biol. 16, 87–96.
71. Winnie, D. (1972) The influence of blood flow water net flux on the absorption of tritiated water from the jejunum of the rat. Arch. Exp. Path. Pharmak. 272, 417–421.
72. Ellis, F. (1969) Dose time and fractionation: a clinical hypothesis. Clin. Radiol. 20, 1–7.
73. Fowler, J.F. (1984) 40 years of radiobiology: its impact on radiotherapy. Phys. Med. Biol. 29, 97–113.
74. Thames, H.D., Peters, L.J., Withers, H.R. and Fletcher, G.H. (1983) Accelerated fractionation vs hyperfractionation: rationales for several treatments per day. Int. J. Radiat. Oncol. Biol. Phys. 9, 127–138.
75. Steel, G.G., Adams, G.E. and Horwich, A. (1989) The Biological Basis of Radiotherapy. Elsevier, Amsterdam.
76. Becciolini, A., Castagnoli, P., Arganini, L. and De Giuli, G. (1973) Post-irradiation enzyme activities of rat small intestine: effects of dose fractionation. Radiat. Res. 55, 291–303.
77. Becciolini, A., Cremonini, D., Fabbrica, D. and Balzi, M. (1984) Qualitative and quantitative effects on the morphology of the small intestine after multiple daily fractionation. Acta Radiol. Oncol. 23, 353–359.
78. Becciolini, A., Cremonini, D., Fabbrica, D. and Balzi, M. (1986) Cell proliferation and differentiation in the small intestine after irradiation with multiple fractions. Acta Radiol. Oncol. 25, 51–56.
79. Becciolini, A., et al., unpublished data.
80. Fabbrica, D., Becciolini, A., Cremonini, D. and Benucci, A., (1987) Morphologic and physiologic modifications of rat small intestine after different schedules of irradiation. In: E.M. Fielden, J.F. Fowler, J.H. Hendry and D. Scott (Eds.), Radiation Research, Vol. 1. Taylor and Francis, London, p. 273.
81. Becciolini, A., Cremonini, D., Fabbrica, D. and Balzi, M. (1983) Modification of S-phase cell distribution in the intestinal crypts after multiple daily fractionation. Acta Radiol. Oncol. 22, 441–448.
82. Becciolini, A., Giache, V., Balzi, M. and Morrone, A. (1987) Brush border enzymes after multiple daily fractionation. Radiat. Res. 109, 374–381.
83. Becciolini, A., Giache, V., Balzi, M. and Morrone, A. (1983) Behaviour of lysosomal enzymes in the small intestine after multiple daily fractionation. Strahlentherapie 159, 508–512.
84. Yang, T.C.H., Risius, J. and Tobias, C.A. (1974) Radiation response of neuroblastoma cells *in vitro*. Radiat. Res. 59, 46–47.
85. Wangenheim, K.H. and Howard, A. (1978) Different models of cell sterilisation: cell killing and early differentiation. Radiat. Res. 73, 288–302.

86. Quirk, S.Y. and Robinson, G.B. (1972) Isolation and characterisation of rabbit kidney brush border. Biochem. J. 128, 1319–1322.

87. Goldman, D.R., Schlesinger, H. and Segal, S. (1976) Isolation and characterisation of the brush border fraction from newborn rat renal proximal tubule cells. Biochim. Biophys. Acta, 419, 251–257.

88. Norgaard, T. (1976) Correlation of enzyme histochemical and structural segmentation in the proximal convoluted tubule of the rat kidney. Acta Pathol. Microbiol. Scand. 84, 172–180.

89. Franciolini, F., Becciolini, A., et al., unpublished data.

90. Saito, M. (1972) Daily rhythmic changes in brush border enzymes of the small intestine and kidney of the rat. Biochim. Biophys. Acta 286, 212–215.

91. Franciolini, F., Becciolini, A., Casati, V., Cremonini, D., Giache, V. and Porciani, S. (1979) Circadian activity of rat kidney enzymes. Experientia 35, 582–583.

92. Becciolini, A., Franciolini, F., Giache, V and Porciani, S. (1976) Enzyme activities of the kidney after irradiation. Radiat. Res. 68, 167–170.

93. Franciolini, F., Becciolini, A., Rossi, A., Giache, V., Balzi, M. and Nardino, A. (1979) Early effects in kidney enzyme activities after irradiation. Acta Radiol. Oncol. 18, 209–217.

94. Franciolini, F., Becciolini, A., Torcini, G. and Lanini, A. (1982) The ageing kidney: biochemical and morphological study after irradiation. Strahlentherapie 158, 43–46.

C.S. Potten and J.H. Hendry (Eds.), *Radiation and Gut*

CHAPTER 6

Early and Late Radiation Effects (External Irradiation) on the Gut

J.W. Osborne

Radiation Research Laboratory, University of Iowa, 14 Medical Laboratory, Iowa City, IA 52242, USA

1. INTRODUCTION

Gastrointestinal injury following radiation exposure was recognized early by Walsh [1] and Regaud et al. [2]. Many of the reports since have described the adverse effects of radiotherapeutic procedures in patients where some portion of the gastrointestinal (GI) tract was inadvertently exposed or of necessity was in the radiation field. Other information has been derived from different animal species which were irradiated under a variety of conditions with the objectives of establishing thresholds, documenting the sequence of changes over time, attempting to modulate the response with chemical and physical procedures, characterizing the injury as early or late, and understanding the mechanisms whereby the tissues of interest became damaged, and were able to repair (or attempted to repair) the injury.

In this chapter, discussion of gastrointestinal injury will be largely limited to non-stochastic radiation effects on the oesophagus, stomach, small bowel, and large bowel of animals. Animal selection by investigators has often been a matter of economics or convenience, but it sometimes reflects some unusual feature of the system which offers the opportunity to understand underlying mechanisms and/or provide a result which might lead to effective ways of preventing or repairing radiation damage in humans.

The radiation sensitivity of various parts of the GI tract varies with the type of epithelium in the mucosa and glands, the degree of vascularization, and possibly with other variables [3]. These could include pancreatic secretions, bile, and bacteria.

It is generally reported that the order of decreasing radiosensitivity is duodenum, jejunum, ileum, oesophagus, stomach, colon, and rectum [3]. Roswit et al. [4] placed oesophagus just above the rectum in tolerance.

As would be the case with other tissues, the radiation-induced damage to any portion of the GI tract is influenced by dose, dose rate, radiation quality, fractionation schemes used, and a number of biologic variables.

2. OESOPHAGUS

2.1 General comments

Many clinical papers in the literature describe damage to the oesophagus after irradiation of an oesophageal malignancy or a normal oesophagus which was of necessity in the radiation field. These findings are discussed in Chapter 8. Such studies have typically noted time of appearance, frequency, and severity of oesophagitis, dysphagia, histological changes, and ulceration with or without subsequent perforation or formation of tracheo-oesophageal fistulae.

Desjardins [5] felt that the paucity of information on radiation-induced oesophageal changes was due to lack of interest in studying a fairly radioresistant system. Even though Englestad [6] later described marked histologic changes in oesophagi of irradiated dogs, many subsequent authors, including Warren and Friedman [7], did not consider the oesophagus especially radiosensitive.

In a frequently quoted clinical paper, Seaman and Ackerman [8] highlighted significant clinical and pathological changes in the oesophagus following radiation therapy for cancer of non-oesophageal structures. The clinical responses and changes noted by them described in many subsequent papers by others included sub-sternal "burning", oesophagitis, dysphagia, ulceration, strictures, perforation, and fistulae formation. These complications in humans have provided incentives for investigators to complete related studies in animals directed toward amelioration of effects and an understanding of the mechanisms involved. Oesophageal changes after irradiation for species other than humans have been reported for dogs, rats, mice, opossums, and monkeys.

2.2 Studies with mice

2.2.1 Single doses
In mice thorax-irradiated by Phillips and Margolis [9] using single doses of 12.5–30 Gy, the $LD_{50/20}$ was estimated to be 24.8 Gy with death occurring between 10–20 days and no histologic damage to organs other than the oesophagus and thymus. Oesophageal perforation was considered to be the cause of death. The results of the mouse study by Phillips and Margolis were essentially in agreement with those of Jennings and Arden [10]. Phillips and Ross [11] irradiated the thorax only of mice using doses from about 17.5–40.0 Gy. Deaths were recorded daily for 6 weeks after the last dose. Some mice were kept as long as 6 months and the oesophageal tissue was examined at intervals for histological changes. The LD_{50} was calculated at various times from 2–23 weeks postirradiation. The $LD_{50/28}$ was 26.8 Gy. The cause of death was considered to

be oesophageal denudation with resultant starvation and dehydration. Histologic changes in the oesophagus after 20 Gy and above were similar to those described for the irradiated rat oesophagus by Kurohara and Casarett [12].

Hornsey and Field [13] irradiated the thorax only and patterns of death were recorded. The LD_{50} value for death in 10–40 days was 32 Gy of X-rays.

Tochner et al. [14] used a 12 MeV electron beam to irradiate the entire chest cavity of mice with 24–36 Gy. Animals were kept for survival studies or sacrificed from 5–30 days after irradiation. Weight loss was not altered after these radiation doses.

Hirn-Stadler et al. [15], using a technique for irradiating the mediastinum in mice without including the entire thorax, found that weight loss was a sensitive assay for oesophageal damage. They preferred that parameter over animal lethality as an endpoint for acute oesophagitis.

2.2.2 Modification of injury

As a means of testing the hypothesis of Phillips and Margolis [9], that the oesophagus of the mouse is normally somewhat hypoxic, Hornsey and Field [13] used the hypoxic cell sensitizer misonidazole or the breathing of oxygen during irradiation. It was concluded that hypoxic cells indeed were present.

Tochner et al. [14] irradiated the entire chest cavity of mice with 24–36 Gy. Mice were injected 24 or 2 h prior to irradiation and 6–46 h after irradiation with either indomethacin (a prostaglandin synthetase inhibitor) or the liquid vehicle only. Some modulation of the radiation effect due to drug injection did occur. Survival was modestly influenced at the 30 Gy level and definitely so with 32 Gy. Thus indomethacin provided protection for the oesophagus as indicated by histological changes, weight changes, and survival.

2.2.3 Dose fractionation

Phillips and Margolis [9], irradiated the entire thorax only with about 10–50 Gy of fractionated orthovoltage X-radiation. Within 1 week after 30 Gy, no active basal cells were visible. The epithelium was mainly keratin with a few nuclei. The submucosa was oedematous and a few inflammatory cells were present. However, within 2 weeks regenerating epithelium was seen in some mice, but in others the epithelium was destroyed and massive inflammation was present in the oesophageal wall. Without mentioning incidence and number of animals involved, it was reported that 1 year after 25 Gy, the oesophageal mucosa appeared normal.

Phillips and Ross [11] irradiated the thorax only of mice with 2 or 10 fractions of orthovoltage X-radiation. The time between each of the 2 fractions was 1, 7, 14 or 28 days. The 10 fractions were given in 11 days. The $LD_{50/28}$ was 57.5 Gy given in 10 fractions.

Hornsey and Field [13] irradiated the thorax only with 2, 5 or 10 equal fractions of X-rays, and patterns of death were recorded. The LD_{50} values for death in 10–40 days increased with numbers of fractions up to 71 Gy in 10 fractions.

2.2.4 Neutrons

Using a system for irradiating the thorax described by Phillips and Margolis [9], Phillips et al. [16] found the $LD_{50/28}$ for death due to oesophageal injury following exposure to 15 MeV neutrons to be 6.6 Gy. In comparing this with 300 kVp X-radiation, the RBE was 4.0, a figure quite high for normal tissues at this neutron dose level.

In studies by Hornsey and Field [13] the RBE values for mice irradiated to the thorax only with single doses or up to 10 fractions of neutrons compared to single or fractionated doses of X-rays, ranged from 2.5–2.7. The time course of death was independent of radiation quality.

Michalowski [17] irradiated the thorax only with a single 14 Gy dose of fast neutrons. All but 5 of 149 mice died within 28 days and the remainder succumbed by day 55. In contrast to the findings of Phillips and Ross [11], who concluded that death prior to 28 days was due solely to oesophageal damage, it was observed that peaks of death occurred at days 5, 10, and 20. Michalowski concluded that this finding alone suggested multiple causes of death. Autopsy of the 144 mice which died revealed that ulcerative oesophagitis was present in 66% of the animals and complicated by oesophageal perforation 8% of the time. In a subsequent paper, Michalowski and Burgin [18] repeated their views on the meaning of multiple peaks of death during the 28 day postirradiation period and also noted that in their studies, weight loss was not a reliable predictor of oesophagitis. Kurohara and Casarett [12], like Phillips and Margolis [9] and Phillips and Ross [11], had reached the opposite conclusion.

2.3 Studies in rats

Jennings and Arden [10] gave a single dose of about 30 Gy of orthovoltage X-radiation to only the thorax. Overall mortality was 30%, but would probably have been higher had the rats not been switched from laboratory chow to a liquid diet during the second and third postirradiation weeks. As a result of animals being killed at intervals over several months, the following observations were made:

4 days — submucosal congestion and leucocytic infiltration

6 days — loss of superficial epithelium due to mucosal necrosis

7 days — extensive sloughing of mucosa

10 days — maximal plugging of oesophagus with necrotic mucosal debris, causing dilatation of oesophagus. Also, moderate inflammation adjacent to the necrotic material and in the muscularis.

12 days — accumulation of inflammatory exudate in the lumen

16 days — extensive healing of the epithelium and in some rats, complete re-epithelialization.

20 days — re-epithelialization in most animals. This was the result of cell migration from the ulcer margin and from foci of squamous cells, commonly near oesophageal folds.

25 days — moderate submucosal fibrosis which persisted for weeks and which became more striking after regeneration of the epithelium.

6–12 weeks — prominent submucosal fibrosis. Diverticula with mucosal herniation into a muscularis defect was a common late finding.

In a study with over 1400 animals, Kurohara and Casarett [12] gave single doses of approximately 6, 12, 24, and 36 Gy to only the thoracic region. Animals were sacrificed or autopsied at intervals over a 35-week period. A comprehensive evaluation system was used to score histologic changes in the oesophagus ranging from absence of mitotic figures and maturity of basal cells to extensive areas of severe necrosis with intensive submucosal inflammation. An oesophageal reaction occurred at 2 days occasionally after 6 or 12 Gy and with considerable incidence after 24 Gy. A mild reaction occurred as early as 1 day after 36 Gy. The incidence and degree of reaction increased to a maximum at 6–7 days, particularly after 24 or 36 Gy. After the first week, the incidence and degree of degenerative changes gradually subsided. After week 4, only mild changes were noted. Oesophageal mucosal hyperplasia was apparent at various times from 1–35 weeks, but only in the 24 and 36 Gy dose groups. The authors concluded that severe radiation oesophagitis was the major contributor to mortality during the first 14 days after irradiation. The changes noted for the doses used were consistent with observations reported earlier by Jennings and Arden [10].

2.4 Studies with opossums

2.4.1 Single doses
In 1979, Northway et al. [19] introduced the opossum as an animal model for studying radiation-induced oesophagitis because the model has many features of the human oesophagus. Doses of 0, 15.0, 17.5, 20, and 22.5 Gy of ^{60}Co gamma radiation were given to the entire oesophagus. Pre- and postirradiation evaluations of oesophageal function were made by barium oesophagography, intralumenal manometry, and endoscopy. With all doses, oesophagitis developed within a week; mucosal biopsies taken at endoscopy indicated inflammation and ulceration. Anorexia was evident at 7–10 days in animals which received the three highest doses and persisted at least another week. Changes in motility were noted 4–8 weeks postirradiation in the 17.5, 20, and 22.5 Gy animals. Only the animal receiving the 22.5 Gy dose exhibited narrowing of the lumen, thickening of the oesophageal wall, and some muscle necrosis. Strictures of the oesophagus were not present in any of the animals.

2.4.2 Modification of injury
Having established the opossum as a useful animal model for study of oesophageal injury, Northway and colleagues [20,21] gave indomethacin or prostaglandin E prior to and after irradiation with 22.5 Gy, as in prior experiments, to test the efficacy of pharmacologic intervention in ameliorating oesophagitis and related responses. Indomethacin in doses of 4 mg/kg prevented the

development of severe oesophagitis while 5 or 10 µg/kg of 16,16,dimethyl prostaglandin E_2 made the reaction more severe. Northway et al. [21] also evaluated aspirin and hydrocortisone as radioprotective agents. Both chemicals were effective in decreasing endoscopic and histologic signs of oesophagitis.

2.5 Studies in dogs

2.5.1 Partial body irradiation

Engelstad [6] observed histologic changes after partial body irradiation. He saw degenerative changes and loss of epithelium in the mucosa which except for very high doses, were followed by complete epithelial regeneration.

Sindelar [22], utilizing intraoperative radiation therapy (IORT), gave 0, 20, or 30 Gy of 9 MeV electrons to a 6-cm segment of intra-thoracic oesophagus located in the posterior mediastinum. The dogs were evaluated prior to treatment and at intervals for 3–24 months after IORT. Except for early weight loss, clinical signs during 24 months suggested that very few changes had occurred, even after 30 Gy. However, endoscopy, barium swallows, and autopsy findings revealed inflammation, ulceration, and strictures at various times up to 24 months. At the 20 Gy level, except for mild inflammation, mild fibrosis, and some glandular atrophy, there were no complications.

2.5.2 Fractionated irradiation

Gillette et al. [23] irradiated portions of the oesophagus *in situ* with X-radiation from a 6 MV linear accelerator and assessed the effect of changing dose per fraction on the late response of the organ. In the first series, animals received up to 80 Gy in 2, 3, or 4 Gy per fraction over a period of 4 weeks and were then observed for 6 months. Morphometric methods were used to show that at this time, the submucosal glands occupied a much lower percentage of total tissue than prior to irradiation, while the connective tissue increased in inverse proportion to the change in submucosal glands. In a second series, the animals received 36, 44, or 52 Gy at 4 Gy per fraction in 4 weeks. Oesophagi were examined at 1 month and 3 months after irradiation. As in the first series, the reduction in glandular tissue was accompanied by an increase in the connective tissue component. Higher total doses were required for an isoeffect when smaller doses per fraction were given.

In a similar study primarily designed for another purpose by McChesney-Gillette et al. [24], a large number of dogs received 24–68 Gy in 2, 3, and 4 Gy fractions spaced evenly over a 4 week period. Oesophagi were removed 2 years later and studied histologically. With all dose combinations utilized, the histological changes at 2 years were slight with some atrophy, loss, dilatation, inflammation, and hypertrophy of submucosal glands. Occasionally, there was excessive connective tissue in the lamina propria and focal thinning of the surface mucosa, but no significant changes in the percent tissue components of the oesophagus were noted.

2.6 Studies with monkeys

Ambrus et al. [25] irradiated the upper half of the oesophagus of stump-tailed monkeys with 20 Gy of X-radiation from a 6 MeV linear accelerator. Sodium meclofenamate, a known inhibitor of prostaglandin and leukotriene synthesis, was effective in reducing inflammatory reactions which reached their maximum 3 weeks postirradiation.

2.7 Summary

The results of animal studies are in general agreement with the observations made in patients. With dose regimens ordinarily used for patients, the epithelium responds within days and may show substantial damage and be sloughed before repairing itself by migration and proliferation of surviving foci. The threshold for short-term complications after single doses is about 20 Gy, but is much higher if the dose is fractionated. Dysphagia, oesophagitis, ulceration, and inflammation occur to varying degrees and may cause the subject to have mild-to-great difficulty in swallowing or complete stricture. Perforation or stenosis due to increasing fibrosis may also occur. There has been very little published on the late effects of radiation on the oesophagus, probably because the damaged structures tend to regenerate and normal function is eventually restored. For detailed reviews of radiation-induced oesophageal injury in animals and patients, the reader is referred to Rubin and Casarett [26], Novak et al. [27], Casarett [3], Berthrong and Fajardo [28], and Chowhan [29].

3. STOMACH

3.1 General comments

The human stomach is frequently irradiated in the course of treating a stomach tumour or it may, of necessity, be included in the radiation field during treatment of some other malignancy. Among the undesirable effects clinicians attempt to minimize in irradiated patients are the early effects such as nausea, vomiting, delay in gastric emptying, reduction or destruction of secretory activity, gastritis, loss of epithelium, and induction of ulcers with their possible subsequent perforation, as well as the late effects of blood vessel and connective tissue changes, fibrosis, and stenosis.

Various animal models have been utilized in attempts to establish dose–response relationships and to understand the mechanisms responsible for the many responses of the stomach to different doses of radiation. Elucidation of histological changes after irradiation of the stomach of various species has often constituted the major focus of many investigations. In studies with other primary objectives, histological changes were also assessed after a study of

biopsies taken during or after treatment, or the result of histological preparations of autopsy specimens. Changes in the stomach of animals after irradiation have been reported for dogs, monkeys, rats, mice, and rabbits.

3.2 Studies in mice

3.2.1 Single doses
Helander [30] gave a detailed account of the early effects of X-radiation on
the ultrastructure of mouse gastric fundus glands. Whole body supralethal
doses of orthovoltage X-rays of about 13 Gy were given. Mice were killed 0.5–48
h later and the fundus region of the stomach wall along the greater curvature
prepared for electron microscopy. There were some membrane changes in the
zymogen cells, some relocation of parietal cells and diameter changes in the
secretory granules, but none of these specifically would have been life-threatening. Chen and Withers [31] used an *in situ* cloning technique to assay the
dose-survival relationship of gastric stem cells in irradiated mice and estimated the D_0 to be 1.37 Gy.

3.2.2 Fractionated doses
Hirose [32] gave about 90 Gy of X-radiation in 6 equal fractions of 15 Gy each
separated by a week or 100 Gy in 5 equal fractions separated by a week to the
stomach region of otherwise lead-shielded mice. The histological changes in
animals sacrificed when they were moribund were similar to those noted in
other authors' reports. The main findings were marked atrophy of mucosa,
severe ulceration, replacement or covering of atrophic or ulcerous mucosa with
squamous epithelium, squamous metaplasia of glands, atypical regeneration
and atypical hyperplasia of glands, and development of carcinoma. The injury
to the gastric mucosa of rats receiving 60 Gy in three equal fractions separated
by weekly intervals was more severe than noted in mice. Peritonitis due to
perforative gastric ulcers and infections was prominent in the first 11 weeks.
Mucosal atrophy increased with time postirradiation. By five weeks, ulcers
which perforated all layers of the forestomach were noted. Of special interest
were the large abscesses and bony metaplasia in the submucosa 5–7 weeks
postirradiation. In contrast to the mouse study described earlier, atypical
hyperplasia of squamous epithelium in the forestomach was not seen in any of
the rats.

Chen and Withers [31] used an *in situ* cloning technique with split-doses,
where the intestine was shielded during the first (larger) dose. In these
experiments, sublethal injury was repaired rapidly, much of it within an hour.
In a group of mice which received 2 Gy every 24 h, followed by an "assay dose"
of 15 Gy, the number of stem cell survivors was essentially the same as in an
animal receiving only the 15 Gy assay dose. Thus, with 2 Gy per day, repair of
sublethal radiation injury and regeneration of surviving cells were sufficient to
maintain the stem cell population.

3.3 Studies in rats

3.3.1 Single whole body doses

Ely and Ross [33] and Goodman et al. [34] reported that whole body irradiation of rats delayed gastric emptying. Both groups utilized a technique still commonly employed — following the progress of a barium meal with serial radiographs.

Myers and Hornsey [35] irradiated rats whole body with various doses of 250 kVp X-rays shortly after the rats finished normal feeding. Subsequently, the weight of the stomach contents was used as an index of stomach clearance. Complete clearance was delayed for 10–12 h by 0.8 Gy of X-rays.

3.3.2 Partial body irradiation

Hulse [36] irradiated various combinations of body volumes of rats with orthovoltage X-radiation seeking to identify an organ or part of the body which was very important in initiating a delay in gastric emptying. Radiation doses nearly equivalent to 0.2–2 Gy were given to various parts of the body and progress of the barium meal followed 30 min to 8 h later. Every radiation dose used had some effect on gastric emptying. Hulse concluded that irradiation of the small intestine and associated structures was the most important factor in producing the delay. In a related paper, Hulse and Mizon [37] found that rats irradiated shortly after eating a barium meal refused to eat a second meal when tested 4–6 weeks later. The strength of this aversion seemed to be related to the severity of the delay in gastric emptying which related to the dose of radiation utilized and the particular tissue volume involved. Total body irradiation was more effective than irradiation of the abdomen. However, in accordance with what Hulse [36] had found earlier, even irradiation of the head and shoulders produced the subsequent aversion just described.

Weshler et al. [38] irradiated the temporarily exteriorized rat stomach with single doses of 3–30 Gy of orthovoltage X-radiation and sacrificed the animals 1–8 weeks later. Three weeks after 5 Gy, free acid and total acid secretion rates were 3–4 times below normal, almost abolished by 7.5 Gy, and undetectable after 9 Gy. Ulceration, inflammation, edema, and mucosal regeneration were minimal at 3 and 5 Gy, and considerable at higher doses. No signs of mucosal regeneration were noted after 25 and 30 Gy.

Buell and Harding [39] described the response of the rat stomach to irradiation of the abdomen with 10 Gy of ^{60}Co-radiation. They considered changes in microcirculatory parameters as indications of degree of inflammation. Gastric plasma volume showed a peak increase at 12 h, gradually declined, but still was significantly above control 24 h after irradiation. Although no change in neutrophil accumulation occurred in the superficial mucosa during a 24-h assessment period, neutrophils were significantly reduced in the deep mucosal region of the stomach antrum after 12 h and remained so for the next 12 h. The morphological changes included mild edema of the lamina propria 8–24 h postirradiation and some isolated foci of vascular congestion. Changes consistent with classical features of inflammation occurred within 12 h after irradiation even though the mucosal epithelium was intact. This suggested that modification of these proinflammatory changes might be possible which in turn could influence the sequence of symptoms normally associated with the gastrointestinal response after irradiation.

Breiter et al. [40] developed a rat model for studying the qualitative and quantitative aspects of early and chronic radiation injuries in the locally irradiated rat stomach. They described in detail their procedure for minimizing exposure to adjacent organs. Single doses of 14–28.5 Gy were given to the stomach. Most animals received a completely absorbable diet for three weeks after irradiation. Scintigraphy was used to estimate gastric transit times. Animals showing severe distress were euthanized, autopsies performed, and tissues saved for histological examinations. The data indicated three different gastric problems with unique latency periods. Observations permitted calculations of an ED_{50} dose for stomach dilatation. For the subacute period, this was estimated to be 19.2 Gy. Functional and histological studies showed that the acute, subacute, and chronic reactions each had a characteristic etiology and histopathology. In the acute period 2–3 weeks after 28.5 Gy, rats expressed hypophagia, cachexia, and dehydration and signs of stomach content regurgitation. Histologically, edema was prevalent throughout the stomach. Different parts of the organ showed varying degrees of hyperkeratinized epithelium, inflammation, depletion and/or degeneration of various cell types, and ulceration. Between 1 and 7 months, animals at all radiation doses were considered to be in the subacute to chronic period. Some were euthanized for humane reasons. Gradual replacement of the gastric epithelium by a multilayered squamous epithelium that was often hyperkeratinized and covered with bacteria was common. After several months, the new layer was occasionally ulcerated and extended to the musculature, which was the sign of a healed ulcer. In the chronic period, about 7 months postirradiation, signs seen in the subacute phase heightened. Stomach walls became stiff and thickened. Regenerating crypts infiltrated the gastric wall and occasionally penetrated the muscularis mucosae and submucosa.

3.3.3 Modification of injury

In the studies by Weshler et al. [38] where the temporarily exteriorised rat stomach was given single doses of 3–30 Gy of orthovoltage X-rays, sucralfate and misoprostol given twice daily during the period of eight weeks following the irradiation provided no influence on progression of damage or repair as measured histologically and macroscopically.

3.4 Studies in rabbits

Engelstad [41], in an extensive study, analyzed the dose–response relationship in 59 rabbits relative to histological changes after single and fractionated doses of X-rays ranging from about 1.25 to 45 Gy delivered to a field which included the stomach. In animals receiving 1.25 to about 10 Gy, zymogen-producing peptic cells were the most sensitive of those present, thus supporting the early findings of Regaud et al. [2]. A dose of 5 Gy was found to be a threshold for damage to these cells. In a sequential study carried out 1–46 days post-irradiation, Engelstad also described the histological changes in stomachs of rabbits receiving about 15 Gy. Irradiation led to cell degeneration and hyperaemia, often increased transudation and leukocytic infiltration, and in some cases, ulceration. Doses of 2.5 and 5 Gy produced demonstrable histological changes and after 10–15 Gy, the changes were considerable. The 15 Gy series presented with frequent ulcerations in the stomach and upon microscopic examination, it was noted that the irradiation-induced ulcer in rabbits and the peptic stomach ulcers in human beings looked very much alike. In the rabbit, the ulcers were always localized on the lesser curvature. Ulcer development proceeded rapidly 2–4 weeks after irradiation and was seen as early as 7 days post-irradiation. In this study, perforation of the stomach occurred frequently, as a rule within 30 days after irradiation. In survivors, 2–3 months after treatment, the ulcers showed a tendency towards healing and epithelialization. A dose of 16 Gy caused death in some animals and doses above 20 Gy produced a high mortality. With doses in this range, the initial reaction after irradiation during the first 24 h consisted of degeneration of the lymph follicles and hyperaemia, a period of very little change, then degenerative and inflammatory changes about 7 days post-irradiation. The degeneration was first noticed and was foremost in the mucous membrane. Other regions, including the lamina propria and muscularis mucosa, were much less sensitive.

3.5 Studies in dogs

3.5.1 Single doses
Dawson [42] gave large single X-ray doses to Pavlov pouches. He studied the changes in the mucous neck cells, the chief cells, and the parietal cells and questioned whether the epithelium itself was injured by the radiation or whether it was indirectly damaged due to a compromised blood supply. In the irradiated pouches, there was hypochlorhydria followed by achlorhydria. The dose to accomplish this was an unusual unit, but proper for the time; it was 155–200% of a dog erythema dose. Dawson also reported that chief cells underwent cytolysis and although parietal cells showed little or no histological injury, they were unable to produce acid. He noticed cell loss and hyperaemia in the mucosa which after regeneration, was thinner but otherwise histologically normal. Irradiation had temporarily stopped fibroblast proliferation which Dawson surmised to be the likely cause of a delay in mucosal repair.

Conard [43] determined the emptying time of the fundic portion of the stomach in normal and total body-γ-irradiated dogs. The normal emptying time, as determined with a roentgenographic technique and a barium meal, averaged 77 min. No delays in emptying were observed 2–8 days postirradiation after about 3 Gy or at 3 days after about 6 Gy. However, at 3 days after about 13 Gy, three animals had significant delays as long as 7 h. However, these last observations were difficult to interpret since symptoms of anorexia, vomiting, diarrhoea, and dehydration were all present. At autopsy, the stomach showed little damage in contrast to that seen in the small and large intestine.

Dubois et al. [44] investigated the relationship between radiation-induced vomiting and gastric emptying in the dog irradiated total body with ^{60}Co γ-radiation. With midline doses of 8 Gy to the abdomen and 6 Gy to the brain, gastric emptying of liquids and solids was suppressed as early as 2 h after radiation exposure. Pre-irradiation administration of domperidone prevented vomiting which usually occurred after irradiation with 8 Gy. Since the drug did not influence delay of gastric emptying, but did prevent vomiting, the authors concluded that the two symptoms were independent phenomena.

Minami [45] simulated in dogs a procedure utilized in Japan for humans with unresectable stomach cancer — delivery of a single dose of 40 Gy of electrons to the stomach of a laparotomized individual. Twenty-six survivors were examined and the postirradiation changes noted 1 h – 9 months later and classified macroscopically. Hyperaemia became progressively severe during the 1–3 week period. During the 4–11 week period, hyperaemia, erosion of mucosa, and ulceration progressed to very severe ulcers which extended to the muscular layer. From 4–9 months, ulcers were very near the myenteric plexus, there was some necrosis in the muscle layer under the ulcer, and an irregular pattern of epithelial regeneration at the centre and edges of the ulcer was noted.

3.5.2 Fractionated and repeated doses

Regaud et al. [2] irradiated dogs with five X-ray doses over a period of 15 months. Although it is not possible to convert the dose into today's units, they found that certain exposures eliminated the crypts and obliterated the chief cells, while sparing the parietal cells. This finding was among the early reports describing the marked but differential effect on the stomach epithelium and pointing to differences in radiosensitivity of the different stomach cell types.

Hueper and Decarhal-Forero [46] irradiated 4 dogs with 3 Gy a day for 5 days per week × 4 successive weeks for a total of 60 Gy. Dogs died between the 9th and 16th week, and in all cases a perforated gastric ulcer was present.

3.6 Studies in monkeys

3.6.1 Single doses

Shea-Donohue et al. [47] evaluated the mucus glycoproteins secreted into the gastric juice of monkeys given 8 Gy of total body radiation. The procedure increased outputs of acidic glycoprotein (AG) and neutral glycoprotein (NG) during a basal period prior to a water load. Such a load normally causes a rise in AG, but this did not occur in irradiated animals. At two days postirradiation, NG output returned to control levels whereas AG output remained suppressed. Thus, irradiation produced changes in the quantity and type of soluble mucus glycoproteins secreted into the gastric juice. The authors speculated that this might compromise the usual protective property of gastric mucus.

In another paper relating to relationships between vomiting and gastric function in total body-irradiated monkeys, Dubois et al. [48] delivered 8 Gy of ^{60}Co γ-radiation, and measured prostaglandin (PG) levels prior to irradiation, at 20 min, and at 2 days after irradiation. Vomiting occurred immediately after irradiation and was accompanied by a suppression of gastric secretion and emptying. In addition, gastric juice concentrations of PGE_2 and PGI_2 increased 20 min after irradiation yet returned to control levels 2 days later. Plasma PG concentrations never changed. In spite of transient changes in PG and acid in gastric juice after irradiation, there were no significant correlations between the two entities. Thus, the role of locally released PG remained obscure.

3.6.2 Modification of injury
Dorval et al. [49] approximated in monkeys given 8 Gy total body the study done by Dubois et al. [48] relative to the relationship between radiation-induced vomiting and stomach function. Pre-irradiation administration of domperidone did not prevent vomiting as it did in the dog [48]. The authors speculated that the disparity may relate to differences in vomiting thresholds of the two species, sensitivity of dopamine receptors to their agonists and antagonists, and/or the permeability of the blood–brain barrier around the vomiting centre to domperidone. In this study, radiation-induced emesis was accompanied by a suppression of gastric emptying and acid secretion. Since electrical control activity in the stomach was slowed, this change may have altered motility which in turn, suppressed gastric emptying.

3.7 Summary

Casarett [3] has provided a comprehensive description of the histopathological effects of radiation on the stomach. His article is the basis for the summary comments which follow. He described the characteristics and locations of the cell types in the three regions of the stomach, and characterized their radiosensitivity and fate. In general, cells in the fundic glands are more sensitive than those in the cardiac and pyloric glands. Within the first 24 h after exposure to a few Gy, the undifferentiated cells of the gastric pits cease mitosis and undergo degeneration. Although this is soon followed by hyperaemia, dilatation of capillaries, and edema of connective tissue, the changes are quickly resolved. With doses of 10–15 Gy, the early changes are more severe and lasting. During the ensuing four days, marked damage is noted and restitution generally occurs. With doses of 20 Gy or more, mucosal damage may be severe and epithelial regeneration delayed considerably. Although most of the damage may involve the mucosa, the reaction may be severe enough to involve the muscular coats and cause haemorrhage and peritonitis. Ulcers may occur as early as one week or as late as two months after irradiation. Epithelial damage is implicated in the early transient superficial mucosal ulcers, but deeper ulceration is likely the consequence of vascular and connective tissue damage. Scarring and healing of ulcers may occur within a few months, but perforation, cicatrization, and stenosis of the stomach within 6–24 months are possibilities. With doses above 30 Gy, the changes described become exaggerated and lead to serious problems. A reduction in acid and pepsin secretion is related to severity of epithelial damage and may persist for months to years. The late effects of irradiating the stomach would generally include progressive fibroatrophy of the gastric mucosa, impairment of gastric motility and capacity, and dyspepsia. Atrophic gastritis would be the result of increasing mucosal fibrosis, while stenosis could occur as a result of fibrosis following marked reactions to a high dose.

The reader is also referred to comprehensive reviews by Berthrong and Fajardo [28] and Rubin and Casarett [26] for further information.

4. SMALL INTESTINE

4.1 General comments

Several different animal models have been utilized for the study of intestinal damage. These include total body or abdomen exposure, various partial body schemes, and temporary exteriorization of all or part of the gastrointestinal tract. With total body exposure, a particular radiation-producing source is used to irradiate the entire body as uniformly as possible. The animal may be situated a fixed distance from a single source, placed between opposed sources, rotated under a source, or irradiated for 50% of the total exposure in the prone position followed by 50% of the exposure in the supine position or vice-versa. The abdomen usually includes the volume between the xiphoid process and the pubic symphysis. Partial body irradiation schemes vary widely, but an area of known size is irradiated with the remainder of the body shielded. Organs other than those of greatest interest are of necessity sometimes in the volume irradiated.

Two animal models which allow localized exposure of small intestine and especially utilized for late effects studies were pioneered by Peck and Gibbs [50] and Hauer-Jensen et al. [51]. In the first case, a 15 mm length of mouse jejunum, in continuity with the remainder of the intestine, is immobilized by attachment to the peritoneal surface of the ventral abdominal wall. This permits local irradiation with single or multiple radiation exposures. The second model, which also allows for single or repeated irradiation of a particular segment of intestine, involves transposition of an ileal segment in-continuity to the left scrotum of orchiectomized rats. Another procedure which has some variations in terms of amount of gastrointestinal tract irradiated but utilized by a number of investigators (noted in Table 1) is temporary exteriorization during exposure. Each of the procedures besides whole body exposure permits flexibility in the study of early or late effects in the irradiated intestine.

A sizable share of the literature on radiation injury of the gastrointestinal tract involves descriptions of histopathological changes. In a classic comprehensive review, Friedman [52] summarized the salient histopathological changes observed in the irradiated intestine by them and others since the early 1900s and in doing so, paraphrased information from classic papers by Regaud et al. [2], Warren and Whipple [53], and Friedman and Warren [54], among others.

The Friedman review [52] described striking changes in the epithelium as well as the responses of the connective tissue stroma, blood vessels, inflammatory cells, lymphoid structures, muscles, nerves, and serosa. Damage and repair of the epithelium in some cases and severe damage to the mucosa with incomplete repair leading to ulceration were described. In 1942, late changes or delayed reactions in patients were referred to as being reported by "the score" [52]. Ulceration, stenosis, and fistula formation were common; the frequency of their occurrence varied in different patient series. Some lesions were the ulcerating and necrotizing type while others were stenosing and cicatrizing. Whether the lesion was predominantly ulcerative or cicatrizing, secondary inflammatory processes were typically involved. The mucosa was often eroded leading to partial or total destruction of the surface epithelial layer. Mucoid degeneration in surviving epithelium was observed. Typical changes in connective tissue included swelling of collagen resulting in an afibrillar cellular matrix. Such changes were often noted in the mucosa, submucosa, muscularis, serosa, and in the walls of blood vessels and termed fibrosis. Characteristic changes in blood vessels included intimal and medial thickening and perivascular adventitial fibrosis. The intestinal muscle layer characteristically had lesions related to extension of an ulcer, necrosis, inflammation, and scarring as well as some fibrosis, fibre atrophy, vacuolation, and nuclear destruction. Thus, many of the changes which researchers in the last 50 years have also observed and tried to establish the underlying cause or to quantify, were identified quite early by various investigators.

A number of studies to characterize late effects has been completed. Histological studies have often been the main focus. In recent years, attempts have been made to quantify late effects and to consider the possible relationship between acute effects and subsequent late effects.

The general pattern and sequence of early histological changes after exposure of the intestine has been discovered and rediscovered by many investigators. The onset of an alteration, the time before a change such as repair begins (if it occurs), the morphology of crypt and villus cells, the response of the lamina propria, and miscellaneous changes which are dependent upon the particular set of physical and biological factors utilized, have often been noted.

Warren and Whipple [53] described the work done on chronic lesions in the intestine and stomach by Regaud, Nogier, and Lacassagne [2] in dogs as the best piece of experimental work related to gastrointestinal injury reported in the early literature. In their own investigations, Warren and Whipple delivered large amounts of radiation in single doses to the abdomen or the whole body of various laboratory animals in attempts to destroy a sufficient amount of intestinal epithelium to bring about total "intoxication". (Their dose units are not convertible into modern units.) They used a series of dogs, cats, rabbits, guinea pigs, rats, pigeons, reptiles, and amphibians. The onset of symptoms of "intoxication" was about the same in all species — no earlier than 2 days or later than 8 days, with a cluster around 3–4 days. Guinea pigs and rats were somewhat more susceptible to radiation than dogs, cats, and rabbits; birds, frogs and reptiles were very radioresistant. Having demonstrated this universality of intestine susceptibility and its effect on the individual, the authors warned the medical community to "utilize abdominal and pelvic radiation carefully because such injury to the intestinal epithelium is always serious and in some cases irreparable".

4.2 Studies in mice

4.2.1 Single doses

Montagna and Wilson [55] published a truly classic comprehensive cytologic study of changes in the intestinal epithelium of mice after total body X-irradiation. They referred to papers by Bloom and Bloom [56] and Tillotson and Warren [57] as the primary ones which up to 1955 had provided details concerning the progress of events culminating in maximal damage and subsequent repair of the small intestine. Montagna and Wilson described the sequential development of injury and the repair of the intestinal mucosa beginning one-half hour after exposure, at hourly intervals up to 96 h, and then daily from 5–15 days after irradiation. Mice received lethal doses of X-rays, either about 10 or 5.5 Gy. The first group died within 4–7 days at a time when the crypts were largely repaired, but the villi were badly damaged. The second group showed minor lesions on the mucosa on the 2nd and 3rd day which were repaired by the 4th day, but even so, these animals died on the 10th to 21st days, probably from complications of the haematopoietic syndrome. Ten Gy of total body X-irradiation stopped mitotic activity in the crypt cells. As early as 1/2 h later, most of the nuclei in the crypt cells were enlarged and some had undergone karyolysis. By 12 h, nuclear swelling, karyolysis and karyorrhexis were more advanced. Cytoplasmic basophilia were conspicuously reduced and many of the cells died. Sparse and abnormal mitotic activity reappeared at this time. By 48 h, the degenerative processes in the crypt epithelium had passed their peak, except for the Paneth cells, whose nuclei were just beginning to swell. In the cells at the tips of the villi, some nuclei were swollen and the cytoplasm was losing its basophilic staining. By 72 h, Paneth cells had fragmented and been extruded into the lumen. The partially repaired crypts contained some normal cells. By 96 h, many of the crypts appeared to be normal but the epithelium of the villi showed a maximum amount of damage. Thus, the cells of the villi began to show damage 48 or more hours after exposure at times when the cells of the crypt were being repaired. The animals subsequently died when the villi showed their greatest damage but the crypts were largely repaired.

The goblet cells in the crypts and on the villi became progressively larger until about 48 h after X-irradiation. In the crypts of the ileum, staining of the goblet cells became more intense until they degenerated. X-irradiation seemed to hold mucigen in the goblet cells with very little of it being secreted into the gut lumen. Montagna suggested that the stagnated mucigen could imbibe water and distend the cell.

In mice given 5.5 Gy, the progress of the injury was qualitatively similar to those animals receiving 10 Gy, but damage was less severe. After 96 h, all damage had been repaired and the mucosa appeared normal. These animals died later with features including bacteraemia at a time when the morphology of the intestine appeared to be normal. The authors suggested that transient lesions which occurred in the villi from 48–72 h or the shortage of mucus may have facilitated bacterial invasion. In this paper, there are 42 photomicrographs showing the progressive damage and recovery of the cells in the crypts and villi of the small intestine.

Lewis et al. [58], utilizing ultraviolet microscopy to study X-irradiated intestine of mice, noted that although Paneth cells are radioresistant, they have a highly sensitive cytoplasmic component.

Quastler and Hampton [59] studied the effects of radiation on the fine structure of villus epithelial cells of mice. Doses of 2, 8, or 30 Gy were selected to produce slight, severe but reversible, and irreversible damage, respectively. In mice given 10 Gy, the authors studied villus epithelial cells of three "classes" — those present at the time of irradiation, those that were proliferating in the crypts at the time of exposure but had since migrated to the villi, and a third type which was proliferative at the time of irradiation and remained so through one or two abortive attempts at proliferation. Class 1 cells looked grossly normal with light microscopy, class 2 cells had enlarged nuclei, and the third type had large and unpolarized nuclei. Fine structure effects on class 1 cells included defects in microvillar membranes with all doses used. A few mitochondria were abnormal and irregularly-shaped nuclei were seen after 30 Gy. Cells of classes 2 and 3 from villi of mice receiving 30 Gy were qualitatively the same, but showed different degrees of response relative to shortening of microvilli, their irregularity, and to mitochondrial changes.

Hugon et al. [60] described the ultrastructure of duodenal crypt cells during the first 24 h after a total body dose of 13.5 Gy of X-rays. After 30 min, there was a dissociation of the triple-layered membrane of the microvilli and by 24 h, the whole border had atrophied. At this time, there were also swollen mitochondria with rupture of cristae. After 90 min, dense lysosome-like bodies and multivesicular bodies were numerous and many nuclei were irregular. At 3 h after irradiation, cytoplasmic inclusions were numerous. These cytolysosomes were also the cause of distorted nuclei since the inclusions were close to the nuclear membrane. By 24 h, most of the stem cells showed atrophy of microvilli and many of the nuclei were enlarged and multi-lobated. At this time, however, only a few cytolysosomes were still in the cytoplasm and many of the mitochondria had a normal appearance. During the 24-h period studied, the centrosomes were normal and the goblet, Paneth, and enterochromaffin cells showed only small changes in morphology.

Hugon et al. [61] extended their earlier study by noting the progression over several days of ultrastructural lesions in duodenal crypts of whole body irradiated mice which received 13.5 Gy of X-rays. The high cylindrical epithelium of stem cells was reduced to a flat cuboidal epithelium with atrophied microvilli. Ribosomes were reduced in number, mitochondria were irregular, and pale nuclei with condensed nucleoli were present. The Paneth cells were abnormal and the zymogen granules gradually disappeared. Only the Kultchisky cells were nearly intact.

4.2.2 Partial-body irradiation

Withers [62] irradiated the abdomen of mice with a dose of 6.6 Gy which reduced cell survival in the duodenal crypts to about 5% of normal. A macrocolony assay was used to quantify the regeneration of the surviving clonogenic jejunal cells. This was accomplished by measuring the relative cellular survival from a second dose of 14.1 Gy given at various times after the first dose of 6.6 Gy. In this study, every macrocolony was considered to have arisen from a single surviving cell. Crypt degeneration appeared early after irradiation and by 36 h, there was extensive disorganization and cell loss. The villi remained long and the epithelial covering showed little change. Sixty h after irradiation, there was evidence of regeneration in the crypts. The villi were shortened and the density of the cells lining their surface greatly reduced. Most of the villus shortening occurred from about 48 h onward and resulted from the failure of the crypts to replace old cells as they were lost from the tips of the villus. In the intestinal wall 96 h after irradiation, the crypts were larger than in the non-irradiated gut, mitotic activity was marked, and migration of cells from crypt to villus recommenced.

4.2.3 Neutrons

Lesher and Vogel [63] studied duodenal damage induced by fission neutrons or cobalt-60 gamma rays. The duodenum of mice was compared histologically and cytologically after exposure to 3.5 Gy of fission neutrons or about 10 Gy of cobalt-60 gamma rays, each dose being sufficient to kill 90% of the animals in a 30 day period. The duodenum recovered completely from gamma irradiation and the animals lived beyond a 3.5 – 6 day period which the authors associated with the "intestinal syndrome". With fission neutrons, there was severe damage and less than 50% of the mice lived beyond the 6 day period. The paper described close relationships among the degree of intestinal damage, generalized bacterial infection, and the time of death.

In a scanning electron microscope study, Carr and Toner [64] examined the surface structure of the small intestinal mucosa in mice after total body irradiation with 15–25 Gy, doses considered to be lethal. The villi were normally typically finger-shaped or slightly flattened. Within the first 48 h, little obvious change was seen in the scan. The villi soon appeared to have lost their normal stability and in some cases appeared more flexible or more readily distorted as shown by their tendency to droop and clump together. By 70 h, the villi appeared shorter and tapered more than noted earlier before developing a conical shape. The orderliness of the creases in the villi had been partially lost. There was no evidence of significant fusion of villi or formation of ridges in place of individual discrete villus projections. In the final stages of injury at about 90–100 h after irradiation, the mucosal surface was grossly abnormal and the normal grooves of the villi were lost. Disorganized warty blebs or projections giving a complete irregularity of contour were seen.

Cairnie and Millen [65] gave 16 Gy of X-radiation to mice and quantified the number of crypts in the small intestine. Five days after 16 Gy, the number of crypts was reduced 77%, but 21 days later, the number had increased steadily to levels approaching normal. During this period, the number of villi did not change. The mechanism of increase in crypt number was by budding and fission of repopulated crypts which had become larger than normal.

4.3 Studies in rats

4.3.1 Single doses

Friedman [66] irradiated rats total body with about 10 Gy and sacrificed the animals at regular intervals up to 96 h after irradiation. In control duodena, mitotic figures were abundant in the crypts, and fully developed goblet cells were laden with mucous. Within one-half hour, nuclear swelling and a reduction in mitotic figures were evident in irradiated specimens. Twelve hours later, no mitoses were present, nuclei were quite swollen, and there were vacuolated sacs with "owls eye" nuclei. About 24 h after X-irradiation, crypts contained numerous elements laden with a mucous secretion. Villus cells appeared normal as late as 48 h postirradiation. However, between 48 and 72 h, the villous epithelial cells became abnormally flattened or vacuolated. Clusters of goblet cells that had been in the crypts for about 24 h disappeared. The remaining epithelium also became flattened and subsequently, groups of mucous cells were found at the extreme tips of the villi. These were the result of crypt cells which differentiated in the crypt and migrated to the villus tip slower than usual.

Detrick et al. [67] irradiated the total-body of rats with about 5.25 Gy and did electron microscope studies of intestinal villi from samples taken after 1 h, as well as at 1, 3, 7, 10, 14, and 17 days postirradiation. In agreement with others [64,68], the villi showed little or no change at 1 h or 1 day postirradiation. By day 3, significant changes in a number of features had occurred, but within 4–6 days, substantial recovery had taken place. During the 7–17 day period, incomplete recovery was present as manifested by focal epithelial degeneration accompanied by edema and microscopic haemorrhage.

In Casarett [3] and Eddy and Casarett [69], there are microangiographs depicting blood vessel changes in duodenal microvasculature of the rat after radiation doses of about 10–14 Gy. After mitosis had stopped and proliferating crypt cells began to necrose, vascular obstruction and incomplete patterns of blood circulation were seen during the first 24 h postirradiation. The changes were the result of degenerative and obstructive changes in small blood vessels, edema, inflammatory cell infiltration, and occasional leakage of erythrocytes.

Within 48 h, degenerative and obstructive changes in small blood vessels intensified. In some cases, the severity of the changes increased even further the next 24 h. When epithelial cell regeneration occurred, some evidence of the recovery of the circulation soon followed.

Porvaznik [70] quoted Staehelin et al. [71] as noting that the tight junctions in the small intestine are situated on the lateral surfaces of the cells immediately below the striated border and these barriers make penetration of molecules difficult or impossible. Porvaznik recalled that Walker et al. [72] had shown that aseptic endotoxemia occurred between days 1 and 5 postirradiation at dose levels which did not denude the intestine of epithelial cells. Porvazink reasoned that changes in the tight junctional barriers of intestinal ilea might therefore be involved in the manifestation of aseptic endotoxemia. He used freeze–fracture and lanthanum tracer methods to determine if the tight junction was disrupted by radiation. Discontinuities in this tight junction might allow a pathway for the diffusion of free endotoxic macromolecules and/or bacteria from the intestinal lumen into the systemic circulation. For the study, rats were irradiated total body with 3 Gy or 5 Gy of ^{60}Co γ-radiation and the intestines examined at 1, 3, 5, and 7 days postirradiation. A general measure of the effectiveness of the junctional barrier was ascertained by obtaining the mean depth of the tight junction in the apical-to-basal direction at each time post-irradiation. The data obtained suggested that disruption of tight-junctional barriers between intestinal goblet cells and adjacent enterocytes after whole body irradiation was a possible route for the escape of lumenal contents such as endotoxin.

4.3.2 Partial-body irradiation

Williams et al. [68] irradiated the whole body or all but a loop of exteriorized intestine of rats with a range of X-ray doses. With whole body irradiation, the authors noted that an initial drop in crypt cell mitotic activity was followed by acute cell destruction, abortive mitotic recovery, prolongation of interphase, and final recovery with overshooting. Acute destruction and abortive mitotic recovery were responses of cells presumed to be in late interphase at the time of irradiation. After 9 Gy, epithelial cells covering the villi survived longer than would normally be the case. When the exteriorized intestine was shielded, there was no evidence of cytological change in the irradiated intestine due to shielding and the shielded loop was entirely normal.

Jervis et al. [73] studied the light microscopy of small intestine from rats which received about 20 Gy whole body irradiation or the same dose to the intestine *in situ* or exteriorized. They found that the mucosa of the small intestine of both the whole body and the *in situ* gut-irradiated rats developed the uniform classic lesions of the acute intestinal syndrome. In contrast, the reaction of the exteriorized small bowel was uneven and the pattern of injury not consistent.

Sebes et al. [74] followed the sequence of histopathological changes after X-irradiation of a 3 cm exteriorized segment of rat ileum with a single dose of about 22 Gy. A few animals were sacrificed as late as one year postirradiation. The histological changes in the intestines of rats where the superior mesenteric artery was clamped were compared with those in segments not so treated. Within 20 days, the mucosal surface of the irradiated segment in all animals showed various stages of ulceration, necrosis, and areas of complete denudation of mucosa with the intestinal surface covered by mucous and purulent exudate. The hypoxic state of the small intestine during irradiation not only extended survival of the superior mesenteric artery-clamped animals, but also noticeably delayed the occurrence of the radiation damage to the small bowel mucosa in the acute phase.

Lieb et al. [75] delivered about 12 Gy of X-radiation to the abdomen of rats. They attempted to find a plausible route for the purported fluid and electrolyte loss via the intestine. The approach used was to look for immature "crypt-type" cells on the villus 4 days postirradiation. At one day after irradiation, the ultrastructure of the organelles of the absorptive cells of the ileum and jejunum remained relatively unchanged from control though there appeared to be an aggregation of mitochondria in the apical portion of these cells. Within 48 h, there was a proliferation and dilation of smooth endoplasmic reticulum in both the ileum and jejunum. In addition, a large number of primary lysosomes was observed in the absorptive cells. At 72 h, the jejunum looked the same as 24 h earlier. In the ileum, however, the predominant cell type contained shortened sparse microvilli, an irregularly-shaped nucleus, and mitochondria with dilated vesicular cristae. In sections that were perpendicular to the luminal surface, many of the villus cells were cuboidal rather than columnar. In addition, dilation of the intercellular spaces was evident and many cells had begun to separate from the lamina propria. By 96 h, both the ileum and jejunum contained "abnormal" villus cells and all of these cells appeared to be cuboidal rather than columnar. If a nucleus was present, it was irregularly-shaped and contained a peripherally located polymorphous nucleolus with an elaborate dense reticulum. The early changes in villus epithelium were due primarily to the consequences of cell age vs. delayed mitosis and cell renewal whereas changes at 4 days post-irradiation were probably the result of forcing immature crypt cells onto the villus during the period of mitotic overshoot. As a result, the mucosal surface may have been covered with immature cells that were incapable of active fluid and electrolyte transport. This could manifest itself as fluid and electrolyte loss in the form of diarrhoea which is considered to be a factor in the acute intestinal radiation syndrome. So their findings gave some support to their working hypothesis.

4.4 Studies in rabbits

Friedman and Warren [54] irradiated rabbits with about 40 Gy in 8–10 doses given approximately every other day to a single, anterior abdominal portal of

10×15 cm with the liver and stomach shielded. During the subsequent 2–24 week period, various indices of intestinal damage and regeneration were observed. There was an initial reaction of epithelial cell nuclear swelling, inhibition of mitosis, and a mucous change, followed by mucosal atrophy and then regeneration. These changes were often accompanied by progressive ulceration and inflammation.

4.5 Studies in dogs

Bosniak et al. [76] used angiography to study the blood vessels of the irradiated bowel and attempted to correlate the results with the gross and microscopic pathological observations in short intestinal loops of dogs irradiated with single doses of 15 Gy or 30 Gy. Vascular spasm was marked in the first 14 days; intraarterial papaverine and procaine relieved this condition and allowed the demonstration of hyperaemia in the bowel 5–10 days postirradiation. Angiographic and pathologic findings following 15 Gy and 30 Gy were similar but the changes were more pronounced with the higher dose. In the 5–10 day period, the angiographic changes corresponded to the histological findings of dilated arterioles and capillaries in the mucosa. The angiographic changes the first two weeks were similar for both doses, but the variance in effect was more obvious in the 2–5 week post-irradiation period.

4.6 Modification of injury

Different procedures for irradiating the intestine (or any portion of the gastrointestinal tract) lead to variations in expression of radiation injury. The most common procedure utilizes whole body irradiation. Irradiation of the abdomen by irradiating the entire body volume between the xiphoid process and pubic symphysis is also often used. Alternate modes include various local irradiation schemes of either temporarily exteriorized intestine or a selected portion of the gastrointestinal tract *in situ*. With small intestine, not only is the amount of intestine at risk usually different, the amount of other tissues which modify the overall response is also frequently different, as is the case when a large portion of the stomach, small intestine, or large intestine is shielded.

Most of the existing literature on radiation injury to the small intestine of animals describes mild-to-somewhat severe effects. Even if only some of the features of the complete gastrointestinal syndrome (GIS) are expressed, when the small intestine is prominently involved, authors typically refer to the changes as the "gastrointestinal syndrome". However, the small intestinal damage and associated secondary events which follow may lead to death at times quite different from the 3–5 days associated with a complete GIS (as described in Section 7.2.). With low radiation doses or exposure of only small portions of intestine, the effects may be only temporary and of little consequence.

Studies often utilize a series of radiation doses and document particular changes or death in animals at a specific time or over a specified observation period. The results may be expressed as the effective dose (ED) to produce the effect in X% of individuals over a particular period (days, months, years). For example, $ED_{50/6d}$ means the effective dose which causes a particular change in 50% of treated individuals over a 6-day period. If LD is substituted for ED, this means the lethal dose. Thus, an $LD_{50/6d}$ is a radiation dose which under specified conditions causes 50% lethality in 6 days. Alterations of one or more pre-irradiation or post-irradiation variables typically influences the probability of lethality and/or a change in survival time. Since different investigators seldom use the same protocol or have precisely the same objectives, the results obtained cannot always be rigorously compared.

Just as with induction of a complete gastrointestinal syndrome, the animal species utilized can make a substantial difference in the response of any or all of the gastrointestinal tract to degrees of radiation-induced injury. Other factors are also involved. Values for the frequently used parameters of lethality, survival time, severity of histopathological injury, and functional changes vary as a result of differences in dose, dose rate, and radiation quality. In general, percent lethality increases with dose; survival times are shortened (but seldom below 3.0 days); histopathological expressions such as length of mitotic delay, number of apoptotic bodies, and degrees of epithelial denudation, ulceration and fibrosis all increase with dose (up to a point); and functions such as motility, peristalsis, absorption etc. are markedly influenced. With a single dose and with all other factors kept equal, there is usually a wide range of dose rates where there are no discernible differences in response.

With regard to the influence of radiation quality, the most frequent comparisons to changes caused by X-irradiation are made with neutrons, gamma rays from ^{137}Cs or ^{60}Co, and pions. Comparisons are commonly made by calculation of relative biological effectiveness (RBE) for producing any one of a possible number of responses to irradiation. RBE values for neutrons and pions are generally considerably greater than one and for gamma rays, somewhat less than one.

Procedures mobilized prior to and/or during irradiation which have been shown to influence eventual damage to the intestinal epithelium include local hyperthermia [77,78]; hypoxia from breathing nitrogen [79], blood flow restriction [80,81], or injection of microspheres [82]; administration of chemical agents including radioprotectors [80,83–100]; control of pancreatic secretions [101,102] and bile flow into the gut lumen [103–106]; decontamination of the gut with antibiotics [107–109]; introduction of specific kinds and numbers of bacteria [110]; and perturbation of epithelial cell kinetics by various means including surgery [111].

Procedures employed post-irradiation which have modified the usual sequence of events after a particular radiation dose include surgical removal or relocation of the irradiated segment [112,113]; diversion of bile flow and pancreatic secretions [101–106,114]; administration of antibiotics [115–117];

electrolyte and fluid replacement [117,118]; local cooling [119]; local hyperthermia [77,78]; and administration of adriamycin [120].

4.7 Dose fractionation and protraction

For details of very early fractionation studies, see Chapter 5 of a book by Thames and Hendry [121].

In a classic study by Lesher [122] of the cellular injury produced in four regions of the mouse intestine, gamma-radiation was given continuously at two dose levels, namely 25 Gy/day and 270 Gy/day. Observations were made at intervals from 1/2 h after the beginning of exposure until death. In the 25 Gy/day series, mitosis stopped in the crypts of the duodenum after 4 h, in the jejunum after 6 h, and in the ileum after 8 h. Duodenal crypts were non-existent at 3 days; jejunal and ileal crypts remained an additional 6 and 12 h, respectively. Differentiated villus cells were quite resistant and Paneth cells at the bottom of the crypts less so. As anticipated, mitotically active crypt cells were the most sensitive. Mice died 3.5–5.5 days after partial or complete denudation of the duodenal epithelium. Although the jejunal and ileal epithelia were partly intact at the time of death, intestinal damage probably played a major role in causing death.

In the 270 Gy/day series, where mice died 2–3.5 days postirradiation, mitosis stopped in all segments of the intestine within 30 min after commencement of irradiation. Immediate degeneration of lymphatic tissue occurred and by 8 h, degenerative changes in the connective tissue stroma were noted. Crypts were destroyed within 3 days. In all segments, however, villus length was maintained and denudation did not take place. Intestinal damage was probably not responsible for the deaths which occurred. With these high levels of continuous irradiation, there was no recovery phase. Lesher viewed this as an advantage when following the sequential destruction of crypts, the life span of the mucosal epithelium of the villi, and differences in susceptibility at three levels of the small intestine. This paper [122] contains 33 illustrations of the histological changes in 4 locations of the intestine after irradiation.

An early paper relating to dose fractionation and its relationship to modulation of injury or use as a tool to study recovery from a particular radiation dose was written by Krebs and Brauer [123]. They helped formulate the thinking of that era by stating "the most easily interpreted experiments to measure recovery from radiation injury are those in which a dose of radiation less than sufficient to produce a selected biological effect (the conditioning dose) is given to animals, and then at various times later the additional dose necessary to produce the effect is measured. The difference between the measured test dose and the single dose of radiation which would have been required to produce the same effect initially represents the amount of the conditioning dose remaining at the time of test". Krebs and Brauer also stated what they considered to be widely accepted, namely, the rate of disappearance of injury from a single radiation dose follows an exponential course with time after irradiation.

Krebs and Leong [124] refined the concept of repair and recovery from gastrointestinal injury. Using a split-dose technique in mice, they determined that with X-ray doses near the gastrointestinal LD_{50}, the rate of recovery from radiation injury was exponential with a half-time of 23 min. The amount of repairable injury rose more steeply at lower exposures and tended to level off as the first (conditioning) exposure became large. Repairable injury was about 50% of the exposure for doses up to about 4.7 Gy, but was nearly constant and independent of exposure between 4.7 and 7.0 Gy.

Earlier in this chapter, some examples of radiation dose fractionation and its effect on the outcome of injury in the stomach and oesophagus were given. The vast majority of studies with animal models on the influence of fractionation on early or late effects has been done in mice or rats and have involved the small intestine or large intestine. For many years the focus was on early changes in the epithelium, its loss and subsequent recovery. More recently, investigators have placed more emphasis on the late effects, especially those eventually leading to intestinal obstruction or perforation.

In the early 1960s, it was postulated that the extent of the shoulder on an animal survival curve in split dose studies of acute gastrointestinal injury was related to the amount of sublethal damage repaired in crypt cells. Hornsey and Vatistas [125] formulated what has since been generally accepted, i.e., the radiation dose required to kill 50% of the animals three to four days after whole body X-irradiation can be considered the dose required to reduce the surviving fraction of crypt epithelial cells to a critical level. Whereas the single $LD_{50/4da}$ was found to be about 13 Gy, the total of the split doses needed to produce the same result was up to 30% higher, depending on the size of the first and second doses and the interval between them. Hornsey et al. [126] also did a study similar to that just described, but with 6 MeV neutrons. They examined the effect of fractionation on four day survival of whole-body-irradiated mice after single and split doses. The $LD_{50/4da}$ value for a single dose was about 5.4 Gy, but there was no significant difference in the $LD_{50/4da}$ due to fractionation unless the doses were separated by more than 12 h. They felt that the increase in survivors with fractionation intervals greater than 12 h was probably due to crypt cell repopulation rather than repair of sublethal damage.

In a very comprehensive study, Withers and Elkind [127,128] used single-dose and two-dose techniques and the macrocolony assay to investigate the survival characteristics of crypt cells in X-irradiated mouse jejunum. They irradiated the abdomen only in some animals and temporarily exteriorized 2 cm segments of the jejunum in others. The $LD_{50/5da}$ value for a total split-dose after abdomen-irradiation was always higher than the single dose value of about 10.6 Gy and the difference increased with fractionation intervals up to 24 h. Crypt stem cell survival after single and split doses to the 2 cm segment indicated a broad shoulder on the cell survival curve and substantial recovery during a 24-h inter-fraction interval. Further, regardless of fractionation schedule, the number of crypt stem cells surviving a dose lethal to 50% of the animals within 5 days was about 10,000 per cm of jejunum, thus supporting

the concept stated earlier [125]. In this era, neutrons were considered promis-
ing as a mode of tumour therapy, but the quantification of normal intestinal
injury was lacking. Withers et al. [129] utilized the microcolony assay [130] to
obtain such information. They investigated clonogenic jejunal epithelial cell
survival in mice given single and fractionated total body doses of 14 MeV
neutrons or X-rays. Isoeffect single doses for cell survival at the $LD_{50/5da}$ for
intestinal death led to an RBE estimate of 1.4 for neutrons when compared to
X-rays. In the split-dose experiments, the isoeffect first dose of X-rays was 6.8
Gy and for neutrons, 4.4 Gy. Fractionation intervals for both radiations were 4
and 24 h. For 4 and 24-h X-ray split dose experiments, the doses "recovered"
between fractions 1 and 2 were 1.20 and 3.25 Gy, respectively. For neutrons,
the values were 0.75 Gy and 1.50 Gy, respectively. In comparing neutrons and
X-rays, the final slopes of the dose–response curves were nearly the same.
Although the split-dose experiments demonstrated that the neutron-irradiated
cells had some repair capacity, the amount was much less than for X-rays, as
evidenced by the shoulder of the cell survival curve which was much narrower
than on the X-ray curve. This difference is the basis for RBE values (neutrons/
X-rays) increasing with dose fractionation.

In a related study, the survival of mouse intestinal crypt cells after fractionated
doses of X-rays and 15 MeV neutrons given 5 times each week was measured by
Broerse and Roelse [131] utilizing the microcolony assay. D_0s were 3 Gy and 4 Gy
for X-rays and neutrons, respectively. With increasing doses of neutrons per
fraction (2.2, 2.8, and 3.4 Gy), RBE values declined from a peak value of 2.1.

Hagemann et al. [132] X-irradiated the total body of mice with a split dose
of about 14 Gy. They first gave 6 or 10 Gy and followed at different times with
8 or 4 Gy, respectively. Intestinal crypt survival, which increased substantially
when split doses were separated by less than 4 h, was attributed to repair of
sublethal damage in surviving crypt stem cells. The initial dose of about 10 Gy
was chosen because it had previously given levels of survival on the exponential
portion of both intestinal stem cell and crypt survival curves; the other initial
dose of about 6 Gy had yielded survival levels on the exponential portion of the
cell survival curve, but on the *shoulder* of the crypt survival curve. This study
is a good illustration of the importance of fraction size and interval between
fractions as they influence the complex interactions involving repair of sublethal damage, redistribution of cells in the cell cycle, and compensatory
response of regeneration [133].

Hornsey [134] utilized intestinal macrocolony and microcolony assays to
generate jejunal crypt stem cell survival curves after irradiation of the total
body or a temporarily exteriorized intestinal loop of the mouse. Neutrons (6
MeV at 0.5–1.0 Gy/min), electrons (7 MeV at 60 Gy/min), and X-rays (7 MV at
1 Gy/min) given as a single dose or two fractions were compared. Characteristic
dose–survival curves were obtained with all combinations. Intercomparisons of
D_0 and D_q for the different radiations established the variation in jejunal
sensitivity to the different radiation qualities. $LD_{50/5da}$ values for animal survival corresponded to a surviving cell fraction of 10^{-2}. With doses split by 2 h or

24 h, cell survival curves were similar for both X-rays and neutrons but $LD_{50/5da}$ values were about 1.75 Gy for the 2 h interval and 1.95 Gy for the 24 h interval for X-rays; comparable values for neutrons were considerably less.

Wambersie et al. [135] studied cellular repair and its effectiveness as a function of dose per fraction. They termed death 20–30 days after irradiation of the mouse abdomen "intestinal death". ^{60}Co γ-radiation was utilized in a number of studies where time between doses varied from 1 h to 4 days. LD_{50}s were computed from survival at 5 days or 20 days. They concluded that with a fractionated radiation treatment, the total dose which corresponds to a given effect did not depend much on the number of fractions, provided overall time was kept constant and the doses per fraction were less than 3 Gy. However, when fractions greater than 3 Gy were replaced by additional smaller fractions, the increase in total dose needed to provide an isoeffect depended on the size of the subfraction.

Withers et al. [136] irradiated mice total body with fractionated doses of γ-rays or neutrons given at 3-h intervals and utilized the crypt microcolony assay to determine survival of jejunal crypt stem cells. The following conclusions were reached:

1. Dose–response curves indicate that recovery occurs during fractionation intervals. This can be quantified in terms of "recovered" dose utilizing the expression $[(D_N–D_1)/(N–1)]$ where D_N and D_1 are the doses in N fractions and 1 fraction, respectively, required to produce the same cell survival. With γ-ray doses up to about 4 Gy, approximately 60% of the dose was "recovered". This value decreased at higher doses. With neutron doses of 1–2 Gy, the recovered dose amounted to only about 13% of a particular dose.

2. With increasing γ-ray dose fractionation up to 10 fractions, there was a progressive shift of the survival curves to higher doses for the same range of cellular survival.

3. With neutrons, the 2, 3, and 5 fraction dose–survival curves were almost superimposable, thus indicating very little dose recovery in the 3-h fractionation interval.

4. There were constraints on the fraction size and number, but between 4 Gy and 5.5 Gy/fraction of γ-rays, the RBE for neutrons (with some γ-contamination) compared to γ-rays decreased from 2.80 to 2.34. In a similar study, Withers et al. [137], obtained results much like those just described. Additionally, it was noted that the cell cycle stage at the time of irradiation caused more variation in the response to γ-radiation than it did to neutrons.

As early as 1975, Withers et al. [138] ruled out the use of any general formula to relate the number of dose fractions and treatment duration to the total dose needed for an isoeffect in irradiated mouse jejunal mucosa. With 3-h fractionation intervals and with doses per fraction of about 1–3 Gy, approximately 65% of the sublethal damage from the preceding dose was repaired. With higher doses per fraction, about 45% of the first dose was recovered.

Hendry et al. [139] used the intestinal microcolony assay to measure the damage to jejunal progenitor cells in mice given single doses or up to five daily exposures of X-rays, γ-rays, or 14 MeV neutrons to the whole body. The RBE increased from 1.9 to 2.3 for single doses to extrapolated values of 3.3 for 10 daily fractions and 3.6 for 15 daily fractions.

Hagemann and Concannon [140] examined time/dose relationships in the response of mice to irradiation of only the abdomen. They used 17 time/dose fractionation schedules and determined the radiation exposure and days to 50% mortality for each of the time/dose schedules. Acute intestinal tolerance to fractionated irradiation was extremely dependent upon fraction number and overall treatment time. In a related study, Hagemann [141] estimated small-intestinal cell proliferation in mice after various fractionation schemes using delivery of X-radiation to the abdomen only. Instead of the microcolony assay, he used an assay developed in his laboratory to estimate cell proliferation. The endpoint was tritium radioactivity incorporated per mg wet weight of jejunum following injection of tritiated thymidine. The compensatory epithelial cell response was marked. This was especially true when several daily doses totalling about 10 Gy were given early in the week. After drastic drops in proliferative activity, marked compensation occurred such that cell proliferation averaged over a 7-day week was about normal.

Tepper et al. [142] utilized the jejunal microcolony assay in mice to determine the RBE for protons compared to ^{60}Co γ-radiation after single and fractionated doses. The RBE after single dose irradiation with the "spread out" Bragg peak or the unmodulated portion of the proton beam was 1.19 and 1.13, respectively. Analogous values for a 20 fraction experiment (with 3 h between fractions) were 1.23 and 1.17, respectively.

Maisin et al. [143] studied the histological appearance of intestinal mucosa after irradiating only the abdomen of mice with fractionated ^{60}Co γ-radiation. The basic schemes were 5×2 Gy/week for a total of 60 Gy; 5×2 Gy/week for a total of 30 Gy; and 5×3.5 Gy/week for a total of 52.5 Gy. They scored a number of endpoints in 25 crypt sections per specimen, as well as various indices of cell and nuclear damage and cell proliferation. Intestinal mucosa could tolerate daily doses of 2 Gy for 5–6 weeks. They concluded that this was possible because of a reduction in cell cycle length and a 40% increase in the size of the proliferative compartment. With daily doses of 3.5 Gy, the mucosa could not compensate for cell destruction.

Thames and Withers [144] described their results from the use of "common dose" fractions, i.e., use of the same dose per fraction in a series with different numbers of fractions. They used this approach in conjunction with the microcolony assay of crypt cell survival in whole body-irradiated mice, to show equal effect per fraction. However, with one hour fractionation intervals, repair of sublethal injury was incomplete and equal effect per fraction did not hold.

Thames et al. [145] measured the survival of mouse jejunal crypt cells after multiple doses of ^{60}Co γ-rays were delivered to the total body. Doses were spaced at an 18 h interval for 2 fractions, 6 h for 3 and 4 fractions, and 3 h for 6–16 fractions. At fractional doses in the range of 1.8–5.0 Gy, the average dose "recovered" per interval was approximately 50% of the dose per fraction.

The microcolony assay for estimating crypt stem cell survival has been utilized in many studies, several of which have just been briefly summarized. Three additional ones will now be noted. Huczkowski and Trott [146] irradiated mice total body with fractionated ^{60}Co γ-rays, utilizing dose rates between 1.2 and 0.08 Gy/min to study the radiation effects on jejunal crypt stem cell survival. With alpha/beta analysis, alpha was independent of dose rate and beta decreased with dose rate to approach zero at 0.01 Gy/min. This study confirmed a close correlation between dose-rate effect and fractionation effect. Dewit and Oussoren [147] used clinically relevant doses to irradiate the abdomen of mice with 14 daily doses of 3 Gy each. Animals were observed for up to six months and various indices of early and late injury were documented. The fractionation scheme used circumvented severe acute injury, as assessed by the microcolony assay and other endpoints, but late effects still occurred. Withers et al. [148] used 1, 2, 3, and 5 fractions of neutrons with different energies and found the effects of dose fractionation on surviving epithelial cells in mouse jejunum to be quite small since there was an equal effect per dose fraction.

Hauer-Jensen developed a histopathological injury score system [149] similar to that reported by Black et al. [150] and used the system in a series of split-dose studies of irradiated intestinal segments. The influence of splitting a dose of 23 Gy to temporarily exteriorized rat small bowel with intervals between doses of 4, 8, 24, 48, or 96 h was assessed [151]. Animals were killed 2, 8, and 26 weeks after irradiation. Increasing the fractionation interval from 4 to 96 h reduced late radiation injury. The exteriorization technique was improved upon through the use of a rat model [51] which allowed repeated localized irradiation of an ileal segment without the need for more than one surgical procedure. To accomplish this, the intestine was transposed to the scrotum of a bilaterally orchiectomized rat and then irradiated at intervals as required by the protocol. This same model was used to quantify the enteropathy which followed daily and thrice-daily fractions of 2.8 Gy of X-radiation (total dose of 56 Gy) to an ileal segment [152]. Complications were more severe with the three-fraction per day scheme. Subsequently, the model and the injury score method were used to establish that overall treatment time was the most important factor in the development of chronic radiation enteropathy in rat small bowel treated with 9 fractions of 5.6 Gy each with interfraction intervals of 24, 48, or 72 h [153]. Observations were made 2 and 26 weeks after irradiation.

Peck and Gibbs [154] used 2–15 fractions and various doses per fraction for late effect studies of mouse jejunum irradiated *in situ* utilizing the model they developed for permanent immobilization of 15 mm of intestine. Using alpha/beta analysis, they provided evidence for separate fibrotic tissue responses. One appeared soon after inflammation along with loss of mucosal epithelium and was termed consequential injury; the other was considered a primary late effect which progressively masked consequential injury.

Some summary statements appropriate to this section are as follows:

1. Fractionation lessens the effect of a particular total radiation dose. As in other biological systems, size of fraction, number of fractions, and interval

between fractions are all important.

2. Within limits, increasing the number of fractions causes a progressive shift of survival curves to higher doses for the same range of cellular survival.

3. Fractionation provides a way of quantifying the amount of recovery which has occurred since the prior radiation dose was given. This can be substantial for X or γ-radiation but is quite small for neutrons. Thus the sparing effect of dose fractionation is much less for neutrons than for low LET radiation.

4. When different quality neutron beams are compared to ^{137}Cs or ^{60}Co gamma rays or X-rays (usually 250 or 300 kVp) for their ability to damage the intestine, the RBE values are inevitably different, but they usually range around 3.

5. Since crypt cells have a reduced capacity for repair of neutron damage, the RBE for neutrons compared to X-rays decreases as the size of the dose fraction of neutrons is increased.

6. Repair of sublethal damage in crypt epithelium occurs within a few hours. Soon afterwards, repopulation, perhaps with compensatory proliferation, can occur.

7. Injury score systems for characterizing late effects have been developed.

8. The microcolony assay of Withers and Elkind has remained popular as a clonogenic assay of intestinal stem cell survival after irradiation with single or fractionated doses.

9. Several useful animal models have been developed for studies of late effects in small and large intestine after fractionated doses of radiation.

10. There are differing opinions on the importance of early radiation-induced effects to the subsequent development of late effects in the small and large intestine.

5. LATE CHANGES IN THE IRRADIATED SMALL INTESTINE

5.1 General comments

There is general agreement that late changes in the small bowel can occur in days up to years after irradiation. Almost any or all of the changes listed below can be induced in mammalian species provided the proper combination of physical and biological factors is utilized.

– necrosis	– fibrosis in various intestinal layers
– adhesions	– hypertrophy of the muscularis
– edema	– collagen deposition in connective tissue
– inflammatory reaction	– stricture
– local mucosal ulceration	– obstruction
– atrophy of mucosa	– perforation
– epithelial atypia	– fistula formation
– vascular sclerosis	– perivascular fibrosis

It has been suggested that damage of slowly proliferating cells in non-epithelial tissue eventually causes late expression of injury [155]. Vascular injury leading to edema, collagen formation, and fibrosis is thought to be central to development of late injury [156–158]. Dewit and Oussoren [147] did not claim that damage to microvasculature was the cause of late effects, but they did feel that it could have caused a reduced number of epithelial cells and submucosal edema in irradiated intestine.

Because of persistence or progression of obstruction or degenerative changes in the vasculature and fibrosis of the mucosa and submucosa, mucosal atrophy may remain or progress leading to changes which compromise various body functions and/or lead to constriction or obstruction some years later [156].

In order for late radiation enteropathy to develop, a small percentage of a segment of the intestine must have received a very high single dose or accumulated a nearly equivalent dose in a fractionated series of radiation exposures. The mucosa may or may not appear normal at the time late changes begin to be expressed. Whether or not the severity of early changes in the mucosa has any predictive value for late changes is still a subject of debate, but there is evidence [155] that they are related.

The following general comments on late effects in irradiated intestines are based on extensive descriptions by Casarett [155]. If an irradiated epithelium regenerates quickly, acute ulceration of the mucosa may not occur, but with sufficient dose, it is likely. Even without acute ulceration, atrophy of mucosal glands and disorganization of the mucosa may be present. Concurrently, some degenerative changes in fine vasculature and connective tissue may be in progress. This could become more severe with time and eventually result in secondary degeneration of mucosal glands and ulceration or blockage of blood vessels with resultant massive necrosis of the dependent mucosa. The time of occurrence of the late effects will vary almost inversely with the size of the radiation dose which in turn influences the rate of progression of tissue damage to the vascular and connective tissue systems.

Casarett expressed the strong view that vascular and connective tissue changes, as well as epithelial damage, may not only play a major role in the development of severe radiation-induced lesions such as acute ulceration, but also in the manifestation of delayed lesions such as atrophy, ulceration, infarction, deep necrosis, fistula formation, fibrosis, or stricture formation. The vascular changes can be characterized by the amount of swelling of the endothelial cells which occurs and the degree to which these cells block the lumen of the vessels. There may be an increase in the number of endothelial cells and some clotting in small vessels, thereby obstructing them to some degree. Telangiectasia, hyperaemia, thrombosis, and haemorrhage are commonly associated with acute ulcerating lesions. Hyaline thickening, degeneration, and vacuolization of vessel walls are more prominent in late acute and chronic lesions. Telangiectasia of blood and lymph capillaries also become more prominent with time. Some investigators feel that acute ulceration is not caused primarily by vascular damage; nevertheless, damage to the vasculature and connective tissue appears to influence the course, healing, or tractability of ulcers. Other complicating factors can play a role at various points in development of ulceration. These factors would include chemical and mechanical trauma, and secondary infection.

Rubin and Casarett [156] have provided additional useful comments. Damage to the intestine can range from minimal degenerative changes in the crypt cells and temporary hyperaemia in the intestinal wall, to total necrosis. Recovery can be rapid from epithelial cell regeneration, or involve a slower recovery which mainly involves fibrosis. In the early connective tissue reactions, edema may predominate. Protein as well as exudative fibrin may be precipitated. In more advanced stages, collagen becomes hyalinized with its characteristic swollen, glassy, and afibrillar appearance. The hyaline thickening and edema increases the thickness of the intestinal wall. Edema may also be seen in the walls of arteries followed later by a hyaline change similar to that seen in connective tissue. Fibrin may be deposited and thromboses occur. The local inflammatory process associated with ulceration is usually accompanied by more marked fibrinoid necrosis, thrombosis, and vascular sclerosis.

If the ulceration is moderately acute, the epithelial and connective tissue repair processes which follow would be much like that seen in other types of ulceration. Flat or cuboidal undifferentiated epithelium will grow from the margin of the ulcer; remnants of the glands within the ulcerated area; sometimes proliferate and become hyperplastic. If the doses are high enough, the changes in the vasculature and connective tissue will lead to vacuolization of muscle nuclei and fibres and other nuclear abnormalities. There may be hyaline changes in the muscle fibres associated with edema and gelatinous changes in the interstitial tissue stroma of the muscular layers. Eventually these muscle fibres may become atrophic and the muscles may also fibrose. Rubin and Casarett [156] also note that such changes have been seen below an intact mucosa, but if the mucosa is ulcerated, the reactions including an inflammatory reaction and necrosis of muscle, may be more severe.

5.2 Significant histological changes and subsequent complications

Brief summaries of some late effect studies on irradiated intestine in the last 25 years are listed in Table 1. Effects on the intestine and other abdominal organs were reviewed by Trott and Herman [159].

6. EARLY AND LATE CHANGES IN THE IRRADIATED LARGE INTESTINE

6.1 General comments

Effects of radiation on the large intestine were observed many times in patients early in this century, especially as side effects of radiotherapy of the

TABLE 1

Late effects — small intestine

Species	Technique	Intestine length (cm)	Doses (Gy) and (radiation type)	Observation period	Results	Ref. no.
Mice	E.I. (S)	4.0	12–35 (X) \ 2.5–18 (n)	5 d; 90 d \ 5 d; 90 d	$LD_{50/5}$ = 10.6 Gy; $LD_{50/90}$ = 22.6 Gy \ $LD_{50/5}$ = 5.9 Gy; $LD_{50/90}$ = 11.8 Gy	[160]
Mice	E.I (S,Fx)	4.0	4.9–50 (X) \ 4.9–50 (n)	5 d; 90 d \ 54; 90 d	Fractionation lessened injury; fractionation spared less with neutrons thereby raising RBE	[161]
Mice	PB (abdomen) (S)	all	9 or 11 (X) Primer followed by 5–16 Gy 2, 6, or 12 mos later (X)	2, 6, 12 mos	Crypts lost, but survivors almost normal. Some classic late effects seen	[162]
Mice	TB (S)	all	10 (X) 10 (heavy ions)	12 mos	Ultrastructural study. Breakdown of basal lamina supporting epithelial cells. Some differences in basement membrane thickness around capillaries.	[163]
Mice	PB (Fx)	in situ duodenum	3×14 Fx → 42 (X)	24 h–6 mos after last treatment	Intestinal perfusion transiently reduced 3 mos after exposure. Reduced crypt number and villus atrophy. Submucosal fibrosis and edema observed. Microcirculation may play role in late injury.	[147]
Mice	PB (in situ jejunum) (S)	1.5	3.5–16 (X)	1–70 wks	Intestinal wall stiffness as index of fibrosis, energy recovered during unloading, and histopathology used as indices of late damage	[154]

(continued)

TABLE 1 (*continuation*)

Species	Technique	Intestine length (cm)	Doses (Gy) and (radiation type)	Observation period	Results	Ref. no.
Mice	PB (abdomen) (S,Fx)	all	7.0–17.5 single and 19 or 20.5 in 2 Fx (γ)	2–7 mos	Deaths 28–70 days not due to fibrosis or adhesion; later, mucosa fairly intact. Adhesion formation and fibrosis prominent at 98–140 days. At 168–224 days postirradiation, vascular damage may occur. Scoring system developed.	[164]
Mice	PB (abdomen) (S)	all	16 (γ)	1–8 mos	Surgery, lipopolysaccharide B, or IL-1 given at various times increased incidence of adhesions	[165]
Mice	PB (Fx)	1.5 (*in situ* jejunum)	Up to 50 with different fractional doses and intervals between fractions (X)	3 wks or 4 mos	α/β analysis indicated that stiffness of intestinal wall assay measured a rapidly appearing consequential late effect and a lower threshold true late effect.	[154]
Rats	E.I. (S)	2.5–7.5	30–50 (X)	400 d	Mucosal ulceration; serosal fibrosis; hypoxia extended life span; obstruction in spite of mucosal repair	[166]
Rats	E.I. (S)	4.0	7.5–25.0 (X)	wks	Microsphere-induced hypoxia protected against fibrosis.	[167]
Rats	E.I. (S)	30–40	17–23 (X)	2–50 wks	Developed radiation injury score (RIS) based on 8 parameters. Score inversely related to dose.	[168]
Rats	E.I. (S,Fx)	10	17–29.5 (X) 1,2,3 Fx with 48 h between fractions	8–44 wks	Radiation injury scores highest after 2 Fx	[169]

Species	Technique	Intestine length (cm)	Doses (Gy) and (radiation type)	Observation period	Results	Ref. no.
Rats	E.I. (Fx)	10	23 in 2 Fx with 4–96 h between fractions (X)	2–26 wks	Radiation injury score reduced by increasing time between fractions.	[149]
Rats	E.I. (S,Fx)	10	19–21 single; 25.3–29.5 with 2–3 Fx (X)	2–44 wks	Hydroxyproline concentration as measure of late injury applicable 2–4 wks after irradiation. Other entities more important later.	[169]
Rats	PB (*in situ* ileum) (Fx)	2–3	56 given as 2.8 Gy/Fx for 1, 2, or 3 Fx/day (X)	6 h and 2 wks after last irradiation	New model for studying injury after fractionated irradiation developed. Accelerated fractionation aggravated mucosal damage more than standard procedure. Residual damage at 2 wks greater after accelerated fractionation.	[51]
Rats	E.I. (S)	5	30–50 (X)	14 d; 28 d	Serosal fibrosis induced in gut of all rats. Doses of 30 Gy and above pose a great risk. Epithelium after 30 Gy was atypical; after 40 or 50 Gy, not present.	[170]
Rats	E.I. (S)	3	15–40 (X)	2–10 mos	Radiation injury score used. Radiation doses above 20 Gy cause risks and irreversible complications.	[171]
Rats	PB (Fx)	2–3 (*in situ* ileum)	56 of 2.8 Gy each in 1 or 3 Fx per day (X)	2, 8, or 26 wks after last exposure	Radiation injury scores indicated that total treatment time influenced late complications. Association between acute mucosal damage and chronic injury strongly suggested.	[152]
Rats	PB (Fx)	2–3 (*in situ* ileum)	50.4 in 9 Fx of 5.6 Gy each with interfraction intervals of 24, 48, or 72 h	2 or 26 wks after last exposure	Radiation injury scores indicated that overall treatment time influenced development of late enteropathy and early injury influences severity of late injury.	[153]

(continued)

TABLE 1 (*continuation*)

Species	Technique	Intestine length (cm)	Doses (Gy) and (radiation type)	Observation period	Results	Ref. no.
Dogs	E.I. (S)	short segment	15,30	1–84 d	Microangiography correlated with pathologic observations; arterial narrowing and thromboses prominent.	[76]
Dogs	PB (abdomen) (Fx)	all	30–67.5 (γ) or 10–33.75 (n) 4 Fx/wk for 6 wks	2300 d	Extensive classic deep lesions in duodenum with neutron dose of 22.5 Gy or above. None with photons.	[172]
Dogs	IORT (S)	25 (jejunum)	19.85–45 (11 MeV electrons)	3.9–5.3 yrs	Hyaline degeneration of muscularis in bowel, submucosal fibrosis, blunted villi, hyaline degeneration of muscularis, fistulae.	[173]
Cats	E.I. (S)	25–30	10–30 (X)	4 d–4 mos	Up to 15 Gy, no change in vascular pattern. With 15–30 Gy, restoration of pattern dose-dependent. With 30 Gy, no recovery of mucosal vascular pattern. Reduced vascularity in all bowel layers.	[174]
Cats	E.I. (S)	proximal ileum	15–25 (X)	4 d, 1 mo, 4 mos	Quantitative analysis of 13 histological alterations and bowel thickness.	[175]

E.I. = exteriorized intestine; PB = partial body; S = single dose; Fx = fractionated or fractions; X = X-rays; γ = gamma radiation; n = neutrons; $LD_{50/5}$ = lethal dose to 50% of individuals in 5 days; $LD_{50/90}$ = lethal dose to 50% of individuals in 90 days; IORT = intraoperative radiation therapy.

cervix, bladder, and prostate. Mulligan [176] points this out in a comprehensive review of patient studies plus comments on selected animal studies covering the period 1897–1938. Jackson [177] reviewed the problems in 52 patients who suffered from chronic bowel damage. Hubman [178] also referred to a select group of early clinical papers.

An acute early reaction and a more chronic late reaction have been so termed for many years. These responses in humans and even in highly inbred animals are variable (especially the late reaction) in the time and degree of expression post-irradiation. In the early reaction, in less than 2 weeks, epithelial cell denudation, proctitis, diarrhoea (sometimes bloody), anorexia, nausea and vomiting, abdominal cramps, urgency, tenesmus, and edematous, hyperaemic mucosal changes can all occur if the radiation dose is sufficient [179]. Many or all of these same responses presumably take place in animals, but it is not always possible to document them. The progression of some large bowel changes in animals is readily monitored by endoscopy [180]. For example, a locally limited proctitis characterized by a hyperaemic erosive zone covered with fibrinous exudate and blood clots is clearly observed in this way. These early events usually subside within a matter of a few weeks. However, several weeks may elapse before mice or rats show a worsening of their general condition in which they lose weight, their coat becomes rougher, defecation ceases, the abdomen swells, and the palpable descending colon thickens [180]. Late damage then becomes evident weeks, months, or years later and may constitute a serious problem.

Descriptions of late changes in the large bowel of animals after irradiation are numerous. The tissue and histological endpoints evaluated often include many of the following: mucosal ulceration, colitis cystica profunda (deep displacement of epithelium in the wall of the bowel), atypical epithelial regeneration, submucosal fibrosis, subserosal fibrosis, vascular sclerosis, deep ulcer formation, perforation, fistula formation, adhesions, collagen deposition, and stenosis (obstruction). Black et al. [150] evaluated each of the first five histological abnormalities just listed on a grade 1–3 basis and obtained a composite score which they found useful for an overall quantitation of histological changes in selected radiation exposure situations. Some subsequent investigators [181–183] have utilized a modified version of Black's scoring scheme to quantify histological changes.

Many studies have been directed to the influence of various physical and biologic factors on the progressive development of stenosis in attempts to understand the mechanisms involved and to possibly prevent stenosis from occurring. Several correlations between frequency of stenosis, time of stenosis development, and their relation to factors such as radiation dose, dose per fraction, and interval between fractions have been developed.

Since the sigmoid colon and rectum are the regions of the large bowel most often affected in patients, animal research involving single or fractionated doses to those areas has been popular. Models utilizing mice and rats have been used the most. One frequently used mouse model involves irradiation of a small area encompassing about 2 cm of sigmoid colon, rectum (or both) with the remainder of the animal shielded (many examples noted in Table 2). With one type of technique, unanesthetized mice are restrained in a lucite box and positioned head down; this causes the small intestines to fall to the sides and out of the beam [181,184]. In rats, the most common model also requires that the animal be anaesthetized and hung head down in a vertical position so the other abdominal organs "fall away" from the field of irradiation [178]. With appropriate shielding and collimation, radiographs can be taken to ensure that the desired area is irradiated. Most studies have utilized X- or γ-radiation sources, but neutrons and pions [183] have also been employed (see Table 2).

Whether there is a relationship between acute radiation damage and subsequent late radiation damage to the colon or rectum has been the subject of many investigations, especially in the last two decades. Some workers [185–187] concluded early in their studies that there was a relationship and that chronic radiation injury to the bowel was a consequence of secondary injury which followed chronic atrophy of the epithelium due to radiation damage of the microcirculation in the capillary bed. However, in a similar investigation, by utilizing 18 fractions and a time interval of 10 days between fractions, Breiter and Trott appeared to have produced a late effect independent of acute damage [188]. With this arrangement, there was no demonstrable acute reaction, but at about 160 days after the last fraction, the late effect of deep ulceration was observed. Because of the intestinal bleeding observed during the third phase of treatment, Dewit [189] and Followill et al. [190] questioned whether repair of the rectal epithelium in the Breiter and Trott study [188] was complete at this stage. Dewit [189] suggested that 7–8 fractions of 6–8 Gy at 10 day intervals might have been more appropriate than the scheme used. In the study of van der Kogel et al. [183], two waves of injury were found: one of acute ulceration and the other of slowly progressive submucosal fibrosis, vascular sclerosis, and colitis cystica profunda. The two waves of injury were not necessarily considered to be independent. In fact, the significant influence of overall time on ED_{50} for median survival suggested an important role for the early mucosal response in the delayed reactions. Followill et al. [190] took a slightly different approach to the issue. After critically examining their data and that of others, they concluded that there are two histologically distinct late bowel obstructions with accompanying fibrosis. They considered the early-appearing obstructions to be a consequence of persistent acute mucosal damage and later obstructions to represent a true late effect which occurs in the absence of epithelial denudation.

Obstruction and ulceration are life-limiting. An animal can live only 2–3 days after obstruction occurs. Hubman [191] listed survival times and noted whether obstruction had occurred in individual rats with 2.2 cm of only the rectum irradiated. No animals receiving 15 Gy died of obstruction, but death occurred in all between 185 and 633 days post-irradiation. The author considered death to be due to a combination of events related to ulceration. After 30

Gy, however, all 10 animals in a group had an obstructed rectum and death occurred 32–61 days post-irradiation. Attempts to prevent rectal obstruction following such doses have been modestly successful. Continuous bacterial decontamination or daily local steroid application used singly were ineffective [185,186]. Combining the two treatments delayed the onset of obstruction from a median time of 35 days to 83 days. A low molecular weight, residue-free synthetic diet prevented rectal obstruction as long as the diet was given [187]. van der Kogel [183] also fed a low-residue, fibreless diet to irradiated rats, but this did not prevent obstruction.

In a recent study in rats irradiated to various rectal volumes, chronic damage was determined by clinical observation, rectoscopy, and histopathology [192]. Structural damage as well as functional damage depended very much on the dose distribution in the large bowel. Much less field size effect was seen for ulceration than for rectal obstruction when the length of whole circumference irradiated was reduced or when only half the circumference was irradiated.

6.2 Dose fractionation studies

Various fractionation schemes have been used to study late effects in irradiated large bowel with the regimens often approximating clinically relevant protocols. In some cases, the descriptions which follow are also very briefly noted in Table 2.

Withers and Mason [193] irradiated the total body of mice with 2–20 equal fractions of ^{137}Cs γ-radiation spaced 3 h apart and total doses from 12–52 Gy. From histological sections, surviving epithelial cells per colonic circumference were measured. The total dose required for isoeffect increased when more fractions were used. Repair of sublethal damage (SLD) was nearly complete within 3 h. Since repopulation was negligible, the increase in dose for an isoeffect was therefore almost entirely due to an increase in repair of SLD between dose-fractions.

Hagemann [194] utilized a fractionation scheme and X-irradiation of the abdomen only of mice with about 2 Gy/day in a 5 day week for four weeks. Using uptake of tritiated thymidine per mg of colon as an assay, he demonstrated the compensatory proliferative response of the epithelium after the renewal system "recognized" that epithelial depletion had occurred. With an unusual fractionation scheme, Hamilton [195] X-irradiated a 2 cm length of mouse colon with about 12.5 Gy every six weeks and found that a smaller proportion of crypts was killed each time. She thought it unlikely that the number of cryptogenic cells per crypt increased during the repeated irradiation and therefore attributed the result to a heritable decrease in crypt cell radiosensitivity. Later it was shown that it was likely that the decrease was due to induced hypoxia, considered to be secondary to fibrotic changes and subsequent ischaemia [164]. Injection of the radiosensitiser misonidazole abolished the induced resistance (in the jejunum).

Just as in the Hamilton paper, a large number of investigators irradiated large bowel segments about 2 cm in length and studied early or late effects (or both). Fowler et al. [196] used a circular field and irradiated 2.2 cm of mouse rectum *in situ* without including the small intestine in the field. ^{137}Cs γ-rays and 3.0 MeV neutrons were given as single doses, 2F/24 h, or 5F/4 d. Assessment of histopathology, early body weight loss, ultimate maximum weight achieved, lethality, and proportion of short faeces were all measured 30–360 days post-irradiation. RBE values of about 3.0 for early and late damage up to 70 weeks were about the same.

Terry and Denekamp [184] used a method and endpoints similar to those just described. Single doses and 2, 5, or 10 fractions were used. The sparing effect of fractionation was marked for γ-irradiated mice and almost absent with neutrons. A very high repair increment (11 Gy) was seen after two γ-ray fractions of 20 Gy. With a lower dose/fraction, the proportion of each γ-ray fraction recovered was 50–69% for all assays.

A series of papers from the University of Munich was devoted to studies of radiation on a rat large bowel/rectum model in which the small bowel was excluded from the treatment field. Trott [185] locally irradiated 2.2 cm of rat rectum *in situ* and estimated the LD_{50} for causing rectal obstruction in 200 days. In one series, 2, 3, or 5 fractions were given in one week; in another series, 2, 5, or 20 fractions were given in 20 weeks. The number of fractions had a much greater influence on tolerance than overall treatment time. Splitting a single dose into two fractions with a 24-h interval increased the LD_{50} from 19.5 Gy to 24.5 Gy, thus indicating that 40% of the first dose of 12.25 Gy was "recovered" within 24 h. Kiszel et al. [197] found that extending the intervals between the fractions as well as decreasing the dose per fraction had a pronounced dose-sparing effect on the development of large bowel stenosis in rats which had radiation locally delivered to about 2.4 cm of sigmoid colon. The single dose LD_{50} in 200 days was 20 Gy. After fractionation, LD_{50} values ranged from 25.0 Gy for 2 fractions in one day to nearly 88 Gy after 20 fractions in 28 days. In contrast to other studies, overall treatment time, dose per fraction, and number of fractions all had a significant influence on the chronic radiation tolerance of the large bowel. Breiter et al. [180] irradiated 2.4 cm of rectum in the rat with 2 MeV neutrons or 300 kV X-rays and determined the RBE for 50% rectal obstruction within 200 days. The value was 1.8 for single doses. Total doses of 11–15.5 Gy given as two fractions at 6 h intervals or five fractions at daily intervals yielded RBE values of 2.1 and 3.0, respectively. With a quite different fractionation scheme, but the same rat model, Breiter and Trott [188] gave 18 fractions of X-radiation with fraction sizes of 6, 7, or 8 Gy per fraction over 170 days with a 10 day interval between fractions. Rectal obstruction was thought to occur independently of any clinically detectable acute mucosal damage. The alpha/beta ratio of 9.6 Gy for fractionation data obtained in an earlier study [188] with 1, 2, 3, and 5 fractions in one week, fitted the data well. However, with the prolonged fractionation schedules of this experiment, there was a large deviation from the regression line of reciprocal of total dose vs. dose per fraction. Thus, these results did not conform well to the linear quadratic model.

In a comparison of pi-mesons with X-rays, van der Kogel et al. [183] used up to 10 fractions of each radiation type to irradiate a 2.5 cm segment of rat rectum *in situ*. Late effect endpoints were assessed. $LD_{50/250da}$ values increased as the overall time was increased for the same number of fractions and total dose delivered. The authors felt that this finding of a rise in isoeffective doses for chronic injury indicated that the more delayed types of injury did not develop independently from acute mucosal damage. The RBE of pions for rectal injury was 1.2 for single doses and increased to 1.4–1.5 for doses of 4 Gy per fraction. Substituting a low fibre diet for the regular diet in a 4-fraction experiment made no difference in survival or pathological changes observed.

In a mouse colon study, Followill et al. [190] studied late changes after single or split doses of γ-radiation to 2.5 cm of temporarily exteriorized colon and rectum. They concluded that two types of late obstruction occur in the bowel, one that depends on persistent epithelial denudation (consequential damage) and a true late effect.

In a recent analysis of the fractionation sensitivity of the rat rectum to stenosis, the α/β ratio was deduced to be 2.7 to 6.7 Gy, and there was a significant repopulation effect when treatments were longer than 5 days [198]. The additional dose per day for equal effect was in the range 0.6 to 1.1 Gy, when using dose fractions of 4 Gy. Repair half-time estimates ranged between 1.8 and 5.0 h.

Based on studies with single or fractionated doses of radiation and local irradiation of a specific area of the colon/rectum *in situ*, the following summary statements about experimental studies in animals can be made:

1. About 2.5 cm of rectum/colon is considered an adequate area to irradiate. There is little, if any, damage to the nearby small intestine with the procedures used.

2. Within a series of animals treated alike and with the same radiation dose, the variation in survival times or likelihood of obstruction in individual animals is considerable.

3. Fractionating a dose of X- or γ-radiation will lessen the severity of late effects considerably.

4. A high single dose may produce a severe acute effect in the vasculature and mucosa such that the intestine appears susceptible to the eroding, irritating action of faeces which leads to marked effects in the submucosa and/or subserosa with eventual obstruction.

5. The RBE values for neutrons compared to X-rays for the common late effect endpoints are about 2.0 for single doses. With fractionated radiation, for a particular total dose, there is an increase in RBE with a reduction in dose per fraction. For pions compared to X-rays, the RBE for rectal injury is 1.2 for single doses, but 1.4–1.5 when 4 or 8 fractions are used.

6. A scoring system identical or similar to that of Black et al. [150] is useful for quantitating histological changes associated with late effects.

7. There are some endpoints which indicate that detrimental late effects are developing. Histological endpoints have been described. Body weight loss, ultimate maximum weight, and the proportion of short faeces excreted in a 24-h

period each bears some relationship to the progressive development of important pathological changes.

8. The role of collagen in the development of late effects and the delineation of a true late effect remain as important subjects for further investigation.

Brief summaries of some relevant late effect studies on irradiated large bowel are listed in Table 2.

7. THE GASTROINTESTINAL RADIATION SYNDROME

7.1 General comments

The term "syndrome" refers to a set of associated signs and symptoms in an individual subjected to a certain amount of a particular stressor. In radiobiology, the "acute radiation syndrome" has often been used to note the response to a large dose of radiation rather uniformly delivered to the entire body. Particular radiation syndromes have been characterized by a critical organ, a characteristic radiation dose threshold and latent period, a death threshold and associated time of death, characteristic signs and symptoms, and a major underlying pathology.

Prior to the identification and naming of particular radiation syndromes, different animal species were exposed to total body irradiation, observed at frequent intervals, and the times of death recorded. It became apparent that one could associate times of death with particular radiation dose ranges [203]. This association prompted investigators to focus on the signs and symptoms with some apparent relationship to death at a particular time. With selective shielding of certain organs and volumes of tissue and the utilization of several different dose levels, three major syndromes were identified. These are popularly termed "haematopoietic", "gastrointestinal", and "central nervous system" syndromes [204]. Quastler [205] called the second-named acute intestinal radiation death. These three entities have also been termed sub-syndromes of the acute radiation syndrome [206].

7.2 Complete gastrointestinal syndrome

A complete gastrointestinal syndrome (GIS) will be expressed only if the total body is uniformly irradiated with a single dose of about 10 Gy or above to induce all the characteristic features of the GIS [205]. Radiotherapy patients have not experienced a complete GIS although some have suffered from serious intestinal complications. However, it is likely that many individuals in Hiroshima, Nagasaki, and Chernobyl died from a complete GIS. In animals, this syndrome has been studied in detail by many investigators.

The main features of the complete GIS, a response which includes destruction of the small bowel epithelium as well as damage to the myelopoietic system, have been described in reviews or papers by Quastler [205] and others [207–209]. In his review, Quastler [205] notes that in 1954, Dessauer gave

TABLE 2

Late effects — large intestine

Species	Technique	Intestine length (cm)	Doses (Gy) and (radiation type)	Observation period	Results	Ref. no.
Mice	PB (in situ colon) (S,Fx)	2	12.5 given 1–3 times with 35–40 days between doses (X)	5–43 days after last dose	In young mice, 60% of crypts survived first dose; 30% survived second dose; 55% survived third dose. Numbers different for old and young mice. Unirradiated colon compensated slightly.	[199]
Mice	PB (in situ colon) (S,Fx)	2	12.5	4.5 days post-irradiation	Crypt survival as % of crypts present at time of irradiation increased from 50% after first dose to 90% after sixth dose. Survival curve suggests heritable increase in crypt cell radioresistance.	[195]
Mice	PB (in situ colon, rectum and anus) (S)	2.2	15–32.5 (γ) 5.0–12.5 (n)	2–12 mos.	Endpoints of faecal deformity, body weight, lethality, and quantitative histology method of Black et al. utilized. Late deaths due to stenosis caused by submucosal fibrosis.	[183]
Mice	PB (in situ rectum) (S,Fx)	2.5	Total not stated. 2 or 5 Fx (γ,n)	up to 70 wks	RBEs for early and late damage about the same. RBEs for split doses about 50% higher than for single doses.	[196]
Mice	PB (in situ colon, rectum and anus) (S,Fx)	2.2	Total up to 66 in 1, 2, 5 or 10 Fx (X,n)	15 mos.	Series of assays to characterize early and late effects with LD50, RBE, and α/β values. Fibrosis prominent at 6 mos. Fractionation of γ, but not n, spared injury.	[184]

(continued)

TABLE 2 *(continuation)*

Species	Technique	Intestine length (cm)	Doses (Gy) and (radiation type)	Observation period	Results	Ref. no.
Mice	PB (*in situ* rectum) (S)	1.5	12–28; 16–32 with WR-2721 (X)	3–16 mos	Quantitative histological scoring system used; collagen levels estimated. Histology scores increased with time after 20–28 Gy; scores lowered by WR-2721. Collagen values not useful.	[182]
Mice	PB (*in situ* rectum) (S) In combination with cis-diammine dichloroplatinum (II)	1.8×2.5 cm field	up to 30 (X)	up to 40 wks	≈ 20 Gy is ED50 for lethal rectal stenosis and incidence of anal discharge. Drug enhanced epithelial damage, but not submucosal injury.	[200]
Mice	PB (*in situ* rectum) (S,Fx)	1.9	5–20 in single doses; 10–30 in 2 equal Fx separated by 24 h (X)	up to 84 wks	Collagen synthesis and degradation rates in colon greater than controls 4 and 8 wks postirradiation, but normal after 16 weeks. Amount of collagen did not change, but shifts in isotypes did occur which could lead to abnormalities later.	[201]
Mice	PB (*in situ* colon) (S,Fx)	2.4	15–35 single or 9.75–14.75 separated by 10 d	up to 70 wks	Doses > 20 Gy caused persistent epithelial denudation and obstruction by 4 wks. Doses < 20 Gy and split doses led to crypt cell depletion and repopulation followed by obstruction after 40 wks. Two types of late obstructions occurred, one dependent on epithelial denudation and one not.	[190]

Species	Technique	Intestine length (cm)	Doses (Gy) and (radiation type)	Observation period	Results	Ref. no.
Rats	PB (*in situ*) through 8×16 mm Pb collimator (S,Fx)	rectal area	20–100 in 1–5 fractions (X)	4 mos. or 12 mos.	Severity of 5 histologic abnormalities evaluated and injury score system developed.	[150]
Rats	PB (*in situ* rectum) (S)	2.2	15–30 (X)	700 d	Fibrosis, rectal stricture, obstruction, and death. For obstruction from 30–250 days after irradiation: $ED_{10} = 17.5$ Gy, $ED_{50} = 21.5$ Gy, $ED_{90} = 27.5$ Gy	[178]
Rats	PB (*in situ* rectum) (S)	2.2	15–30 in 2.5 Gy increments (X)	up to 98 wks	LD_{50} for rectal obstruction was 21.5 Gy. % obstruction dose-dependent. Cause of death where no obstruction present not known. After 30 Gy, times of death 32–61 days with 100% obstruction. Characteristics of proctitis cystica profunda, which appears 30 days after 22.5 Gy or more, described.	[191]
Rats	PB (*in situ* rectosigmoid colon) (S,Fx)	2.2	?? 1–20 Fx (X)	at least 12 mos.	Classic gut obstruction. Number of fractions more important than overall treatment time. Chronic radiation damage secondary to necrosis rather than its cause. LD_{50} for obstruction = 19.5 Gy for single dose, and 24.5 Gy for two doses.	[185]

(continued)

TABLE 2 (*continuation*)

Species	Technique	Intestine length (cm)	Doses (Gy) and (radiation type)	Observation period	Results	Ref. no.
Rats	PB (*in situ* sigmoid colon) (S,Fx)	2.4	15–25 single; up to 88 in 2–20 Fx (X)	> 2 years	LD50 for bowel stenosis varied from 20.2–87.8 Gy as a function of number of Fx. Deep ulceration present in all stenosed bowels and may be the result of interaction of primary damage to vascular-connective tissue of submucosa and secondary damage to atrophic mucosa.	[197]
Rats	PB (*in situ* rectum) (S,Fx)	2.2	15–64 in 1, 2, or 5 Fx with overall treatment time up to 28 days (X)	up to 93 wks	ED50 values for obstruction from 27.0–47.5 Gy, depending on number of fractions and overall treatment time.	[202]
Rats	PB (*in situ* rectosigmoid) (S)	2.4	23 (X)	200 d	Progressive bowel obstruction within 8 wks. Antibiotics and diet together delayed onset of ileus. Deep ulcer always observed. Mucosa may be hypertrophied while stromal tissue has severe damage. 23 Gy is an LD90/200 day dose for obstruction.	[186]
Rats	PB (*in situ* rectosigmoid) (S)	2.4	23 (X)	200 d	Residue-free diet altered quality of feces and prevented rectal obstruction; at 42 d, mucosa atrophic and capillary density reduced; submucosa thickened and arteries fibrotic. Removal from diet led to erosion of mucosa, inflammatory reactions, ulceration, then stenosis.	[187]

TABLE 2 (continuation)

Species	Technique	Intestine length (cm)	Doses (Gy) and (radiation type)	Observation period	Results	Ref. no.
Rats	PB (in situ rectosigmoid) (S)	2.4	108–144 in 18 Fx with 10 d between Fx of 6, 7, 8 Gy (X)	200 d after last irradiation	Rectal obstruction occurred 7–173 days after last fraction; incidence 100% in highest dose group and 41% in lowest dose group. ED50/200 days = 120 Gy. Ulcer extended around circumference as in earlier studies, but developed secondary to mucosal atrophy.	[188]
Rats	PB (in situ rectum) (S,Fx)	2.4	8.6 or 12.4 (single) (n) 11 or 15.5 Gy as 2 fractions at 6 h intervals or 5 fractions at daily intervals (n)	200 d	ED50/200d for obstruction around 12 Gy for single and fractionated n; fractionation increased ED50/200d from 20.2 to 38.2 Gy.	[180]
Rats	PB (in situ rectum) (Fx)	2.5	up to 44 for pions in up to 8 Fx; up to 70 for X-rays in up to 10 Fx.	up to 550 d	Transient early proctitis. Chronic rectal injury after 2 mos; some deep ulcerating lesions and fistula formation. After 100 days, ulcers less frequent; fibrosis and vascular sclerosis prominent in non-epithelial layers. Histological scoring system useful. Feeding fibreless diet not useful.	[183]

PB = partial body; S = single dose; Fx = fractionated or fractions; X = X-rays; γ = gamma radiation; n = neutrons; ED10 = effective dose for causing a specific change in 10% of treated individuals; ED50 = effective dose for causing a specific change in 50% of treated individuals; ED90 = effective dose for causing a specific change in 90% of treated individuals; ED50/200d = effective dose for causing a specific change in 50% of treated individuals within 200 days; LD50 = lethal dose for 50% of individuals treated; LD90/200 = lethal dose to 90% of individuals in 200 days; RBE = relative biological effectiveness; α/β = dose in Gy at which the linear and quadratic terms contribute equally to an effect.

credit for the independent discovery of the GIS and its association with a wide radiation dose range to Quastler of the U.S.A., Rajewski of Germany, and Bonet-Maury of France. In brief, the characteristics of the complete GIS are:

1. Mitotic activity ceases in the crypts, the region responsible for supplying new cells for the villi. Normal mitotic activity does not occur before the mucosal epithelium is denuded and the animal dies.

2. Cell migration from crypts to villi is slower than normal as if a feedback system realizes that no new cells are forthcoming.

3. As cell density on the villi decreases, the epithelium of villi becomes progressively denuded. The usual columnar epithelium first takes on a cuboidal appearance followed by a squamous morphology in an attempt to keep the now shortened villi covered.

4. Epithelial cell loss is accompanied by excretion of electrolytes (especially sodium) and water.

5. Haemorrhaging into the bowel lumen is prominent. This change, coupled with denudation of the epithelium, leads to a translucent intestine filled with blood which when excreted produces a very foul unique odour.

6. Prominent changes in gastrointestinal motility and gastric emptying accompany the small bowel changes. At the time of death, the stomach is distended with fluid.

7. Marked changes are seen in other parts of the gastrointestinal tract, but are not as prominent as in the small intestine.

Sequentially, ruffled fur, loss of appetite, gastric retention, increasing lethargy, bloody diarrhoea, loss of epithelial cells and electrolytes, dehydration, and loss of leucocytes are prominent features during the course of GIS development in animals.

When complete denudation of the small intestinal epithelium has occurred, the animals die, as early as 3 days in some species. Details of the variations in responses of different species may be found in several references [207,210–212].

Parameters which have been assessed at intervals during the course of severe gastrointestinal injury or the complete GIS include: water [213,214] and food [215] consumption, excretion of water [214,216,217], serum electrolytes [218–220], electrolyte excretion [214,216,217,220–222], body weight loss [207, 215, 223], intestinal weight loss [224–226], blood volume [227–229], bacterial quality and quantity in the intestine [110,226,230] and blood [110,226,231], and histological changes [55,63,232]. Changes in each of these parameters likely play some role in full expression of the GIS.

As noted earlier, various criteria must be met to induce a complete GIS as described in classic reviews by Quastler [205], Conard [208], Bond [207,212], Rubin and Casarett [156], and Casarett [204]. Lushbaugh [233,234] philosophized on the use of the GIS term as he discussed situations where individuals referred to their results as representative of a complete gastrointestinal syndrome, but in fact only some features of a complete GIS had been observed. Regardless of ones position on the rigor with which the term is used, "gastrointestinal syndrome" conveys considerable information to a reader.

7.3 Modification of a complete gastrointestinal syndrome

Soon after identification and acceptance of the GIS as a definite entity, it was natural to pursue ways to modify the course of events, to understand what was happening, and as a goal, to save the individual from death due to the GIS. A complete GIS is quite refractory to agents or procedures used pre- or postirradiation, but modest improvement in survival times was achieved by bile duct ligation [103], shielding and bone marrow therapy [235], fluid, antibiotic, and plasma therapy postirradiation [118], water-electrolyte antibiotic therapy [117], antibiotics [109,236], and cholic acid administration [237]. When at least part of the intestine or a major portion of the gastrointestinal tract is shielded by any one of a number of procedures, modification of the progression of changes and in some cases, survival, is possible.

Investigators do not always utilize exactly the same biological material or physical factors in their studies. Besides the difference in species, sex, weight and physiological state of the animal, the procedure varies (irradiated whole body, abdomen, exteriorized intestine, partial body, etc.). Further, the radiation quantity, quality, and fractionation scheme (if any) are typically different. Lastly, the portion of the gastrointestinal tract analyzed is not the same in all studies. The majority of studies do not involve a complete GIS. Therefore, the bulk of existing literature on gastrointestinal injury relates to modest-to-severe effects in animals which express many of the features of the GIS and for convenience a particular author refers to the changes as the "gastrointestinal syndrome".

7.4 Factors related to the cause of death in the complete gastrointestinal syndrome

After discovery of the complete GIS and closely related responses to irradiation, several different approaches to understanding the progression of changes and the cause(s) of death was (were) taken. In a rather short time span, the radiation dose necessary for inducing a complete GIS in many species became known and the life expectancy under such conditions established [207]. This was followed by attempts to identify the critical biological changes and to establish their relative importance to the welfare of the animal. In the course of such studies, it became clear that the integrity of the small intestinal epithelium was very important and that when total loss of the epithelium occurred, it was followed within hours by death of the animal, independent of species [207]. In germfree mice, where epithelial cell denudation occurred in irradiated animals several days later than in irradiated conventional mice, this same relationship was true [238–242].

A very impressive feature of the GIS was the development of severe diarrhoea, indicating that loss of water and electrolytes was important. Animals attempted to compensate for water loss by drinking excessive amounts [213, 214], but whether they really excreted life-threatening amounts of water and electrolytes via urine and/or faeces remained to be determined.

Jackson et al. [214] undertook a study of faecal and urinary excretions of sodium, potassium, and water in fasting rats given about 15 Gy of whole-body X-irradiation. They found that the total mean postirradiation sodium loss was about 1.50 meq. Removing that amount from fasting non-irradiated rats by means of intraperitoneal dialysis with glucose solutions caused death within 24 h, prompting the conclusion that rats suffering from a complete GIS lost amounts of sodium within days after irradiation which were sufficient to cause death. Lushbaugh et al. [216] thought that such a study would be more complete if water and electrolyte loss could be determined at more time periods after exposure. They used ^{22}Na, ^{42}K, and tritiated water studies to characterize sodium, potassium, and water loss in rats given total body doses of about 7–80 Gy. They concluded that sodium loss plays no primary role in the complete GIS and that loss of electrolyte-containing fluids into the GI tract is only a terminal phenomenon secondary to denudation of the intestinal mucosa. Lushbaugh revisited this issue at a special symposium on gastrointestinal injury [234] and included some new data on loss of ^{24}Na originally produced *in situ* by irradiating the animal with neutrons. His conclusion remained the same — "electrolyte loss is not the critical biochemical lesion in the GI syndrome".

Additional investigators became interested in the question of electrolyte loss. Bouckaert [218] investigated the compartmental distribution of sodium in rats given about 10 Gy or 17 Gy to the abdomen only. Under these conditions, which produced some features of a complete GIS, Bouckaert utilized radiotracer techniques and concluded that there was a reduction in total body sodium after irradiation as well as an abnormal distribution of the ion. He hypothesized that irradiation caused formation of a "trap" where sodium could accumulate and escape excretion while playing no role in metabolic processes. If this was the case, it would explain radiosodium retention and decreased exchangeable sodium after irradiation. Gits and Gerber [220] pursued the electrolyte loss question further. With rats given about 20 Gy whole-body X-irradiation, there was an increase in both GI tract and faecal content of Na$^+$ during the GIS. However, the measured increase of about 0.3 meq was considered insufficient to be the sole cause of death. In comparing their results with those of Jackson et al. [214], Gits and Gerber reported that 1.5 meq Na$^+$ can be drained via a bile duct cannula without ill effects and that Na$^+$ replacement is not an effective therapy unless glucose is also given and/or the radiation dose is near the minimum to cause a complete GIS.

As another approach to the importance of sodium, Forkey et al. measured net transport of sodium at 24 h post-surgery in bile duct-ligated and sham-operated rats irradiated with up to 15 Gy [221]. They found that the presence of bile was not a prerequisite for intestinal leakage after irradiation and the presence of bile acids in the intestines of sham-operated animals did not significantly increase sodium leakage across the intestine. They concluded that in the GIS, although bile acids do not influence intestinal transport, sodium-rich bile is not reabsorbed and therefore could contribute to body losses.

From the time of very early studies, bacteria common to the lower intestinal tract have been found in the blood and organs of animals after total body X-irradiation [53,243,244] and antibiotic therapy has been effective [244] where radiation doses were below the threshold for the GIS. In an early study [231], doses which produced the GIS in mice yielded no bacteraemia and antibiotics were ineffective. A much more recent paper by Geraci et al. [226] also concluded that enteric bacteria do not play a role in the GIS, suggesting that antimicrobial therapy would be ineffective for individuals dying of a complete GIS.

Several studies have shown that mortality in irradiated animals with intestinal injury is reduced by antibiotic therapy [107,116,117,230,245]. Inoculation of bacteria increased mortality of irradiated animals [110].

Studies with germfree mice have provided some useful information. McLaughlin et al. found that when germfree mice, monocontaminated mice, and conventional mice were irradiated with a dose in the GIS range (about 9.5 Gy), all animals died, but germfree mice lived almost 10 days longer than the other two types [238]. In similar experiments, Matsuzawa and Wilson [240] found that germfree mice lived, on average, 7.3 days compared to 3.5 days for conventional mice and the increased life span correlated well with the increased life span of the epithelial cells.

Geraci et al. [217] brought several issues pertinent to GI injury to focus. They simultaneously measured body and organ fluid compartments and plasma sodium concentrations in irradiated-conventional, GI-decontaminated, bile duct-ligated, and bile duct-cannulated rats at different times after various doses of γ-radiation. In addition, the total Na excreted between 48 and 84 h postexposure was measured in animals destined to die from intestinal radiation injury. This thorough study provides a series of interrelated conclusions. To quote, "As a result of the radiation-induced breakdown of the intestinal mucosa, there is lethal loss of water and Na in the form of diarrhoea. This loss of fluid and electrolytes from the plasma is associated with hemoconcentration and reductions in the extracellular fluid space (ECFS) and the interstitial space (ISS) which are sufficient to reduce tissue perfusion leading to irreversible hypovolemic shock and death. All of the lost extracellular fluid and 60% of ECFS Na are excreted. The remaining ECFS Na loss may be redistributed to the intracellular space (ICS) with an equivalent amount of ICS potassium being excreted. It is uncertain whether this redistribution of Na from the ECFS is a consequence of hypovolemic shock or a direct effect of radiation on cellular membrane permeability to Na."

In a useful review article, Geraci et al. [246] made a thorough analysis of the prime factors which have been evaluated in attempts to understand the etiology of the complete GIS. As they pointed out, there is still disagreement concerning the primary physiological changes leading to full expression of the GIS and death. The mechanisms which have been most frequently proposed as the primary ones are: (1) enteric bacteria and/or their toxins which may enter the blood due to loss of the intestinal mucosa causing lethal infection, toxaemia, and accelerated fluid loss (via diarrhoea); (2) bile acids act on the radiation-damaged intestinal mucosa to cause excess fluid and electrolyte loss; (3) there is excessive fluid and electrolyte loss from plasma to the intestinal lumen due to direct radiation damage in the mucosa; and (4) major changes in compartmentalization of fluid and electrolytes occur as a result of whole body changes in vascular and cellular membrane permeability. The reader is referred to this article for details and a summary of how all these factors could play a role in the complete GIS. In brief, Geraci et al. believe that sepsis and endotoxemia do not play a role in the complete GIS. In spite of some very clever experiments by several investigators, the importance of bile is not fully understood. Fluid and electrolyte loss across the denuded intestine appears to be the major influence. Changes in whole body compartmentalization of fluid and electrolytes also appear to be important.

Bond et al. stated in 1965 that death from the GIS reflects the synergism of effects from damage to several tissues, especially the gastrointestinal epithelium and the myelocytic renewal system of the bone marrow [207]. This has been re-emphasized more recently by Mason et al. [247]. Using specific pathogen-free defined-flora mice and 12–22 Gy of ^{60}Co gamma radiation to the whole or partial body, they found the following:

1. Acute lethality is associated with different numbers of surviving crypt stem cells, depending on secondary influences such as concomitant bone marrow depletion or bacterial content of gut.

2. When haemopoietic function is maintained by total abdominal irradiation or reconstitution by bone marrow grafting, animal survival is related to different absolute numbers of surviving crypt stem cells.

Thus the gastrointestinal response in these unconventional mice is modulated considerably by the haemopoietic system.

References

1. Walsh, D. (1897) Deep tissue traumatism from roentgen ray exposure. Brit. Med. J. 2 (July 31), 272–273.

2. Regaud, C., Nogier, T. and Lacassagne, A. (1912) Sur les effects redoutables des irradiations entendues de labdomen et sur les lesions du tuke digestif determinées par les rayons de Roentgen. Arch. Élect. Méd. 21, 321–334.

3. Casarett, G.W. (1980) In: Radiation histopathology, vol. 1, CRC Press, Boca Raton, pp. 107–108, 113–116; 124–130.

4. Roswit, B., Malsky, S.J. and Reid, C.B. (1972) Radiation tolerance of the gastrointestinal tract. In: J.M. Vaeth (Ed.), Frontiers of Radiation Therapy and Oncology, Vol. 6. University Park Press, Philadelphia, pp. 160–181.

5. Desjardins, A.U. (1931) Action of roentgen rays and radium on the gastrointestinal tract. Am. J. Roentgenol. 26, 151–190; 337–370; 495–510.

6. Engelstad, R.B. (1934) Über die wirkungen der röntgenstrahlen auf ösophagus und trachea. Acta. Radiol. 15, 608–614.

7. Warren, S. and Friedman, N.B. (1942) Pathology and pathologic diagnosis of radiation lesions in the gastro-intestinal tract. Am. J. Path. 18, 499–513.

8. Seaman, W.B. and Ackerman, L.V. (1957) The effect of radiation on the esophagus. Radiology 68, 534–541.

9. Phillips, T.L. and Margolis, L. (1972) Radiation pathology and the clinical response of lung and esophagus. In: J.M. Vaeth (Ed.), Frontiers of Radiation Therapy and Oncology, Vol. 6. University Park Press, Philadelphia, pp. 254–273.

10. Jennings, F.L. and Arden, A. (1960) Acute radiation effects in the esophagus. Arch. Pathol. 69, 407–412.

11. Phillips, T.L. and Ross, G. (1974) Time–dose relationships in the mouse esophagus. Radiology 113, 435–440.

12. Kurohara, S.S. and Casarett, G.W. (1972) Effects of single thoracic x-ray exposure in rats. Radiat. Res. 52, 263–290.

13. Hornsey, S. and Field, S.B. (1979) The effects of single and fractionated doses of x-rays and neutrons on the oesophagus. Europ. J. Cancer 15, 491–498.

14. Tochner, Z., Barnes, M., Mitchell, J.B., Orr, K., Glatstein, E., and Russo, A. (1990) Protection by indomethacin against acute radiation esophagitis. Digestion 47, 81–87.

15. Hirn-Stadler, B., Wbra, F., Fowler, J.F., and Rojas, A. (1991) Response of the mouse mediastinum to single and fractionated X-rays. Br. J. Radiol. 64, 740–746.

16. Phillips, T.L., Barschall, H.H., Goldberg, E., Fu, K., and Rowe, J. (1974) Comparison of RBE values of 15 MeV neutrons for damage to an experimental tumour and some normal tissues. Europ. J. Cancer 10, 287–292.

17. Michalowski, A.S. (1981) Gastro-intestinal lesions in thorax-irradiated mice. Brit. J. Radiol. 54, 713.

18. Michalowski, A. and Burgin J. (1982) Duodenal ulcers as an abscopal effect of thoracic irradiation in mice. In: K.H. Karcher, H.D. Kogelnik and G. Reinartz (Eds.), Progress in Radio-oncology II. Raven Press, New York, pp. 105–110.

19. Northway, M.G., Libshitz, H.I., West, J.J., Withers, H.R., Mukhopadhyay, A.K., Osborne, B.M., Szwarc, I.A. and Dodd, G.D. (1979) The oppossum as an animal model for studying radiation esophagitis. Radiology 131, 731–735.

20. Northway, M.G., Libshitz, H.I., Osborne, B.M., Feldman, M.S., Mamel, J.J., West, J.H. and Szwarc, I.A. (1980) Radiation esophagitis in the opossum: radioprotection with indomethacin. Gastroenterology 78, 883–892.

21. Northway, M.G., Eastwood, G.L., Libshitz, H.I., Feldman, M.S., Mamel, J.J. and Szwarc, I.A. (1982) Antiinflammatory agents protect opossum esophagus during radiotherapy. Digest. Dis. Sci. 27, 923–928.

22. Sindelar, W.F., Hoekstra, H.J., Kinsella, T.J., Barnes, M., DeLuca, A.M., Tochner, Z., Pass, H.I., Kranda, K.C. and Terrill, R.E. (1988) Response of canine esophagus to intraoperative electron beam radiotherapy. Int. J. Radiat. Oncol. Biol. Phys. 15, 663–669.

23. Gillette, E.L., Hoopes, P.J., and Ensley, B.A. (1986) Response of canine oesophagus to change in dose per fraction. Br. J. Cancer 53 Suppl., 37–38.

24. McChesney-Gillette, S., Gillette, E.L., Shida, T., Boon, J., Miller, C.W. and Powers, B.E. (1992) Late radiation response of canine mediastinal tissues. Radiother. Oncol. 23, 41–52.

25. Ambrus, J.L., Ambrus, C.M., Lillie, D.B., Johnson, R.J., Gastpar, H. and Kishel, S. (1984) Effect of sodium meclofenamate on radiation induced esophagitis and cystitis. J. Medicine 15, 81–92.

26. Rubin, P. and Casarett, G.W. (1968) Alimentary tract: esophagus and stomach. In: Clinical Radiation Pathology, Vol. 1. WB Saunders, Philadelphia, pp. 153–192.

27. Novak, J.M., Collins, J.T., Donowitz, M., Farman, J., Sheahan, D.G. and Spiro, H.M. (1979) Effects of radiation on the human gastrointestinal tract. J. Clin. Gastroenterol. 1, 9–39.

28. Berthrong, M. and Fajardo, L. (1981) Radiation injury in surgical pathology. Am. J. Surg. Path. 5, 153–178.

29. Chowhan, N.M. (1990) Injurious effects of radiation on the esophagus. Am. J. Gastroenterol. 85, 115–120.

30. Helander, H.F. (1965) Early effects of x-irradiation on the ultrastructure of gastric fundus glands. Radiat. Res. 26, 244–262.

31. Chen, K.Y. and Withers, H.R. (1972) Survival characteristics of stem cells of gastric mucosa in C3H mice subjected to localized gamma irradiation. Int. J. Radiat. Biol. 21, 521–534.

32. Hirose, F. (1969) Induction of gastric adenocarcinoma in mice by localized x-irradiation. GANN 60, 253–260.

33. Ely, J.O. and Ross, R.M. (1947) Some physiological responses of rats to neutron irradiation. In: E. McDonald (Ed.), Neutron Effects on Animals. Williams & Wilkins, Baltimore, pp. 142–151.

34. Goodman, R.D., Lewis, A.E., and Schuck, E.A. (1952) Effects of x-irradiation on gastrointestinal transit and absorption availability. Am. J. Physiol. 169, 242–247.

35. Myers, R. and Hornsey, S. (1982) Effects of radiation on stomach clearance. Br. J. Radiol. 55, 705.

36. Hulse, E.V. (1966) Gastric emptying in rats after part-body irradiation. Int. J. Radiat. Biol. 10, 521–532.

37. Hulse, E.V. and Mizon, L.G. (1967) Radiation-conditioned aversion in rats after part-body x-irradiation and its relationship to gastric emptying. Int. J. Radiat. Biol. 12, 515–522.

38. Weshler, Z., Ligumski, M., Tochner, Z., Kopolovic, J., Carmeli, F. and Rachmilewitz, D. (1988) Functional and morphological alterations following irradiation of isolated rat stomach: a model for estimation of radiation injury. Pharmac. Ther. 39, 85–87.

39. Buell, M.G. and Harding, R.K. (1989) Proinflammatory effects of local abdominal irradiation on rat gastrointestinal tract. Dig. Dis. Sci. 34, 390–399.

40. Breiter, N., Trott, K.-R. and Sassy, T. (1989) Effect of x-irradiation on the stomach of the rat. Int. J. Radiat. Oncol. Biol. Phys. 17, 779–784.

41. Engelstad, R.B. (1938) The effect of roentgen rays on the stomach in rabbits. Am. J. Roentgenol. 40, 243–263.

42. Dawson, A.B. (1925) Histological changes in the gastric mucosa (Pawlow pouch) of the dog following irradiation. Am. J. Roentgenol. 13, 320–326.

43. Conard, R.A. (1956) Effect of gamma radiation on gastric emptying time in the dog. J. App. Physiol. 9, 234–236.

44. Dubois, A., Jacobus, J.P., Grissom, M.P., Eng, R.R. and Conklin, J.J. (1984) Altered gastric emptying and prevention of radiation-induced vomiting in dogs. Gastroenterol. 86, 444–448.

45. Minami, A. (1977) Histologic changes in the canine stomach following massive electron beam irradiation. Strahlentherapie 153, 415–422.

46. Hueper, W.C. and DeCarvajal-Forero, J. (1944) The effects of repeated irradiation of the gastric region with small doses of roentgen rays upon the stomach and blood of dogs. Am. J. Roentgenol. 52, 529–534.

47. Shea-Donohue, T., Danquechin-Dorval, E., Montcalm, E., El-Bayar, H., Durakovic,

A., Conklin, J.J. and Dubois, A. (1985) Alterations in gastric mucus secretion in rhesus monkeys after exposure to ionizing radiation. Gastroenterol. 88, 685–690.

48. Dubois, A., Dorval, E.D., Steel, L., Fiala, N.P., and Conklin, J.J. (1987) Effect of ionizing radiation on prostaglandins and gastric secretion in rhesus monkeys. Radiat. Res. 110, 289–293.

49. Dorval, E.D., Mueller G.P., Eng, R.R., Durakovic, A., Conklin, J.J. and Dubois, A. (1985) Effect of ionizing radiation on gastric secretion and gastric motility in monkeys. Gastroenterol. 89, 374–380.

50. Peck, J.W. and Gibbs, F.A. Jr. (1987) Assay of premorbid murine jejunal fibrosis based on mechanical changes after X irradiation and hyperthermia. Radiat. Res. 112, 525–543.

51. Hauer-Jensen, M., Poulakos, L. and Osborne, J.W. (1988) Effects of accelerated fractionation on radiation injury of the small intestine: a new rat model. Int. J. Radiat. Oncol. Biol. Phys. 14, 1205–1212.

52. Friedman, N. (1942) Effects of radiation on the gastrointestinal tract, including the salivary glands, the liver and the pancreas, in Effects of radiation on normal tissues, Arch. Path. 34, 749–787.

53. Warren, S.L. and Whipple, G.H. (1923) Roentgen ray intoxication. IX. Intestinal lesions and acute intoxication produced by radiation in a variety of animals. J. Exp. Med. 38, 741–752.

54. Friedman, N.B. and Warren, S. (1942) Evolution of experimental radiation ulcers of the intestine. Arch. Path. 33, 326–333.

55. Montagna, W. and Wilson, J.W. (1955) A cytologic study of the intestinal epithelium of the mouse after total-body X irradiation. J. Nat. Cancer Inst. 15, 1703–1735.

56. Bloom, W. and Bloom, M.A. (1954) Histological changes after irradiation. In: A. Hollander (Ed.), Radiation Biology, Vol. I: High energy radiation, Part II. McGraw-Hill, New York, pp. 1091–1143.

57. Tillotson, F.W. and Warren, S. (1953) Nucleoprotein changes in the gastro-intestinal tract following total-body roentgen irradiation. Radiology 61, 249–260.

58. Lewis, Y.S., Quastler, H.. and Svihla, G. (1958) Ultraviolet microscopy of X-irradiated intestine. J. Nat. Cancer Inst. 21, 813–823.

59. Quastler, H. and Hampton, J.C. (1962) Effects of ionizing radiation on the fine structure and function of the intestinal epithelium of the mouse. Radiat. Res. 17, 914–931.

60. Hugon, J., Maisin, J.R. and Borgers, M. (1965) Changes in ultrastructure of duodenal crypts in X-irradiated mice. Radiat. Res. 25, 489–502.

61. Hugon, J., Maisin, J.R. and Borgers, M. (1966) Delayed ultrastructural changes in duodenal crypts of X-irradiated mice. Int. J. Rad. Biol. 10, 113–122.

62. Withers, H.R. (1971) Regeneration of intestinal mucosa after irradiation. Cancer 28, 75–81.

63. Lesher, S. and Vogel, H.H. Jr. (1958) A comparative histological study of duodenal damage produced by fission neutrons and Co^{60} gamma-rays, Radiat. Res. 9, 560–571.

64. Carr, K.E. and Toner, P.G. (1972) Surface studies of acute radiation injury in the mouse intestine. Virchows Archiv (Cell Pathol.) 11, 201–210.

65. Cairnie, A.B. and Millen, B.H. (1975) Fission of crypts in the small intestine of the irradiated mouse. Cell Tissue Kinet. 8, 189–196.

66. Friedman, N.B. (1945) Cellular dynamics in the intestinal mucosa: The effect of irradiation on epithelial maturation and migration. J. Exp. Med. 81, 553–557.

67. Detrick, L.E., Latta, H., Upham, H. and McCandless, R. (1963) Electron-microscopic changes across irradiated rat intestinal villi. Radiat. Res. 19, 447–461.
68. Williams, R.B. Jr., Toal, J.N., White, J. and Carpenter, H.M. (1958) Effect of total-body X radiation from near-threshold to tissue-lethal doses on small-bowel epithelium of the rat. I. Changes in morphology and rate of cell division in relation to time and dose. J. Nat. Cancer Inst. 21, 17–61.
69. Eddy, H.A. and Casarett, G.W. (1968) Intestinal vascular changes in the acute radiation intestinal syndrome. In: M.F. Sullivan (Ed.) Gastroinestinal Radiation Injury. Excerpta Medica, Amsterdam, pp. 385–395.
70. Porvaznik, M. (1979) Tight junction disruption and recovery after sublethal γ irradiation. Radiat. Res. 78, 233–250.
71. Staehelin, L.A., Mukerjee, T.M., and Williams, A.W. (1969) Freeze-etch appearance of the tight junctions in the epithelium of small and large intestine of mice. Protoplasma 67, 165–184.
72. Walker, R.I., Ledney, G.D., and Galley, C.B. (1975) Aseptic endotoxemia in radiation injury and graft-vs-host disease. Radiat. Res. 62, 242–249.
73. Jervis, H.R., Donati, R.M., Stromberg, L.R. and Sprinz H. (1968) Effect of exposure conditions on the production of radiation lesions in rat small intestine. Proc. Soc. Exp. Biol. Med. 127, 948–952.
74. Sebes, J.I., Zaldivar, R. and Vogel, H.H. Jr. (1975) Histopathologic changes induced in rats by localized X-irradiation of an exteriorized segment of the small intestine. Strahlentherapie 150, 403–410.
75. Lieb, R.J., McDonald, T.F. and McKenney, J.R. (1977) Fine-structural effects of 1200-R abdominal X irradiation on rat intestinal epithelium. Radiat. Res. 70, 575–584.
76. Bosniak, M.A., Hardy, M.A., Quint, J. and Ghossein, N.A. (1969) Demonstration of the effect of irradiation on canine bowel using in vivo photographic magnification angiography. Radiology 93, 1361–1368.
77. Merino, O.R., Peters, L.J., Mason, K.A., Withers, H.R. (1978) Effect of hyperthermia on the radiation response of the mouse jejunum. Int. J. Radiat. Oncol. Biol. Phys. 4, 407–414.
78. Hume, S.P. and Marigold, J.C.L. (1981) The response of mouse intestine to combined hyperthermia and radiation: the contribution of direct thermal damage in assessment of the thermal enhancement ratio. Int. J. Radiat. Biol. 39, 347–356.
79. Hornsey, S. (1970) The effect of hypoxia on the sensitivity of the epithelial cells of the jejunum. Int. J. Radiat. Biol. 18, 539–546.
80. Prasad, K.N., Kollmorgen, G.M., Kent, T.H. and Osborne, J.W. (1963) Protective effect of β-mercaptoethylamine and mesenteric vessel clamping on intestine-irradiated rats. Int. J. Radiat. Biol. 3, 257–269.
81. Peterson, C.E., Eddy, H.A. and Patterson, W.B. (1977) Hypoxic protection of canine jejunum from radiation injury. Surgical Forum 28, 426–428.
82. Forsberg, J.O., Jung, B. and Larsson, B. (1978) Mucosal protection during irradiation of exteriorized rat ileum. Acta Radiologica Oncology 17, 485–496.
83. Maisin, J.R., Novelli, G.D., Doherty, D.G., Congdon, C.C. (1960) Chemical protection of the alimentary tract of whole-body X-irradiated mice. Int. J. Radiat. Biol. 2, 281–293.
84. Schwartz, E.E. and Shapiro, B. (1961) Radiation-induced changes in the gastrointestinal function of mice and their prevention by chemical means. Radiology 77, 83–90.

85. Concannon, J.P., Summers, R.E., Cole, C., Weil, C., Kopp, U. and Sigdestad, C.P. (1970) Effects of X radiation and actinomycin D on intestinal epithelium of dogs. Radiology 97, 157–164.

86. Maisin, J.R. and Lambiet-Collier, M. (1972) Influence of radioprotectors on the regeneration of the mucosa of the small intestine of mice exposed to a low dose of X-irradiation. Int. J. Radiat. Biol. 21, 57–63.

87. Sigdestad, C.P., Connor, A.M., Scott, R.M. (1975) The effect of WR-2721 on intestinal crypt survival. Radiat. Res. 62, 267–275.

88. Sigdestad, C.P., Connor, A.M., Scott, R.M. (1975) Chemical radiation protection of the intestinal epithelium by mercaptoethylamine and its thiophosphate derivative. Int. J. Radiat. Oncol. Biol. Phys. 1, 53–60.

89. Sigdestad, C.P., Connor, A.M., Scott, R.M. (1976) The effect of WR-2721 on intestinal crypt survival from fission neutrons. Radiat. Res. 65, 430–439.

90. Tseng, V.L.Y., Bybee, J.W. and Osborne, J.W. (1978) Intestinal crypt survival after X irradiation of the rat small intestine under conditions of radioprotection. Radiat. Res. 74, 129–138.

91. Connor, A.M. and Sigdestad, C.P. (1978) Combined effect of procarbazine and ionizing radiation on mouse jejunal crypts. Chemotherapy 24, 368–373.

92. Moore, J.V. and Hendry, J.H. (1978) Response of murine jejunal crypts to single doses of cyclophosphamide and radiation. Int. J. Radiat. Oncol. Biol. Phys. 4, 415–419.

93. Ross, G.Y., Phillips, T.L. and Goldstein, L.S. (1979) The interaction of irradiation and adriamycin in intestinal crypt cells. Int. J. Radiat. Oncol. Biol. Phys. 5, 1313–1315.

94. Phelps, T.A. and Blackett, N.M. (1979) Protection of intestinal damage by pretreatment with cytarabine (cytosine arabinoside). Int. J. Radiat. Oncol. Biol. Phys. 5, 1617–1620.

95. Dethlefsen, L.A. and Riley, R.M. (1979) The effects of adriamycin and X-irradiation on the murine duodenum. Int. J. Radiat. Oncol. Biol. Phys. 5, 507–513.

96. Moore, J.V. and Broadbent, D.A. (1980) Survival of intestinal crypts after treatment by adriamycin alone or with radiation. Br. J. Cancer 42, 692–696.

97. Halberg, F.E., LaRue, S.M., Rayner, A.A., Burnel, W.M., Powers, B.E., Chan, A.S., Schell, M.C., Gillette, E.L. and Phillips, T.L. (1991) Intraoperative radiotherapy with localized radioprotection: Diminished duodenal toxicity with intraluminal WR2721. Int. J. Radiat. Oncol. Biol. Phys. 21, 1241–1246.

98. Delaney, J.P., Bonsack, M.E. and Felemovicius, I. (1994) Misoprostol in the intestinal lumen protects against radiation injury of the mucosa of the small bowel. Radiat. Res. 137, 405–409.

99. Hanson, W.R. (1995) Modification of radiation injury to the intestine by eicosanoids and thiol radioprotectors, Chapter 13. In: A. Dubois, G.L. King and D. Livengood (Eds.), Radiation and the Gastrointestinal Tract. CRC Press, Boca Raton, FL, pp. 169–181.

100. Weiss, J.F., Landauer, M.R., Gunter-Smith, P.G. and Hanson, W.R. (1995) Effect of radioprotective agents on survival after acute intestinal radiation injury; Chapter 14. In: A. Dubois, G.L. King, and D. Livengood (Eds.), Radiation and the Gastrointestinal Tract. CRC Press, Boca Raton, FL, pp. 183–199.

101. Morgenstern, L., Patin, C.S., Krohn, H.L. and Hiatt, N. (1970) Prolongation of survival in lethally irradiated dogs. Arch. Surgery 101, 586–589.

102. Hauer Jensen, M., Sauer, T., Berstad, T. and Nygaard, K. (1985) Influence of

pancreatic secretion on late radiation enteropathy in the rat. Acta Radiologica Oncology 24, 555–560.

103. Jackson, K.L. and Entenman, C. (1959) The role of bile secretion in the gastrointestinal radiation syndrome. Radiat. Res. 10, 67–79.

104. Sullivan, M.F. (1962) Dependence of radiation diarrhoea on the presence of bile in the intestine. Nature 195, 1217–1218.

105. Sullivan, M.F., Hulse, E.V. and Mole, R.H. (1965) The mucus-depleting action of bile in the small intestine of the irradiated rat. Br. J. Exp. Pathol. 66, 235–244.

106. Gorizontov, P.D., Fedorovskii and Lebedeva, G.A. (1965) Role of bile in development of the gastrointestinal syndrome in very acute forms of radiation sickness. Arkhiv. Patologii. 27, T107–T110.

107. Linkenheimer, W.H. and Berger, H. (1961) The effect of continuous antibiotic feeding on X-irradiation mortality in mice. Proc. Soc. Exp. Biol. Med. 108, 676–680.

108. Geraci, J.P., Jackson, K.L. and Mariano, M.S. (1985) Effect of *Pseudomonas* contamination or antibiotic decontamination of the GI tract on acute radiation lethality after neutron or γ irradiation. Radiat. Res. 104, 395–405.

109. Mastromarino, A. and Wilson, R. (1976) Antibiotic radioprotection of mice exposed to supralethal whole-body irradiation independent of antibacterial activity. Radiat. Res. 68, 329–338.

110. Hatch, M.H., Chase, H.B., Fenton, P.F., Montagna, W. and Wilson, J.W. (1952) Response of X-irradiated mice to intravenous inoculation of intestinal bacteria. Proc. Soc. Exp. Biol. Med. 80, 632–635.

111. Sigdestad, C.P., Osborne, J.W. and Levine, D.L. (1969) The influence of prior intestinal resection on survival time of intestine-irradiated rats. Int. J. Radiat. Biol. 15, 65–73.

112. Osborne, J.W. (1956) Prevention of intestinal radiation death by removal of the irradiated intestine. Radiat. Res. 4, 541–546.

113. Osborne, J.W. (1962) Modification of intestinal radiation death by surgical means. Radiat. Res. 17, 22–33.

114. Geraci, J.P., Dunston, S.G., Jackson, K.L., Mariano, M.S., Holeski, C. and Eaton, D.L. (1987) Bile loss in the acute intestinal radiation syndrome in rats. Radiat. Res. 109, 47–57.

115. Gonshery, L., Marston, R.Q. and Smith, W.W. (1953) Naturally occurring infections in untreated and streptomycin-treated X-irradiated mice. Am. J. Physiol. 172, 359–369.

116. Webster, J.B. (1967) The effect of oral neomycin therapy following whole-body X-irradiation of rats. Radiat. Res. 32, 117–124.

117. Taketa, S.T. (1962) Water-electrolyte and antibiotic therapy against acute (3- to 5-day) intestinal radiation death in the rat. Radiat. Res. 16, 312–326.

118. Conard, R.A., Cronkite, E.P., Brecher, G. and Strome, C.P.A. (1956) Experimental therapy of the gastrointestinal syndrome produced by lethal doses of ionizing radiation. J. Appl. Physiol. 9, 227–233.

119. Gude, W.D., Upton, A.C. and Odell, Jr., T.T. (1959) Modification of radiation-induced intestinal injury in rats by chilling after irradiation. Int. J. Radiat. Biol. 1, 247–255.

120. Burholt, D.R., Hagemann, R.F., Cooper, J.W., Schenken, L.L. and Lesher, S. (1975) Damage and recovery assessment of the mouse jejunum to abdominal X-ray and adriamycin treatment. Brit. J. Radiology 48, 908–912.

121. Thames, H.D. and Hendry, J.H. (1987) Fractionation in Radiotherapy. Taylor &

Francis, London.

122. Lesher, S. (1957) Cytologic changes in the mouse intestine under daily exposure to gamma rays. J. Nat. Cancer Inst. 19, 419–449.

123. Krebs, J.S. and Brauer, R.W. (1963) Comparative accumulation of injury from X-, gamma and neutron irradiation — the position of theory and experiment. In: Proceedings of a Symposium "Biological Effects of Neutron and Proton Irradiations IAEA at Brookhaven National Laboratory, Upton, NY, pp. 347–364.

124. Krebs, J.S. and Leong, G.F. (1970) Effect of exposure rate on the gastrointestinal LD_{50} of mice exposed to ^{60}Co gamma rays or 250 kVp X-rays. Radiat. Res. 42, 601–613.

125. Hornsey, S. and Vatistas, S. (1963) Some characteristics of the survival curve of crypt cells of the small intestine of the mouse deduced after whole body X irradiation. Br. J. Radiol. 36, 795–800.

126. Hornsey, S., Vatistas, S., Bewley, D.K. and Parnell, C.J. (1965) The effect of fractionation on four day survival of mice after whole-body neutron irradiation. Br. J. Radiol. 38, 878–880.

127. Withers, H.R. and Elkind, M.M. (1968) Dose-survival characteristics of epithelial cells of mouse intestinal mucosa. Radiology 91, 998–1000.

128. Withers, H.R. and Elkind, M.M. (1969) Radiosensitivity and fractionation response of crypt cells of mouse jejunum. Radiat. Res. 38, 598–613.

129. Withers, H.R., Brennan, J.T. and Elkind, M.M. (1970) The response of stem cells of intestinal mucosa to irradiation with 14 MeV neutrons. Br. J. Radiol. 43, 796–801.

130. Withers, H.R. and Elkind, M.M. (1970) Microcolony survival assay for cells of mouse intestinal mucosa exposed to radiation. Int. J. Radiat. Biol. 17, 261–267.

131. Broerse, J.J. and Roelse, H. (1971) Survival of intestinal crypt cells after fractionated exposure to X-rays and 15 MeV neutrons. Int. J. Radiat. Biol. 20, 391–395.

132. Hagemann, R.F., Sigdestad, C.P. and Lesher, S. (1971) Intestinal crypt survival and total and per crypt levels of proliferative cellularity following irradiation: Fractionated X-ray exposures. Radiat. Res. 47, 149–158.

133. Withers, H.R. (1975) The four Rs of radiotherapy. In: J.T. Lett and H. Adler (Eds.), Advances in Radiation Biology, Vol. 5. Academic Press, New York, pp. 241–271.

134. Hornsey, S. (1973) The effectiveness of fast neutrons compared with low LET radiation on cell survival measured in the mouse jejunum. Radiat. Res. 55, 58–68.

135. Wambersie, A., Dutreix, J., Gueulette, J., and Lellouch, J. (1974) Early recovery for intestinal stem cells, as a function of dose per fraction, evaluated by survival rate after fractionated irradiation of the abdomen of mice. Radiat. Res. 58, 498–515.

136. Withers, H.R., Chu, A.M., Mason, K.A., Reid, B.O., Barkley, Jr., H.T. and Smathers, J.B. (1974) Response of jejunal mucosa to fractionated doses of neutrons or γ-rays. Europ. J. Cancer 10, 249–252.

137. Withers, H.R., Mason, K., Reid, B.O., Dubravsky, N., Barkley, Jr., H.T., Brown, B.W. and Smathers J.B. (1974) Response of mouse intestine to neutrons and gamma rays in relation to dose fractionation and division cycle. Cancer 34, 39–47.

138. Withers, H.R., Chu, A.M., Reid, B.O. and Hussey, D.H. (1975) Response of mouse jejunum to multifraction radiation. Int. J. Radiat. Oncol. Biol. Phys. 1, 41–52.

139. Hendry, J.H., Major, D. and Greene, D. (1975) Daily D-T neutron irradiation of mouse intestine. Radiat. Res. 63, 149–156.

140. Hagemann, R.F. and Concannon, J.P. (1975) Time/dose relationships in abdominal

irradiation: a definition of principles and experimental evaluation. Br. J. Radiol. 48, 545–555.

141. Hagemann, R.F. (1976) Intestinal cell proliferation during fractionated abdominal irradiation. Br. J. Radiol. 49, 56–61.

142. Tepper, J., Verhey, L., Goitein, M. and Suit, H.D. (1977) *In vivo* determinations of RBE in a high energy modulated proton beam using normal tissue reactions and fractionated dose schedules. Int. J. Radiat. Oncol. Biol. Phys. 2, 1115–1122.

143. Maisin, J., Wambersie, A., Lambiet-Collier, M. and Gueulette, J. (1977) Intestinal proliferation after multiple fractions of gamma irradiation. Radiat. Res. 71, 338–354.

144. Thames, Jr., H.D. and Withers, H.R. (1980) Test of equal effect per fraction and estimation of initial clonogen number in microcolony assays of survival after fractionated irradiation. Br. J. Radiol. 53, 1071–1077.

145. Thames, Jr., H.D., Withers, R., Mason, K.A. and Reid, B.O. (1981) Dose-survival characteristics of mouse jejunal crypt cells. Int. J. Radiat. Oncol. Biol. Phys. 7, 1591–1597.

146. Huczkowski, J. and Trott, K.R. (1987) Jejunal crypt stem-cell survival after fractionated γ-irradiation performed at different dose rates. Int. J. Radiat. Biol. 51, 131–137.

147. DeWit, L. and Oussoren, Y. (1987) Late effects in the mouse small intestine after a clinically relevant multifractionated radiation treatment. Radiat. Res. 110, 372–384.

148. Withers, H.R., Mason, K.A., Taylor, J.M.G., Kim, D.K. and Smathers, J.B. (1993) Dose–survival curves, alpha/beta ratios, RBE values, and equal effect per fraction for neutron irradiation of jejunal crypt cells. Radiat. Res. 134, 295–300.

149. Hauer Jensen, M., Sauer, T., Devik, F. and Nygaard, K. (1983) Effects of dose fractionation on late roentgen radiation damage of rat small intestine. Acta Radiol. Oncol. 22, 1–4.

150. Black, W.C., Gomez, L.S., Yuhas, J.M. and Kligerman, M.M. (1980) Quantitation of the late effects of X-radiation on the large intestine. Cancer 45, 444–451.

151. Hauer-Jensen, M., Sauer, T., Reitan, J.B. and Nygaard, K. (1986) Late radiation enteropathy following split-dose irradiation of rat small intestine. Acta Radiol. Oncol. 25, 203–206.

152. Hauer-Jensen, M., Poulakos, L. and Osborne, J.W. (1990) Intestinal complications following accelerated fractionated X-irradiation. An experimental study in the rat. Acta Oncologica 29, 229–234.

153. Langberg, C.W., Waldron, J.A., Baker, M.L. and Hauer-Jensen, M. (1994) Significance of overall treatment time for the development of radiation-induced intestinal complications. Cancer 73, 2663–2668.

154. Peck, J.W. and Gibbs, F.A. (1994) Mechanical assay of consequential and primary late radiation effects in murine small intestine: alpha/beta analysis. Radiat. Res. 138, 272–281.

155. Casarett, G.W. (1980) In: Radiation Histopathology, Vol. I. CRC Press, Boca Raton, FL, pp. 115.

156. Rubin, P. and Casarett, G.W. (1968) In: Clinical Radiation Pathology, Vol. I. W.B. Saunders Co., Philadelphia, pp. 217–229.

157. Withers, H.R., Peters, L.J., and Kogelnik, H.D. (1979) The pathobiology of late effects of irradiation. In: R.E. Meyn and H.R. Withers (Eds.), Radiation Biology in Cancer Research. Raven Press, New York, pp. 439–447.

158. Hopewell, J.W. (1979) The importance of vascular damage in the development of late radiation effects in normal tissues. In: R.E. Meyn and H.R. Withers (Eds.), Radiation Biology in Cancer Research. Raven Press, New York, pp. 449–459.

159. Trott, K.R. and Herman, T. (1991) Radiation effects on abdominal organs. Chapter 11 in: E. Scherer, C. Streffer and K. Trott (Eds.), Radiopathology of Organs and Tissues. Springer-Verlag.

160. Geraci, J.P., Jackson, K.L., Christensen, G.M., Parker, R.G., Fox, M.S. and Thrower, P.D. (1974) The relative biological effectiveness of cyclotron fast neutrons for early and late damage to the small intestine of the mouse. Europ. J. Cancer 10, 99–102.

161. Geraci, J.P., Jackson, K.L., Christensen, G.M., Thrower, P.D. and Weyer, B.J. (1977) Acute and late damage in the mouse small intestine following multiple fractionations of neutrons or X-rays. Int. J. Radiat. Oncol. Biol. Phys. 2, 693–696.

162. Reynaud, A. and Travis, E.L. (1984) Late effects of irradiation in mouse jejunum. Int. J. Radiat. Biol. 46, 125–134.

163. Fatemi, S.H., Antosh, M., Cullan, G.M. and Sharp, J.G. (1985) Late ultrastructural effects of heavy ions and gamma irradiation in the gastrointestinal tract of the mouse. Virchows Archiv B (Cell Pathol.) 48, 325–340.

164. McBride, W.H., Mason, K.A., Davis, C., Withers, H.R. and Smathers, J.B. (1989) Adhesion formation in experimental chronic radiation enteropathy. Int. J. Radiat. Oncol. Biol. Phys. 16, 737–743.

165. McBride, W.H., Mason, K., Withers, H.R. and Davis, C. (1989) Effect of interleukin 1, inflammation, and surgery on the incidence of adhesion formation and death after abdominal irradiation in mice. Cancer Res. 49, 169–173.

166. Osborne, J.W., Prasad, K.N. and Zimmerman, G.R. (1970) Changes in the rat intestine after X-irradiation of exteriorized short segments of ileum. Radiat. Res. 43, 131–142.

167. Forsberg, J.O., Jiborn, H. and Jung, B. (1979) Protective effect of hypoxia against radiation induced fibrosis in the rat gut. Acta Radiologica Oncol. 18, 65–75.

168. Hauer-Jensen, M., Sauer, T., Devik, F. and Nygaard, K. (1983) Late changes following single dose roentgen irradiation of rat small intestine. Acta Radiol. Oncol. 22, 299–303.

169. Hauer-Jensen, M., Sauer, T., Sletten, K., Reitan, J.B. and Nygaard, K. (1986) Value of hydroxyproline measurements in the assessment of late radiation enteropathy. Acta Radiol. Oncol. 25, 137–142.

170. Poulakos, L., Elwell, J.H., Osborne, J.W., Urdaneta, L.F., Hauer-Jensen, M., Vigliotti, A.P., Hussey, D.H. and Summers, R.W. (1988) Intraoperative irradiation in a rat model: Histopathological changes in irradiated segments of duodenum. J. Surg. Oncol. 38, 130–135.

171. Poulakos, L., Elwell, J.H., Osborne J.W., Urdaneta, L.F., Hauer-Jensen, M., Vigliotti, A.P., Hussey, D.H. and Summers, R.W. (1990) The prevalence and severity of late effects in normal rat duodenum following intraoperative irradiation. Int. J. Radiat. Oncol. Biol. Phys. 18, 841–848.

172. Zook, B.C., Bradley, E.W., Casarett, G.W. and Rogers, C.C. (1983) Pathologic effects of fractionated fast neutrons or photons on the pancreas, pylorus and duodenum of dogs. Int. J. Radiat. Oncol. Biol. Phys. 9, 1493–1504.

173. Sindelar, W.F., Tepper, J.E., Kinsella, T.J., Barnes, M., DeLuca, A.M., Terrill, R., Matthews, D., Anderson, W.J., Bollinger, B.K. and Johnstone, P.A.S. (1994) Late effects of intraoperative radiation therapy on retroperitoneal tissues, intestine,

and bile duct in a large animal model. Int. J. Radiat. Oncol. Biol. Phys. 29, 781–788.

174. Eriksson, B. (1982) Microangiographic pattern in the small intestine of the cat after irradiation. Scand. J. Gastroenterol. 17, 887–895.

175. Eriksson, B., Johnson, L. and Rubio, C. (1982) A semiquantitative histological method to estimate acute and chronic radiation injury in the small intestine of the cat. Scand. J. Gastroenterol. 17, 1017–1024.

176. Mulligan, R.M. (1942) The lesions produced in the gastro-intestinal tract by irradiation. Am. J. Pathol. 18, 515–527.

177. Jackson, B.T. (1976) Bowel damage from radiation. (Proc.) Royal Society of Medicine 69, 683–686.

178. Hubman, F.-H. (1981) Effect of X irradiation on the rectum of the rat. Br. J. Radiol. 54, 250–254.

179. Summers, R.W. and Hayek, B. (1993) Changes in colonic motility following abdominal irradiation in dogs. Am. J. Physiol. 264, G1024–G1030.

180. Breiter, N., Kneschaurek, P., Burger, G., Huczkowski, J. and Trott, K.R. (1986) The r.b.e. of fast fission neutrons (2 MeV) for chronic radiation damage of the large bowel of rats after single dose and fractionated irradiation. Int. J. Radiat. Biol. 49, 1031–1038.

181. Terry, N.H.A. Denekamp, J. and Maughan (1983) RBE values for colo-rectal injury after caesium 137 gamma-ray and neutron irradiation. I. Single doses. Br. J. Radiol. 56, 257–265.

182. Ito, H., Meistrich, M.L., Barkley, H.T. Jr., Thames, H.D. Jr. and Milas, L. (1986) Protection of acute and late radiation damage of the gastrointestinal tract by WR-2721. Int. J. Radiat. Oncol. Biol. Phys. 12, 211–219.

183. van der Kogel, A.J., Jarett, K.A., Paciotti, M.A. and Raju, M.R. (1988) Radiation tolerance of the rat rectum to fractionated X-rays and pi-mesons. Radiother. Oncol. 12, 225–232.

184. Terry, N.H.A. and Denekamp, J. (1984) RBE values and repair characteristics for colo-rectal injury after caesium 137 gamma-ray and neutron irradiation. II. Fractionation up to ten doses. Br. J. Radiol. 57, 617–629.

185. Trott, K.-R. (1984) Chronic damage after radiation therapy: Challenge to radiation biology. Int. J. Radiat. Oncol. Biol. Phys. 10, 907–913.

186. Trott, K.-R., Breiter, N. and Spiethoff, A. (1986) Experimental studies on the pathogenesis of the chronic radiation ulcer of the large bowel in rats. Int. J. Radiat. Oncol. Biol. Phys. 12, 1637–1643.

187. Breiter, N. and Trott, K.-R. (1986) The pathogenesis of the chronic radiation ulcer of the large bowel in rats. Br. J. Cancer 53 (Suppl. VII), 29–30.

188. Breiter, N. and Trott, K.-R. (1986) Chronic radiation damage in the rectum of the rat after protracted fractionated irradiation. Radiother. Oncol. 7, 155–163.

189. Dewit, L. (1987) Prevention of acute radiation damage in the rat rectum by protracted fractionated irradiation. Radiother. Oncol. 8, 369–370.

190. Followill, D.S., Kester, D. and Travis, E.L. (1993) Histological changes in mouse colon after single- and split-dose irradiation. Radiat. Res. 136, 280–288.

191. Hubman, F.-H. (1982) Proctitis cystica profunda and radiation fibrosis in the rectum of the female Wistar rat after X irradiation: A histopathological study. J. Pathology 138, 192–204.

192. Trott, K.R., Tamon, S., Sassy, T. and Kiszel, Z. (1995) The effect of irradiated volume on the chronic radiation damage of the rat large bowel. Strahlenther. Oncol. (in press).

193. Withers, H.R. and Mason, K.A. (1974) The kinetics of recovery in irradia⁺ᵈd colonic mucosa of the mouse. Cancer 34, 896–903.
194. Hagemann, R.F. (1979) Compensatory proliferative response of the colonic epithelium to multi-fraction irradiation. Int. J. Radiat. Oncol. Biol. Phys. 5, 69–71.
195. Hamilton, E. (1979) Induction of radioresistance in mouse colon crypts by X-rays. Int. J. Radiat. Biol. 36, 537–545.
196. Fowler, J.F., Parkins, C.S., Denekamp, J., Terry, N.H.A., Maughan, R.L. and Travis, E.L. (1982) Early and late effects in mouse lung and rectum. Int. J. Radiat. Oncol. Biol. Phys. 8, 2089–2093.
197. Kiszel, Z., Spiethoff, A. and Trott, K.-R. (1984) Large bowel stenosis in rats after fractionated local irradiation. Radiotherapy and Oncology 2, 247–254.
198. Dubray, B.M. and Thames, H.D. (1994) Chronic radiation damage in the rat rectum: an analysis of the influences of fractionation, time, and volume. Radiother. Oncol. 33, 41–47.
199. Hamilton, E. (1978) Cell proliferation and ageing in mouse colon. I. Repopulation after repeated X-ray injury in young and old mice. Cell Tissue Kinet. 11, 423–431.
200. Dewit, L., Oussoren, Y. and Bartelink, H. (1987) Early and late damage in the mouse rectum after irradiation and cis-diamminedichloroplatinum(II). Radiother. Oncol. 8, 57–69.
201. Martin, S.G., Stratford, M.R.L., Watfa, R.R., Miller, G.G. and Murray, J.C. (1992) Collagen metabolism in the murine colon following X irradiation. Radiat. Res. 130, 38–47.
202. Kal, H.B., Litjens, I.W.M. and Fieret E. (1986) Rectum obstruction in rats after local irradiation. Strahlentherapie und Onkologie 162, 772–774.
203. Bond, V.P., Fliedner, T.M. and Archambeau, J.O. (1965) The cellular basis of radiation-induced lethality. The radiation syndrome. In: Mammalian Radiation Lethality. Academic Press, New York, pp. 101–114.
204. Casarett, G.W. (1980) Radiation syndromes. In: Radiation Histopathology, Vol. II. CRC Press, Boca Raton, FL, pp. 133–151.
205. Quastler, H. (1956) The nature of intestinal radiation death. Radiat. Res. 4, 303–320.
206. Cerveny, T.J., MacVittie, T.J. and Young, R.W. (1989) Acute radiation syndrome in humans. In: Col. R. Zajtchuk (Sr. Ed.), Textbook of Military Medicine, Part I, Volume 2. Medical Consequences of Nuclear Warfare. TMM Publications, Falls Church, VA.
207. Bond, V.P., Fliedner, T.M. and Archambeau, J.O. (1965) Mammalian Radiation Lethality. Academic Press, New York.
208. Conard, R.A. (1956) Some effects of ionizing radiation on the physiology of the gastrointestinal tract: A review. Radiat. Res. 5, 167–188.
209. Handford, S.W. (1960) The acute radiation syndrome in dogs after total-body exposure to a supralethal dose of ionizing radiation ($Co^{60}LD_{100/88\ hours}$). Radiat. Res. 13, 712–725.
210. Vriesendorp, H.M. and van Bekkum, D.W. (1984) Susceptibility to total body irradiation. In: J.J. Broerse and T.J. MacVittie (Eds.), Response of Different Species to Total Body Irradiation. Martinus Nijhoff Publishers, Boston, p. 44.
211. Wilson, B.R. (1969) Recovery mechanisms in the GI tract — species and strain differences. In: V.P. Bond and T. Sugahara (Eds.), Comparative Cellular and Species Radiosensitivity. Igaku Shoin Ltd., Tokyo, pp. 281–285.
212. Bond, V.P. (1969) The gastrointestinal syndrome. In: V.P. Bond and T. Sugahara

(Eds.). Comparative Cellular and Species Radiosensitivity. Igaku Shoin Ltd., Tokyo, pp. 235–243.

213. Nims, L.F. and Sutton, E. (1952) Weight changes and water consumption of rats exposed to whole-body X-irradiation. Am. J. Physiol. 171, 17–21.

214. Jackson, K.L., Rhodes, R. and Entenman, C. (1958) Electrolyte excretion in the rat after severe intestinal damage by X-irrradiation. Radiat. Res. 8, 361–373.

215. Smith, D.E., Tyree, E.B. (1954) Influence of X-irradiation upon body weight and food consumption of the rat. Am. J. Physiol. 177, 251–260.

216. Lushbaugh, C.C., Sutton, J. and Richmond C.R. (1960) The question of electrolyte loss in the intestinal death syndrome of radiation damage. Radiat Res. 13, 814–824.

217. Geraci, J.P., Jackson, K.L. and Mariano, M.S. (1987) Fluid and sodium loss in whole-body-irradiated rats. Radiat. Res. 111, 518–532.

218. Bouckaert, A. (1969) Sodium metabolism disturbances after lethal abdominal irradiation in the rat. Atomkernenergie 14, 440–442.

219. Bouckaert, A. and Cantraine, F. (1969) Electrolyte distribution spaces in abdomen-irradiated rats. Atomkernenergie 14, 223–225.

220. Gits, J. and Gerber, G.B. (1973) Electrolyte loss, the main cause of death from the gastrointestinal syndrome? Radiat. Res. 55, 18–28.

221. Forkey, D.J., Jackson, K.L. and Christensen, G.M. (1968) Contribution of bile to radiation-induced sodium loss via the rat small intestine. Int. J. Radiat. Biol. 14, 49–57.

222. Keyeux, A. and Dunjic, A. (1975) The modification of sodium excretion after abdominal irradiation. A dose–effect relationship study in the rat. Int. J. Radiat. Biol. 28, 335–343.

223. Smith, W.W., Ackermann, I.B. and Smith, F. (1952) Body weight, fasting and forced feeding after whole body X-irradiation. Am. J. Physiol. 168, 382–390.

224. Conard, R.A. (1954) Dose dependence and sequential changes in mouse small intestinal weight induced by ionizing radiation. Proc. Soc. Exp. Biol. Med. 86, 664–668.

225. Kay, R.E. and Entenman (1959) Weight, nitrogen, and DNA content of small intestine mucosa of rats exposed to X-rays. Am. J. Physiol. 197, 13–18.

226. Geraci, J.P., Jackson, K.L. and Mariano, M.S. (1985) The intestinal radiation syndrome: sepsis and endotoxin. Radiat. Res. 101, 442–450.

227. Swift, M.N. and Taketa, S.T. (1958) Effect on circulating blood volume of partial shielding of rat intestine during X-irradiation. Radiat. Res. 8, 516–525.

228. Lukin, L. (1957) The effects of total-body X-irradiation on blood volume in splenectomized dogs. Radiat. Res. 7, 150–160.

229. Lukin, L. and Gregersen, M.I. (1957) Premortal blood volumes in splenectomized dogs after total-body X-irradiation. Radiat. Res. 7, 161–166.

230. Rosoff, C.B. (1963) The role of intestinal bacteria in the recovery from whole body radiation. J. Exp. Med. 118, 935–943.

231. Osborne, J.W., Bryan, H.S., Quastler, H. and Rhoades, H.E. (1952) X-irradiation and bacteremia. Studies on roentgen death in mice, IV. Am. J. Physiol. 170, 414–417.

232. Potten, C.S. (1990) A comprehensive study of the radiobiological response of the murine (BDF1) small intestine. Int. J. Radiat. Biol. 58, 925–973.

233. Lushbaugh, C.C. (1969) Theoretical and practical aspects of models explaining "gastrointestinal death" and other lethal radiation syndromes. In: V.P. Bond and

T.Sugahara (Eds.), Comparative Cellular and Species Radiosensitivity. Igaku Shoin Ltd., Tokyo, pp. 288–297.

234. Bond, V.P., Osborne, J.W., Lesher, S., Lushbaugh, C.C. and Hornsey, S., (1968) Mechanism of intestinal radiation death. In: M.F. Sullivan (Ed.), Gastrointestinal Radiation Injury. Excerpta Medica, Amsterdam, pp. 351–373.

235. Taketa, S.T., Swift, M.N. and Bond, V.P. (1959) Modification of radiation injury in rats through gastrointestinal tract shielding and bone marrow therapy. Am. J. Physiol. 196, 987–992.

236. Hendry, J.H., Potten, C.S. and Roberts, N.P. (1983) The gastrointestinal syndrome and mucosal clonogenic cells: Relationships between target cell sensitivities, LD_{50} and cell survival, and their modification by antibiotics. Radiat. Res. 96, 100–112.

237. Mastromarino, A.J. and Wilson, R. (1976) Increased intestinal mucosal turnover and radiosensitivity to supralethal whole-body irradiation resulting from cholic acid-induced alterations of the intestinal microecology of germfree CFW mice. Radiat. Res. 66, 393–400.

238. McLaughlin, M.M., Dacquisto, M.P., Jacobus, D.P. and Horowitz, R.E. (1964) Effects of the germfree state on responses of mice to whole-body irradiation. Radiat. Res. 23, 333–349.

239. Matsuzawa, T. (1965) Survival time in germfree mice after lethal whole body X-irradiation. Tohoku J. Exp. Med. 85, 257–263.

240. Matsuzawa, T. and Wilson, R. (1965) The intestinal mucosa of germfree mice after whole-body X-irradiation with 3 kiloroentgens. Radiat. Res. 25, 15–24.

241. Wilson, R., Bealmear, P. and Matsuzawa, T. (1968) Acute intestinal radiation death in germfree and conventional mice. In: M.F. Sullivan (Ed.), Gastrointestinal Radiation Injury. Excerpta Medica, Amsterdam, pp. 148–158.

242. Tsubouchi, S. and Matsuzawa, T. (1973) Correlation of cell transit time with survival time in acute intestinal radiation death of germ-free and conventional rodents. Int. J. Radiat. Biol. 24, 389–396.

243. Chrom, Sv.A. (1935) Studies on the effects of roentgen rays upon the intestinal epithelium and upon the reticuloendothelial cells of the liver and spleen. Acta Radiol. 16, 641–660.

244. Miller, C.P., Hammond, C.W. and Tompkins, M. (1950) The incidence of bacteremia in mice subjected to total body X-irradiation. Science 111, 540–541.

245. Spratt, Jr., J.S., Heinbecker, P. and Saltzstein, S. (1961) The influence of succinylsulfathiazole (sulfasuxidine) upon the response of canine small intestine to irradiation. Cancer 14, 862–874.

246. Geraci, J.P., Jackson, K.L. and Mariano, M.S. (1988) Protection against the physiological derangements associated with acute intestinal radiation injury. Pharmac. Ther. 39, 45–57.

247. Mason, K.A., Withers, H.R., McBride, W.H., Davis, C.A. and Smathers, J.B. (1989) Comparison of the gastrointestinal syndrome after total-body or total-abdominal irradiation. Radiat. Res. 117, 480–488.

C.S. Potten and J.H. Hendry (Eds.), *Radiation and Gut*

CHAPTER 7

Effects of Irradiation on the Supportive Tissues of the Gastrointestinal Tract

B.E. Powers and E.L. Gillette

Department of Radiological Health Sciences, Colorado State University, Fort Collins, CO 80523, USA

1. INTRODUCTION

The effects of irradiation on the supportive tissues of the gastrointestinal tract include damage to the connective tissue stroma, blood and lymphatic vessels, smooth muscle and peripheral nervous tissue. This damage is usually a late developing occurrence. The role that histologically observed damage plays with regard to the late developing clinical syndromes of chronic radiation ulcer, stenosis, obstruction, perforation, fistula formation, or adhesion formation is not clearly understood, but is likely to be significant.

In humans, the most frequent location for development of late radiation induced gastrointestinal injury is the lower portion of the intestine, especially the colon and rectum. The reasons for this are twofold. First, the lower portion of the abdominal cavity is more frequently irradiated for cancers involving the uterus, ovaries, cervix, prostate gland and urinary bladder [1–3]. Second, the mobility of the small intestine versus the immobility of the large intestine, results in the large intestine consistently receiving each delivered radiation dose, while the small intestine may move out of the radiation field on exposure to subsequent doses [1,3,4].

There are risk factors that have been shown to increase the incidence of late radiation effects in the gastrointestinal tract. The most important of these is prior surgery in the abdomen. The possible mechanism may involve the development of adhesions after surgery which cause portions of the bowel to become immobile and subsequently be subjected to repeated radiation exposures [1–6]. Another possibility is that surgery may induce inflammation which may potentiate the radiation effect through release of tissue cytokines. In support of this latter theory is that preexisting inflammatory conditions in the abdominal cavity is another risk factor associated with an increased incidence of late radiation effects. Other potential risk factors include hypertension, diabetes mellitus and other cardiovascular diseases [1,4–6].

There are numerous animal models that have been developed to study the late effects of irradiation on the gastrointestinal tract. Most of these models are in rodent systems, although a few studies involve larger animals such as the cat and dog. Because the gastrointestinal tract is so sensitive to acute radiation effects, whole abdominal irradiation is usually not suitable for the study of late effects. Therefore usually specific portions of the intestinal tract are studied separately, such as the stomach, portions of the small intestine, or the colon and rectum. Single doses have been used in most studies as fractionated irradiation is difficult to reproduce in small animals, especially if it involves mobile portions of the intestinal tract. Some models include exteriorizing portions of the intestine to avoid acute deaths due to inclusion of too much intestine in the radiation field, or affixing portions of the intestine to the abdominal wall or into the scrotal sac of castrated animals so that fractionated radiation doses can be delivered. In most instances it is difficult to give enough radiation dose to produce late effects without producing acute effects which may complicate interpretation of results and influence the development of late effects [3].

While there are not as much data regarding the late effects of irradiation on the supportive tissue of the gastrointestinal tract compared to the acute effects on intestinal mucosa, there are detailed observations from material derived from humans with late radiation complications as well as numerous experimental animal studies investigating these late effects. Even though the gastrointestinal tract is not as sensitive regarding late as opposed to early radiation reactions, the late effects are often of more concern as they are not transient and they are difficult to manage clinically. If surgery is necessary to manage a late radiation effect in the intestinal tract, the postoperative mortality may be as high as 25%. If not fatal, late complications can cause significant morbidity [2,3].

2. MORPHOLOGICAL CHANGES

The morphological changes reported in humans and experimental animals with radiation complications of the supportive tissue of the gastrointestinal tract involve lesions in the connective tissue, blood vessels and lymphatics, smooth muscle and peripheral nerves.

2.1 Connective tissue

The most common late effect of irradiation on the connective tissue of the gastrointestinal tract is fibrosis [1,3–7]. In humans, fibrosis of the mucosal lamina propria, the submucosa and subserosa has been observed in the stomach, small intestine, caecum and colon 2 months to 30 years after irradiation. Usually edema precedes or occurs concurrently with the fibrosis. The submucosal area usually has the most pronounced fibrosis with abundant hyalinized collagen and atypical fibroblasts with irregular large nuclei and abundant cytoplasm. If an overlying radiation induced ulcer is present, there is more extensive fibrosis and abundant granulation tissue around the ulcer which usually extends into the submucosa and may extend deeper into the muscle. Associated with the granulation tissue and necrotic debris of the ulcer there is an infiltrate of inflammatory cells including neutrophils, lymphocytes, plasma cells and macrophages. The serosa is usually less severely fibrotic and may be covered by fibrinous or fibrous masses [1,2,6].

In the rat stomach 7 or more months after 14 to 23 Gy, the stomach wall was observed to be thickened and have a hyalinized submucosa. Higher doses up to 28.5 Gy were associated with earlier deaths and submucosal edema with mucosal ulceration [8].

In a study of irradiated small intestine in mice, there was stenosis of the lumen with increased collagen in the lamina propria around the epithelial crypts and increased collagen in the submucosa 2 to 9 months after 9 to 16 Gy [9]. Similarly mice given 9 to 11.5 Gy to the abdomen had an increased submucosal area due to edema at 6 months, and collagen at 2, 6, and 12 months [10]. In the rat small intestine after 19 and 21 Gy, fibrosis occurred in the subserosa at 2 to 8 weeks but regressed and increased in the submucosa at 8 weeks and longer. Transmural fibrosis developed secondary to mucosal ulcers at 21 to 24 Gy [11,12]. Rats given single doses of 15 to 40 Gy to the duodenum developed intestinal wall fibrosis and serosal thickening beginning at 2 months after irradiation that was present with or without mucosal ulcers. These lesions were more severe at doses of 20 Gy and above [13]. Similarly cats given 15, 20 or 25 Gy to the ileum had significant submucosal thickening by fibrosis at 1 and 4 months after 25 Gy only [14]. Dogs given 30 Gy to the duodenum developed submucosal fibrosis 6 months later that was more severe if associated with mucosal ulcers (Fig. 1) [15], and dogs given doses above 17.5 Gy and examined at earlier time intervals were found to have mucosal fibrosis by 4 months [16]. In dose fractionation studies, narrowing of the small bowel of mice with diffuse submucosal edema but not fibrosis was observed at 3 to 6 months after 42 Gy given in 3 Gy fractions [17]. Rats developed small intestinal fibrosis starting at 2 weeks after 17 to 56.0 Gy in 1, 2, or 3 fractions [18,19,20], and they had fibrosis at 26 weeks after 28 to 67.2 Gy in 5.6 Gy or 4.2 Gy fractions [12].

The colorectum of mice irradiated with 8 to 34 Gy in a single dose had narrowing of the lumen with submucosal thickening caused by edema and fibrosis [21,22,23]. Fibrosis began at 3 months and progressed with time, and edema began at 21 days and persisted to 6 months after 22 Gy. The amount of connective tissue increased with increasing dose. Fibrosis was seen to be more severe in cases in which there was also mucosal ulceration but it was also present in the absence of ulceration. The serosal surface was also thickened and fibrotic [21,22]. Similarly, mice given 15 to 35 Gy as single doses and split doses up to 29.5 Gy to the colorectal area developed acute changes within 30 days and chronic changes at 4 to 48 weeks. Acute changes at doses above 20 Gy consisted of ulcers with attendant inflammation, edema and fibrosis in the submucosal

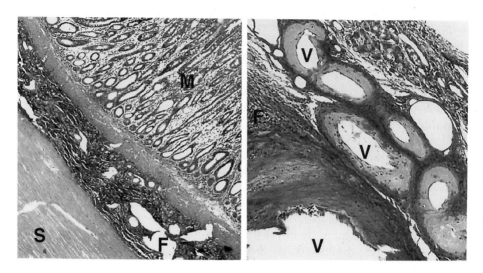

Fig. 1. Section of duodenum from a dog 6 months after 30 Gy single dose. Left panel: the mucosa (M) is intact and the smooth muscle (S) of the intestinal wall is normal. There is mild fibrosis (F) of the submucosa which is slightly thicker and more dense than normal. Right panel: adventitial vessels (V) have subendothelial fibrin formation, fibrinoid necrosis of the media and perivascular fibrosis (F).

to serosal surface. In mice surviving 20 Gy or above acutely, chronic changes consisted of persistent deep ulcers with inflammation, edema and fibrosis involving most of the intestinal wall. In some mice given 20 Gy or most mice given less than 20 Gy or split doses, the mucosa was intact at 5 months but the submucosa was fibrotic, and at 12 months there was even more increased collagen in the lamina propria and submucosa [24]. Rats given 23 Gy single dose to the colorectum also developed submucosal edema and fibrosis 30 to 60 days later [25] and rats given 15 to 30 Gy developed submucosal edema early and fibrosis with up to 8 times normal thickness 30 to 100 days later [26,27]. The fibrosis was present in the absence of mucosal ulceration, but it was more severe and accompanied by inflammation and necrosis if an ulcer was present [25,26]. Serosal fibrosis was present in cases with mucosal ulceration [25] but otherwise it was mild [27]. Submucosal necrosis and extensive serosal fibrosis in association with mucosal ulceration and inflammation was also seen in the colorectum of rats within 200 days with an LD_{50} dose of 20.2 Gy [28]. Rats given 20 to 100 Gy in 1, 2, 5 and 10 fractions to the colorectum had submucosal hyalinized collagen that was more extensive at 12 versus 4 months. Fibrosis was more severe with increased doses and larger fraction sizes and mucosal ulcers were associated with the more severe lesions [29]. Using fractionated irradiation of 6, 7, or 8 Gy fractions 10 days apart to a total of 108 to 148 Gy to the rat colorectum, late rectal ulcers with fibrosis, inflammation and subserosal fibrosis were observed. In some cases the mucosa was intact but atrophic and increased fibrous connective tissue in the lamina propria, submucosal edema, submucosal fibrosis to 5 times normal thickness and subserosal fibrosis was present [30]. Similarly rats receiving various doses up to 80 Gy in 4 to 10 fractions to the colorectal area developed chronic injury at 2 months characterized by deep ulcers with inflammation and fibrosis or late injury at over 100 days characterized by submucosal and serosal fibrosis [31].

Adhesion formation characterized by fibrous connective tissue adhering the abdominal organs to one another may also occur as a late effect following irradiation to the abdomen. In mice given 7 to 17.5 Gy single dose, adhesions developed at doses above 13.5 Gy between 98 and 224 days after irradiation. The adhesions especially involved the large intestine near the caecum and occurred in 8.3 to 26.2% of the mice. Adhesions were characterized by fibrosis with inflammation and breakdown of the serosal layer [32,33]. Adhesions were also seen in mice given 9 and 11.5 Gy single doses or 42 Gy in 3 Gy fractions to the small intestine [10,17]. Perirectal fibrotic adhesions were also observed in mice after 25 to 34 Gy to the colorectum [21,23], and in rats given 20 Gy to the colorectum [28].

2.2 Blood vessels and lymphatics

Changes in blood vessels and lymphatics are a commonly reported manifestation of late radiation injury to the gastrointestinal tract [1,3–5,7,34]. In humans, capillary telangiectasia, dilated lymphatics, hyalinized arterioles, intimal fibrosis of vessels, and obstructive blood vessel changes have been observed in the submucosa of the stomach. In the small intestine, atrophic or absent lymphatics and telangiectasia in the lamina propria have been described. In addition to submucosal vessel changes similar to that in the stomach, early endothelial swelling, thrombosis of small vessels, atypical large endothelial cells, foamy intimal plaques, medial fibrinoid necrosis of arterioles, perivascular fibrosis, and occasionally venules with intimal changes or thrombi may be present. Vascular lesions similar to those in the submucosa may also occur in the tunica muscularis and serosal layers. Similar vascular lesions are also found in the caecal appendage and colorectum of humans after irradiation [1–3,6,7].

In the rat stomach, large vessels with fibrinoid and hyalinized changes and occasionally thrombosis in the mucosa, submucosa and subserosa occurred 1 to 7 months after a single dose of 16 to 28.5 Gy [8].

Vascular sclerosis was present in mouse jejunum given single doses of 9 to 16 Gy [9] and dilated lymphatics and vessels were seen after 11.5 Gy [10]. In mice after 42 Gy in 3 Gy fractions to the small intestine, focal haemorrhages and infarctions occurred in some cases after 6 months. At 3 to 6 months, markedly dilated and hyalinized vessels were in the submucosa associated with edema and infarction [17]. Rats given 15 to 40 Gy in single or fractionated doses to the small intestine developed congested lymphatics and vascular sclerosis [12,13,18–20] and cats given 15, 20 or 25 Gy developed perivascular fibrosis at 4 months [14]. Dogs given 30 Gy to the duodenum developed perivascular fibrosis, intimal proliferation, fibrinoid necrosis of arterioles, and subendothelial fibrin formation (Fig. 1) [15].

Mice irradiated in the colorectal area using 8 to 34 Gy in single doses had narrowed arterioles with thickened walls, hyaline degeneration of arterioles and dilated arterioles and venules in the submucosa and serosa. Dilated vessels and submucosal edema were seen at 21 days after 16 to 22 Gy while at 49 days and longer, vasoocclusive changes and perivascular fibrosis were noted [21,22]. In another study of mice given 20 to 35 Gy in single doses to the colorectum, vessel fibrosis, vascular thickening or occlusion occurred 30 days or longer after irradiation [24]. Rats given 23 Gy as a single dose to the colorectal area had necrosis of the arteries, intimal proliferation of small arteries and hyalinoid damage to vessels 30 to 60 days later in the presence or absence of radiation induced ulcers [25]. Similarly rats given 15 to 30 Gy to the colorectum had endothelial proliferation, adventitial fibrosis, hyalinization and thickening of vessel walls and lumen narrowing of small arteries, especially 2 months after 20 Gy or higher. Lymphatic cysts developed early but were absent later [27]. Thrombosed vessels were also seen in rats with deep ulcers at 200 days after around 20 Gy to the colorectum [28]. Similarly in the colorectum of rats given multiple total doses up to 80 Gy in 4 to 10 fractions, late vascular injury was observed in the submucosa, muscularis and serosa at 100 days or longer [31]. Vascular changes of hyalinization, thickening, fibrinoid necrosis, intimal foam cells and narrowed vessels, especially in the submucosa were seen in rat colorectum after 15 to 100 Gy in 1, 2, 5, and 10 fractions [26,29]. In the rat colorectum after 108 to 148 Gy in 6, 7, or 8 Gy per fraction 10 days apart, late ulcers developed and were accompanied by degenerate vessels 7 to 173 days after irradiation. In some cases the mucosa was intact but there were telangiectatic vessels in the lamina propria with a 46% decrease in capillary density. Thrombosed and thickened, degenerate vessels were also seen in the submucosa and subserosa [30].

2.3 Smooth muscle

Morphological changes in the smooth muscle of the gastrointestinal tract are not reported commonly after irradiation. Fibrosis may involve the muscularis mucosa or muscularis of the stomach, small intestine or colon and vessels changes as described above may be observed in the muscle layers. Occasionally deep radiation ulcers may extend into the muscularis and cause more extensive damage including necrosis and fibrosis. Occasionally cystically dilated mucosal glands may extend into the muscle layers, usually in the colon, similar to colitis cystica profunda [1,2].

There are no reports of histologically observed muscle damage to the irradiated stomach of experimental animals. In mice given 13.5 to 17.5 Gy single dose to the abdomen, fibrosis of the outer muscle wall of the small intestine was associated with adhesion formation [32]. Muscle hypertrophy and fibrosis of the muscularis mucosa of the small intestine of mice was present after 9 or 11.5 Gy [10]. The muscle wall of cat ileum was thickened 4 months after 25 Gy [14]. Occasionally the muscle layers of the small intestine may be invaded by glandular proliferations, indicating ileitis cystica profunda [3,12,13,18,19].

Mice irradiated with a dose of 8 to 34 Gy given as single doses had necrosis and inflammation of the smooth muscle layers of the colorectum associated with deep ulcers. In other areas the muscle was observed to be disorganized with irregularly shaped myocytes and some myocytes had vacuolar cytoplasmic degenerative changes after 16 or 22 Gy [21]. In another study in mice, muscle fibrosis in the colorectum was also seen after single doses of 20 Gy or more and were associated with ulcers. Occasionally muscle vacuolation was observed after 20 Gy in the absence of ulcers [24]. Scarring of the muscularis was also seen in rats given 23 Gy single dose [25] or given 80 Gy in 4 to 10 fractions [31] to the colorectal area. Muscle necrosis and absence of the muscularis mucosa was observed in association with deep radiation ulcers in the colorectum of rats after single doses of around 20 Gy [28] and after fractionated doses of 108 to 148 Gy given in 6,7,or 8 Gy fractions 10 days apart [30]. In addition, mucosal glands may be observed in the deep muscle layers, typical of colitis cystica profunda, after irradiation in mice and rats [21,24,26,27,29–31].

2.4 Peripheral nerves

Morphological evidence of damage to the nerve fibres and ganglia of the myenteric plexus has occasionally been noted in humans after irradiation to the gastrointestinal tract. Fibrosis and degeneration of the myenteric plexus and ganglia has been reported in the stomach and small intestine [1]. In one study, 27 of 33 patients receiving 30.5 to 87.5 Gy in fractions developed symptoms of chronic radiation enteropathy and had increased nerve fibres in the lamina propria of the surgically resected small and large intestine. Also increased numbers of ganglion cells and atypical ganglion cells were observed in the lamina propria. In addition, neuroendocrine cells were present in the lamina propria of irradiated patients but not in normal intestine [34].

Few studies in experimental animals have reported lesions in the peripheral nerves of the gastrointestinal tract. In rabbits irradiated with 80 or 120 Gy to the ileum, there was destruction of the intermuscular plexus and degeneration and decrease in ganglion cells [35].

3. FUNCTIONAL CHANGES

Functional changes reported in humans and experimental animals with radiation complications of the supportive tissue of the gastrointestinal tract may include alterations in the connective tissue, blood vessels and lymphatics, smooth muscle and peripheral nerves. In some cases the correlation of a functional alteration with a specific morphologic tissue change may be difficult.

3.1 Connective tissue

In humans with late radiation complications, narrowing of the bowel lumen with functional obstructions may be the result of fibrosis in the connective tissue of the gastrointestinal tract. This may occur in the presence or absence of mucosal ulcers. Rarely perforations or fistulas may occur [1,4–7].

Similarly in experimental animals with late radiation complications, the morphological changes of edema and fibrosis of the connective tissue may result in bowel narrowing and obstructions. Obstructions of the stomach have not been reported but narrowing and increased rigidity of the small intestine in mice occurred 6 months after doses up to 42 Gy in 3 Gy fractions [17]. The LD_{50} for late small intestinal death in mice was 22.6 Gy single doses and 45.5 Gy in 9.1 Gy per fraction at 90 days [36]. Tensile testing of irradiated segments of the mouse jejunum irradiated to 9 to 16 Gy revealed an increased elastic stiffness with increased dose. The reduced circumference of the bowel lumen correlated with increased stiffness [9]. Rats developed stenosis and duodenal obstructions 20 to 80 days after a 20 to 40 Gy single dose, but few died after 15 Gy [13]. In rats the LD_{50} for small intestinal obstruction secondary to fibrosis or fistula formation was about 22 Gy (Fig. 2) [12,18]. Hydroxyproline measurements after 19 and 21 Gy to the small intestine in rats were significantly increased and correlated with subserosal fibrosis at 2 and 8 weeks but at greater than 8 weeks hydroxyproline measurements were not increased and did not correlate with the submucosal fibrosis that was present [11].

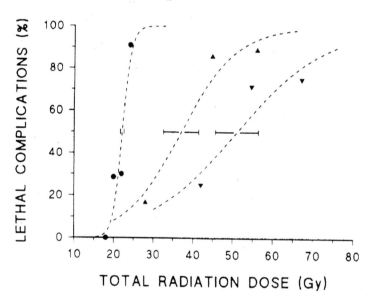

Fig. 2. Dose response curves for the frequency of complications after irradiation of the rat small intestine. Circle = single dose, triangle = 5.6 Gy per fraction, upside-down triangle = 4.2 Gy per fraction. Reprinted with permission from Langberg et al. [12].

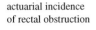

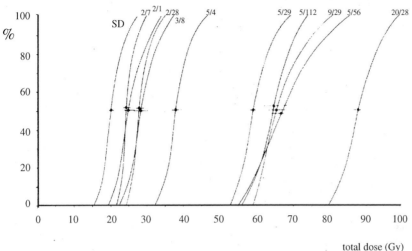

Fig. 3. Dose response curves for the frequency of obstruction after irradiation of the rat colon. Curves are labelled with the first number indicating the number of fractions and the second number the overall treatment time in days; SD = single dose. Reprinted with permission from Kiszel et al. [28].

After irradiation of the colorectal area of mice lethal functional obstructions developed at 40 weeks with an ED_{50} of 20.3 Gy single dose [21]. In another study of mice obstructions of the colorectum occurred at 8 weeks after 27 and 35 Gy, at 16 to 29 weeks after 20 to 24 Gy and at 48 weeks after 18 Gy single dose. All of the mice receiving greater than 20 Gy eventually developed obstructions. Early developing obstructions were associated with mucosal ulcers, while late developing obstructions were not [24]. Using faecal deformity as a functional measurement of colorectal fibrosis in mice, dose response curves were generated at 6, 10 and 16 months after irradiation [23]. Measurements of hydroxyproline content in irradiated mouse rectum showed an increase in the amount of hydroxyproline per mg wet weight but not per 5 mm length of rectum [37]. In 90% of rats given 23 Gy single dose, colorectal obstructions developed 30 to 60 days after irradiation and all were associated with mucosal ulcers [25]. Stenosis of the colorectum developed in rats at 200 days after irradiation with an LD_{50} of 20.2 Gy and all were associated with deep ulcers (Fig. 3) [28]. In another study, rectal obstruction occurred with an ED_{50} of 21.5 Gy at 150 days after irradiation of the rat colorectum [26,27].

3.2 Blood vessels and lymphatics

Morphologic changes in the blood vessels in humans with late radiation complications to the gastrointestinal tract are common, and a few studies document the functional consequences of the lesions. Angiography in humans with intestinal irradiation injury reveal degenerative and occlusive changes reducing vascular volume [38,39]. Occasionally gut infarction with complete necrosis of the entire bowel segment occurs which is likely due to complete dysfunction and obstruction of the vascular supply [1].

Similarly in experimental animals there have been studies measuring the function of the vasculature. The stomach vasculature has not been evaluated functionally after irradiation. In mice after doses up to 42 Gy in 3 Gy fractions to the small intestine there was a transient decrease in blood perfusion at 3 months that was normal at 6 months after irradiation. However, at 6 months there were also focal areas of haemorrhage and bowel infarction, indirectly implying focal complete obstruction of the vasculature [17]. In cat ileum 4 days after 10 to 30 Gy there were areas of avascularity, occluded vessels and filling defects microangiographically. At 1 to 4 months the mucosa regenerated after 10 to 15 Gy with a normal vascularity, but at doses of 25 to 30 Gy there was decreased vascularity with a lack of mucosal regeneration [40,41]. In irradiated canine small intestine there was early vascular leakage, vasodilation and increased blood flow and later degenerative and obliterative changes [42,43]. In another study of irradiated mouse rectum an increased amount of blood in the rectum was present 5 days after irradiation, was normal by 21 days and decreased by 49 days after irradiation. There was a biphasic increase in vascular permeability occurring at 1 to 3 weeks and again at 3 to 6 months after irradiation [22].

Indirect evidence of intestinal functional vascular damage was demonstrated by increased radioresistance of mouse small intestine mucosa to 8 to 16 Gy after a previous dose of 9 to 11.5 Gy 2, 6, or 12 months earlier. The increased radioresistance was thought to be due to hypoxia secondary to vascular damage. Furthermore, misonidazole abolished the increased radioresistance [10]. These results were repeated in a similar study in mice showing increased resistance to 11.5 Gy 2 months after a previous dose of 11.5 Gy [44].

3.3 Smooth muscle and peripheral nerves

Morphologic changes are infrequently reported to involve the smooth muscle or peripheral nerves of the gastrointestinal tract in humans, and direct functional assessment of these tissues is even less frequent [1,3]. In one study in which irradiated bowel had increased nerve fibres, ganglion cells and neuroendocrine cells in the lamina propria, it was speculated that these changes could affect intestinal motility and mucosal secretions and contribute to some of the symptoms of radiation injury [34]. Increased intestinal transit times have been reported in humans after abdominal irradiation [45,46].

In experimental animals there are reports that may suggest functional abnormalities of smooth muscle or nerves. In rats, stomach dilation with delayed gastric emptying time developed 1 to 7 months after irradiation. The ED_{50} for this gastroparesis was 19.2 Gy [8]. In rabbits irradiated to the ileum, the frequency of antiperistaltic propagation and dysrhythmia of electric discharge increased with increasing dose. The motile function of the intestine increased at doses up to 80 Gy but decreased at doses over 120 Gy and decreased at later times after 80 Gy [35]. In dogs, total abdominal irradiation with a dose of 22.5 Gy in 9 fractions caused increased frequency of giant migrating contractions in the small intestine and colon and increased retrograde giant contractions in the small intestine within hours or days after irradiation. A direct activation of neural or neuro-immune pathways by irradiation was speculated as histologic changes are minimal at this time [45].

4. PATHOGENESIS

The pathogenesis of lesions developing in the supportive tissues of the gastrointestinal tract is not completely understood, nor is the role of the supportive tissues in late developing radiation effects on the mucosal tissue (atrophy and ulceration) agreed upon. Furthermore the relative roles of the supportive tissues and mucosa in the clinical expression of late radiation effects of the gastrointestinal tract is not clear. The major difficulties are determining if damage to the vasculoconnective tissue results in late mucosal atrophy and ulceration or if radiation damage to stem cells in the mucosa lead to persistent or late mucosal atrophy and ulceration with subsequent changes in the vasculoconnective tissue.

In humans the pathogenesis of late gastric ulcers is uncertain but is thought to be due to damage to the vasculoconnective tissue [2,6]. It has been proposed that the late developing radiation induced ulcers of the small and large intestine are secondary to damage to the vasculature which results in fibrosis of the connective tissue and ischemia to the mucosa with subsequent mucosal atrophy and ulceration [1–7,47]. However, late ulcers may also be due to early ulcers that never heal [3]. Complete intestinal necrosis and infarction is even more strongly linked to late radiation damage to the vasculature [1,7].

In experimental animals the pathogenesis of late gastric ulcers is also uncertain. The pathogenesis of late developing ulcers in the small and large intestine of experimental animals after irradiation is also a matter of debate. Based on experimental data, it has been proposed that there may be at least 2 different mechanisms leading to late mucosal ulceration, depending on dose. With higher doses, there is rapid mucosal damage which may be too extensive to completely heal in which case the late observed ulceration is really a consequence of a persistent acute effect. Associated with these ulcers, there is extensive inflammation, fibrosis and vascular lesions, all of which may be secondary to the ulceration and inflammation [9,12,18,20,21,24,30,31,48]. Support for this concept is that overall treatment time significantly increases late developing complications, implicating a role for rapidly proliferating mucosal cells influencing late developing changes [20,48]. With lower radiation doses, the acute mucosal affects may heal and the late developing ulcers may be secondary to mucosal damage due to ischemia caused by radiation damage to the vasculature with attendant fibrosis [2,9,15,21,24,30,40]. Support for this later theory is that in some studies with lower radiation doses the mucosa is observed to be intact, although atrophic, yet there is still extensive connective tissue fibrosis and numerous vascular lesions [21,24,30]. It has been suggested that early after irradiation the increased vascular permeability and leakage observed correlates with dilated vessels and submucosal edema seen histologically [3,17,22]. This earlier edema may resolve into dense fibrosis [3]. The second wave of increased vascular permeability observed may be due to endothelial cell loss and vessel thrombosis and occlusion which would also correlate with the decreased blood volume and decreased vascularity that is present [3,22,40].

The influence of diet on the development of late radiation ulcers provides some further support for the theory that these late ulcers are secondary to damage to the vasculoconnective tissue. In rats given a residue free diet, ulcers did not develop after 23 Gy while those rats receiving standard diet and 23 Gy to the colorectum did develop ulcers. Furthermore, rats on a residue free diet remained free of clinical obstructions, yet when changed to standard diet they developed obstructions and ulcerations. From these studies it was concluded that the mechanical abrasion caused by faecal pellets resulted in late mucosal ulceration, and that the mucosa was more susceptible to this damage because of damage to the vasculature with subsequent fibrosis and ischemia to the mucosa [25]. In another study, however these dietary modifications did not influence the occurrence of radiation ulcers, although the diet in this later study was not completely residue free [31].

The development of clinically observed obstructions in both humans and experimental animals is usually believed to be due to the extensive fibrosis that develops causing narrowing of the intestinal lumen, but when there is ulceration present, it is still not resolved whether the fibrosis was present prior to the development of the ulceration or occurred in response to the ulceration. In the presence of ulcers, the fibrosis may often be more extensive [1,7,9,21]. There are numerous instances, however where obstructions occur due to marked thickening of the intestinal wall with fibrosis, yet the mucosa is still intact and ulcers are not present [9,21,24,30]. The fibrosis is thought to develop subsequent to the edema secondary to vascular damage [2,3,17,21,22] which could be possibly due to decreased fibrinolysis causing persistent fibrin accumulation that is organized into fibrous connective tissue [3]. Intestinal fibrosis may also be caused by radiation induced altered collagen orientation [9], decreased collagen degradation or absorption, altered glycosaminoglycans, malfunction of irradiated fibroblasts, or obstruction of lymphatics with accumulation of debris [3]. One study however, suggested that fibrosis was due to tissue atrophy rather than increased production as hydroxyproline content was increased per wet weight but not per length of rectum [37].

Recently there has been interest in the potential role of cytokines in the development of late radiation lesions. In one study in humans treated with irradiation prior to removal of the colon for colon cancer, an increase in transforming growth factor-beta was observed in the tissues of 4 of 6 patients. This growth factor was observed in the adjacent tissues not involved with cancer but included in the radiation field, and was specifically localized to thickened vessels and macrophages and lymphocytes in the stroma. As transforming growth factor-beta is a strong promoter of fibrosis, it was postulated that this growth factor may have a significant role in the development of late connective tissue fibrosis following radiation therapy [49]. Comparable studies of transforming growth factor-beta in the gastrointestinal tract of experimental animals have not been reported.

As prior surgery appears to increase the risk for late radiation damage in the gastrointestinal tract, the role of inflammation and cytokines in the development of adhesions was investigated in mice. Surgery prior to irradiation caused a significant increase in the number of adhesions following whole abdominal irradiation compared to mice which had no prior surgery. Intraperitoneal injection of interleukin-1 caused a similar increase in the number of adhesions that developed after irradiation. From these studies it was concluded that cytokines released during surgery played a significant role in the development of adhesion following irradiation, and that this effect may be mediated through the action of interleukin-1 on the vasculature and on the regulation of fibrin formation [33].

The pathogenesis of radiation effects on the smooth muscle and nerves in the intestine is uncertain. The fibrosis that may involve these structures probably has a similar pathway of development as fibrosis of the submucosal and serosal layers [1,3,8]. The cause for the increased nerve fibres and ganglions cells noted in one study was suggested to reflect a disturbance in migration of neurons and hyperplasia of nerve fibres and ganglion cells as may also be seen after trauma or severe inflammatory bowel diseases [34]. The pathogenesis for the apparent damage to the autonomic nervous system in rats resulting in gastroparesis is not known [8]. In rabbits the morphologic degenerative changes in the nerve plexus and ganglion cells were thought to be responsible for the abnormalities in the motile function of the intestine [35].

5. TOLERANCE DOSES, DOSE FRACTIONATION AND CHEMOTHERAPY

In humans, the incidence of late gastrointestinal tract radiation complications, which presumably are mostly due to damage to the supportive tissue, is about 1 to 5% but may be as high as 36% [1,3–6]. The tolerance doses for a 50% late radiation induced complication of the gastrointestinal tract are estimated to be 45 to 55 Gy for the stomach, 60 to 65 Gy for the small intestine and about 80 Gy for the colorectal region at 5 years after treatment [1,6]. For a 5% late complication rate at 5 years, the tolerance doses are about 45 Gy for the stomach and intestine and about 55 Gy for the rectum [1,6]. In the case of intraoperative radiation therapy for pancreatic cancer, a portion of the duodenum may be subjected to large single doses. The complication rate for late duodenal injury is about 20 to 25% [15,50] and the tolerance is estimated to be between 17 and 20 Gy single dose [13,50]. Fraction size is important in the development of late radiation complications. In one study, patients received 40 Gy to the abdomen and the late intestinal complication rate was 25% if fraction size was 3.3 Gy and 8% if the fraction size was 2.5 Gy [51].

From experimental studies, the tolerance doses of late gastrointestinal radiation injury are mostly determined after single dose exposures. The ED_{50} for single dose late radiation complications in rodents is 19.2 Gy for the stomach [8], 22.0 to 22.6 Gy for the small intestine [12,18,36] and 20.2 to 22.0 Gy for the colorectum [21,26–28,31]. Relatively less information is available regarding the effects of dose fractionation in experimental models although it is clear that smaller doses per fraction cause increased tolerance [3,12,17,28–31,36]. Increased time between fractions and longer overall treatment time also increases tolerance in the small intestine and colorectum [3,28,31,46]. For late injury in the mouse small intestine the ED_{50} was 25.2 Gy in 12.6 Gy fractions, 30.4 Gy in 10.1 Gy fractions, and 45.5 Gy in 9.1 Gy fractions [36]. The LD_{50} for late complications in the rat small intestine was 37.0 Gy in 5.6 Gy fractions and 51.0 Gy in 4.2 Gy fractions (Fig. 2) [12]. In the rat rectum the ED_{50} for late injury was 38 Gy in 9.5 Gy fractions and 53 Gy in 5.3 Gy fractions [31] and in the colon the LD_{50} varied from 25.0 Gy in 12.5 Gy fractions to 87.8 Gy in 4.4 Gy fractions (Fig. 3) [28]. In most studies regarding dose fractionation, the data do not fit the linear quadratic model well [2,28,30]. Estimates of the α/β ratio in the small intestine and colorectum vary from 2 to 10.7 Gy [2,3,12,31]. The difficulties in fitting late complication data to the linear quadratic model as well as the unexpected influence of treatment time on late effects is probably due to a overlapping of early and late effects with more severe early effects influencing the incidence of late effects [2,3,6,12,24,31,48].

Tolerance doses and late complications rates are affected by a variety of factors. There is an increased risk of late complications following previous abdominal surgery, pelvic inflammatory disease, vascular diseases, diabetes mellitus or hypertension [1–6]. In one study of Hodgkin's disease patients the risk of late intestinal complications was 23% if there was prior surgery versus 7% without prior surgery [51]. The influence of the volume of intestinal tract irradiated is also of importance [2,4]. A decrease of irradiated length of intestine from 50 to 10 mm increases tolerance by a factor of 2 [2]. The incidence of severe late bowel complication was 3–10% after pelvic irradiation versus 33% with pelvic plus retroperitoneal irradiation [4,52]. Detailed volume studies in experimental animals have not been done. However, volume effects are apparent as rodents given whole abdominal irradiation have increased deaths at 10 to 13 Gy single dose [3,32], versus 20 to 23 Gy if only portions of the intestine are irradiated [18,21,26–28,36]. However, the deaths due to whole abdominal irradiation are due to acute reactions whereas if only portions of intestine are irradiated the deaths are due to late reactions [3].

The effects of chemotherapy on the incidence of late radiation effects on the gastrointestinal tract are not clearly understood. Cisplatin and 5-fluorouracil may cause increased early intestinal reactions, but cisplatin does not apparently cause increased late effects in humans [2]. 5-Fluorouracil may have caused an increased incidence of late effects in people treated for rectal carcinoma [53], or if used with high dose but not low dose irradiation for pancreatic cancer [54]. Adriamycin, actinomycin-D and methotrexate may also cause increased radiation complications [4,5]. In experimental animals cisplatin caused increased early mortality in mice after small intestinal irradiation but did not affect the apparent late effects [44]. Cisplatin also did not affect the incidence of late rectal stenosis in mice but did affect some of the early mucosal reactions [21,22]. The radioprotector WR2721 has been shown to increase survival and decrease histologic reactions in irradiated mice rectum with a protection factor of 1.3 to 1.5 [37]. Similarly WR2721 given intraluminally into the duodenum of dogs protected the intestine, but not the pancreas from radiation damage following intraoperative irradiation to 30 Gy [15]. Preliminary data in humans showed no severe late intestinal complications following WR2721 plus irradiation to the pelvis for rectal cancer versus about 5% complications with irradiation without WR2721 [55].

6. CONCLUSIONS

The major effect of irradiation on the supportive tissues of the gastrointestinal tract is fibrosis with subsequent obstruction which is a severe complication following radiation therapy. While the sensitivity of the small intestine to late effects is somewhat greater than the sensitivity of the large intestine, the large intestine, due to its immobility, may receive a higher dose during a course of fractionated radiation therapy which, coupled with greater trauma from intestinal contents, leads to a higher incidence of fibrosis and subsequent obstruction.

In animal studies, single doses greater than 15 Gy were accompanied by a high risk of severe vascular injury, fibrosis, adhesions and functional obstruction. The time to development of lesions did not vary markedly between segments of the intestine but higher doses caused an earlier appearance of lesions. Damage to smooth muscle or peripheral nerves is infrequent but may occur after single doses of greater than 20 Gy. Sparing of fibrosis, vascular damage and functional obstruction was achieved by dose fractionation. In humans, functional injury is likely to occur with a greater than 5% incidence with total doses in excess of 45 Gy given in 2 Gy fractions.

The pathogenesis of fibrosis and subsequent obstruction has not been clearly defined, but appears to be due to injury to the vasculature as well as possibly a direct response of connective tissue to irradiation. The release of cytokines by radiation damage to tissues may play an important role in the development of fibrosis. The resultant fibrosis is enhanced when mucosal ulceration occurs as an early or persistent effect of irradiation. The combination of ulceration and fibrosis makes it difficult to devise radiation schemes to reduce the probability for intestinal injury short of reducing volume and excluding the intestine from the field of irradiation.

Reducing dose per fraction would reduce the direct injury to supportive structures, but might increase the acute response and therefore lead to greater incidence due to development of mucosal ulceration and subsequent fibrosis. Larger doses per fraction are likely to increase the overall incidence of late effects. Larger doses per fraction as might be given with high dose rate brachytherapy or large single doses of intraoperative radiation therapy are useful only if the total volume can be reduced significantly or if sensitive structures can be removed from the radiation field. While this protects sensitive tissues, it significantly increases the probability of injury to muscle, vessels and nerves that cannot be excluded from the radiation field.

The combination of surgery and chemotherapy can enhance the probability of severe gastrointestinal radiation injury. Cytokines released due to direct radiation injury associated with those released following surgery may be important in the development of fibrosis. The use of modifiers of the activity of some cytokines might lead to a decreased incidence of radiation injury. The radioprotector WR2721 has had a local effect on reducing both mucosal and supportive tissue injury following irradiation. This may be a practical means of reducing the possibility of injury with intraoperative radiotherapy or high dose rate brachytherapy, but would likely be of limited value with fractionated radiation therapy.

References

1.   Berthrong, M. and Fajardo, L.F. (1981) Radiation injury in surgical pathology, Part II. Am. J. Surg. Pathol. 5, 153–178.
2.   Trott, K.R. and Herrmann, T. (1991) Radiation effects on abdominal organs. In: E. Scherer, C. Streffer and K.R. Trorr (Eds.), Radiopathology of Organs and Tissues. Springer-Verlag, New York, pp. 313–346.
3.   Hauer-Jensen, M. (1990) Late radiation injury of the small intestine. Acta Oncologica 29, 401–415.
4.   Kinsella, T.J. and Bloomer, W.D. (1980) Tolerance of the intestine to radiation therapy. Surg. Gynecol. Obst. 151, 273–283.
5.   Nussbaum, M.L., Campana, T.J. and Weese, J.L. (1993) Radiation-induced intestinal injury. Clinics in Plastic Surg. 20, 573–580.
6.   Becciolini, A. (1987) Relative radiosensitivities of the small and large intestine. In: J.T. Lett and K.I. Altman (Eds.), Advances in Radiation Biology, Vol. 12, Academic Press, New York, pp. 83–128.
7.   Casarett, G.W. (1980) Alimentary Tract. In: G.W. Casarett (Ed.), Radiation Histopatholgy, Vol. I, CRC Press Inc., Boca Raton, pp. 107–133.
8.   Breiter, N., Trott, K. and Sassy, T. (1989) Effect of x-irradiation on the stomach of the rat. Int. J. Radiat. Oncol. Biol. Phys. 17, 779–784.
9.   Peck, J.W. and Gibbs, F.A. (1987) Assay of premorbid murine jejunal fibrosis based on mechanical changes after x-irradiation and hyperthermia. Rad. Res. 112, 525–543.

10. Reynaud, A. and Travis, E.L. (1984) Late effects of irradiation in mouse jejunum. Int. J. Radiat. Biol. 46, 125–134.

11. Hauer-Jensen, M., Sauer, T., Sletten, K., Reitan, J.B. and Nygaard, K. (1986) Value of hydroxyproline measurements in the assessment of late radiation enteropathy. Acta. Radiol. Oncol. 25, 137–142.

12. Langberg, C.W., Sauer, T., Reitan, J. B., and Hauer-Jensen, M. (1992) Tolerance of rat small intestine to localized single and fractionated irradiation. Acta Oncol. 31, 781–787.

13. Poulakos, L., Elwell, J.H., Osborne, J.W., Urdaneta, L.F., Hauer-Jensen, M., et al. (1990) The prevalance and severity of late effects in normal rat duodenum following intraoperative irradiation. Int. J. Radiat. Oncol. Biol. Phys. 18, 841–848.

14. Eriksson, B., Johnson, L. and Rubio, C. (1982) A semiquantitative histological method to estimate acute and chronic radiation injury in the small intestine of the cat. Scand. J. Gastroenterol. 17, 1017–1024.

15. Halberg, F.E., LaRue, S.M., Rayner, A.A., Burnel, W.M., Powers, B.E., et al. (1991) Intraoperative radiotherapy with localized radioprotection: diminished duodenal toxicity with intraluminal WR2721. Int. J. Radiat. Oncol. Biol. Phys. 21, 1241–1246.

16. Ahmadu-Suka, F., Gillette, E.L., Withrow, S.J., Husted, P.W., Nelson, A.W. and Whiteman, C.E. (1988) Pathologic response of the pancreas and duodenum to experimental intraoperative irradiation. Int. J. Radiat. Oncol. Biol. Phys. 14, 1197–1204.

17. Dewit, L. and Oussoren, Y. (1987) Late effects in the mouse small intestine after a clinically relevant multifraction ated radiation treatment. Rad. Res. 110, 372–384.

18. Hauer-Jensen, M., Sauer, T., Devik, F. and Nygaard, K. (1983) Late changes following single dose roentgen irradiation of rat small intestine. Acta Radiologica Oncol. 22, 299–303.

19. Hauer-Jensen, M., Sauer, T., Devik, F. and Nygaard, K. (1983) Effects of dose fractionation on late roentgen radiation damange of rat small intestine. Acta Radiologica Oncol. 22, 381–384.

20. Hauer-Jensen, M., Poulakos, L. and Osborne, J.W. (1990) Intestinal complications following accelerated fractionated x-irradiation: an experimental study in the rat. Acta Oncol. 29, 229–234.

21. Dewit, L., Oussoren, Y. and Bartelink, H. (1987) Early and late damage in the mouse rectum after irradiation and *cis*-diamminedichloroplatinum (II). Radiother. Oncol. 8, 57–69.

22. Dewit, L. and Oussoren, Y. (1987) Vascular injury in the mouse rectum after irradiation and *cis*-diamminedichloroplatinum (II). Br. J. Radiol. 60, 1037–1040.

23. Terry, N., Denekamp, J. and Maughan, R.L. (1983) RBE values for colo-rectal injury after caesium 137 gamma-ray and neutraon irradiation. I. Single doses. Br. J. Radiol. 56, 257–265.

24. Followill, D.S., Kester, D. and Travis, E.L. (1993) Histological changes in mouse colon after single and split dose irradiation. Rad. Res. 136, 280–288.

25. Trott, K., Breiter, N. and Spiethoff, A. (1986) Experimental studies on the pathogenesis of the chronic radiation ulcer of the large bowel in rats. Int. J. Radiat. Oncol. Biol. Phys. 12, 1637–1643.

26. Hubmann, F.H. (1981) Effect of X irradiation on the rectum of the rat. Br. J. Radiol. 54, 250–254.

27. Hubmann, F.H. (1982) Proctitis cystica profunda and radiation fibrosis in the

rectum of the female Wistar rat after X irradiation: a histopathological study. J. Pathol. 138, 193–204.

28. Kiszel, Z., Spiethoff, A. and Trott, K. (1984) Large bowel stenosis in rats after fractionated local irradiation. Radiother. Oncol. 2, 247–254.
29. Black, W.C., Gomez, L.S., Yuhas, J.M. and Kligerman, M.M. (1980) Quantitation of the late effects of X-radiation on the large intestine. Cancer 45, 444–451.
30. Breiter, N. and Trott, K. (1986) Chronic radiation damage in the rectum of the rat after protracted fractionated irradiation. Radiother. Oncol. 7, 155–163.
31. van der Kogel, A.J., Jarrett, K.A., Paciotti, M.A. and Raju, M.R. (1988) Radiation tolerance of the rat rectum to fractionated X-rays and pi-mesons. Radiother. Oncol. 12, 225–232.
32. McBride, W.H., Mason, K.A., Davis, C., Withers, H.R. and Smathers, J.B. (1989) Adhesion formation in experimental chronic radiation enteropathy. Int. J. Radiat. Oncol. Biol. Phys. 16, 737–743.
33. McBride, W.H., Mason, K.A., Withers, H.R. and Davis, C. (1989) Effect of interleukin 1, inflammation, and surgery on the incidence of adhesion formation and death after abdominal irradiation in mice. Cancer Res. 49, 169–173.
34. Hirschowitz, L. and Rode, J. (1991) Changes in neurons, neuroendocrine cells and nerve fibres in the lamina propria of irradiated bowel. Virchows Archiv. A. Pathol. Anat. 418, 163–168.
35. Deguchi, H. (1991) An experimental study on the effect of irradiation on motility of the small intestine. J. Smooth Muscle Res. 27, 35–54.
36. Geraci, J.P., Jackson, K.L., Christensen, G.M., Thrower, P.D. and Weyer, B.J. (1977) Acute and late damage in the mouse small intestine following multiple fractionations of neutrons or X-rays. Int. J. Radiat. Oncol. Biol. Phys. 2, 693–696.
37. Ito, H., Meistrich, M.L., Barkley, H.T., Thames, H.D. and Milas, L. (1986) Protection of acute and late radiation damage of the gastrointestinal tract by WR-2721. Int. J. Radiat. Oncol. Biol. Phys. 12, 211–219.
38. Deneker, H., Holmdahl, K.H., Lunderguist, A., Olivecrona, H. and Tyler, V. (1972) Mesenteric angiography in patients with radiation injury of the bowel after pelvic irradiation. Am. J. Radiol. 114, 476–481.
39. Carr, N.D., Pullen, B.R., Hasleton, P.S. and Shofield, P.F. (1984) Microvascular studies in human radiation bowel disease. Gut 25, 448–454.
40. Eriksson, B. (1982) Microangiographic pattern in the small intestine of the cat after irradiation. Scand. J. Gastroenterol. 17, 887–895.
41. Eriksson, B., Johnson, L. and Lundquist, P.G. (1983) Ultrastructural aspects of capillary function in irradiated bowel. An experimental study in the cat. Scand. J. Gastroenterol. 18, 473–480.
42. Bosniak, M.A., Hardy, M.A., Quint, J. and Ghossein, N.A. (1969) Demonstration of the effect of irradiation of canine bowel using in vivo photographic magnification angiography. Radiology 93, 1361–1368.
43. Cockerham, L.G., Doyle, T.F., Trumbo, R.B. and Nold, J.B. (1984) Acute post-irradiation canine intestinal blood flow. Int. J. Radiat. Biol. 45, 65–72.
44. Julia, A.M., Bachaud, J.M., Canal, P. and Daly, N.J. (1991) Radiosensitivity of jejunal mucosa after whole abdomen irradiation and CDDP pretreatment. Int. J. Radiat. Oncol. Biol. Phys. 20, 343–345.
45. Erickson, B.A., Otterson, M.F., Moulder, J.E. and Sarna, S.K. (1994) Altered motility causes the early gastrointestinal toxicity of irradiation. Int. J. Radiat. Oncol. Biol. Phys. 28, 905–912.

46. LaManna, M., Parker, J., Wolodzko, J., Zekavat, P. and Popky, G. (1985) Radionuclide esophageal and intestinal transit time scintigraphy in patients undergoing radiation therapy. Radiat. Med. 3, 13–16.

47. MacCannell, K. (1993) Gastrointestinal inflammation: focus on the vascular endothelium. Can. J. Physiol. Pharmacol. 71, 65–66.

48. Langberg, C.W., Waldron, J.A., Baker, M.L. and Hauer-Jensen, M. (1994) Significance of overall treatment time for the development of radiation-induced intestinal complications. Cancer 73, 2663–2668.

49. Canney, P.A. and Dean, S. (1990) Transforming growth factor beta: a promoter of late connective tissue injury following radiotherapy? Br. J. Radiology 63, 620–623.

50. Kawamura, M., Kataoka, M., Fujii, T., Itoh, H., Ishine, M., et al. (1992) Electron-beam intraoperative radiation therapy (EBIORT) for localized pancreatic carcinoma. Int. J. Radiat. Oncol. Biol. Phys. 23, 751–757.

51. Gallez-Marchal, D., Fayolle, M., Henry-Amar, M., Le Bourgeois, J.P., Rougier, P. and Cosset, J.M. (1984) Radiation injuries of the gastrointestinal tract in Hodgkin's disease: the role of exploratory laparotomy and fractionation. Radiother. Oncol. 2, 93–99.

52. Withers, H.R. and Romsdahl, M.M. (1977) Post-operative radiotherapy for adenocarcinoma of the rectum and rectosigmoid. Int. J. Radiat. Oncol. Biol. Phys. 2, 1069–1074.

53. Danjoux, G.E. and Catton G.E. (1979) Delayed complications in colo-rectal carcinoma treated by combination radiotherapy and 5-fluorouracil — ECOG pilot study. Int. J. Radiat. Oncol. Biol. Phys. 5: 311–315.

54. Moertel, C.G., Childs, D.S., Reitmeier, R.J., et al. (1969) Combined 5-fluorouracil and supervoltage radiation therapy of locally unresectable gastrointestinal cancer. Lancet 2, 865–868.

55. Kligerman, M.M., Liu, T., Liu, Y., Scheffer, B., He, S. and Zhang, Z. (1992) Interim analysis of a randomized trial of radiation therapy of rectal cancer with and without WR-2721. Int. J. Radiat. Oncol. Biol. Phys. 22, 799–802.

C.S. Potten and J.H. Hendry (Eds.), *Radiation and Gut*

CHAPTER 8

Radiation Effects on the Human Gastrointestinal Tract

J. Barber and R.D. James

Department of Clinical Oncology, Christie Hospital NHS Trust, Manchester, UK

1. RADIATION EFFECTS ON THE GASTROINTESTINAL TRACT

1.1 Introduction

Information on the effects of radiation upon the human gut are available from both clinical data, some experimental data and a limited series of data from the atomic bomb explosions and nuclear accidents [1]. The human gastrointestinal tract frequently receives ionising radiation in clinical practice during the treatment of tumours within the abdomen or pelvis. However tumours of the gut itself are often resectable by surgery with a minimum of morbidity, and this is usually the treatment of choice. Treatment of these tumours by radiotherapy is limited by the narrow therapeutic ratio which exists between most bowel tumours and the normal bowel mucosa, and there are also technical problems with mobility of bowel and the difficulty in defining a target volume. Hence most of the clinical data on radiation induced bowel changes are usually as a result of the bowel unavoidably appearing in the treatment volume during the treatment of a nearby structure — for example, carcinoma of the cervix uterus.

1.2 Comparison of radiation effects upon normal and diseased bowel

It is not always possible to extrapolate the radiation tolerance of bowel involved by tumour to normal undiseased bowel. Tumours themselves may produce abnormalities of the gut which could be confused with radiation damage. Although a true 'malignant' enteropathy is extremely rare, it is recognised that there are a variety of pathophysiological changes occurring in the gastrointestinal mucosa of severely ill patients which may mimic the effects of radiation [2]. Another complicating condition is that known as diversion colitis, where a section of bowel which has been disconnected from the faecal stream following a defunctioning colostomy can become inflamed, giving rise to a bloody discharge and cramping abdominal pains. Histologically it may progress to ulceration and sometimes stricture formation [3]. This condition is caused by the depletion of short chain fatty acids which are a major energy source for the colonic epithelium.

1.3 Biopsy studies

The experimental data in man are limited by ethical considerations, and the relative inaccessibility of the gut to biopsy, although with modern endoscopic techniques this is much less of a problem. The acute pathological reactions of the mucosa may be followed by endoscopic biopsy during and immediately after radiation, and several groups have performed serial biopsy studies (e.g. stomach [4–7], small bowel [8], and rectum [9]) and these are described under the subsequent paragraphs.

1.4 Clinical data

There is over 70 years of experience of irradiating the bowel in clinical practice both with external beam radiation and with brachytherapy sources. Variations in radiation quality, and the time, dose and fractionation pattern have been wide, and this has generated a large body of information. Despite this, interpretation of the data is difficult, due to its diverse nature and the lack of formal clinical trials. As the quality of these data varies so much between the different sites in the gut they will be dealt with in turn by site.

2. EFFECTS OF RADIATION ON THE STOMACH

2.1 Acute effects of radiation upon the stomach

Unpleasant clinical toxicities result from delivering radiotherapy to the stomach, even at low doses. Initially persistent nausea, vomiting, anorexia and dyspepsia occur. The nausea generated by gastric irradiation is more severe than that caused by irradiation of other portions of the gastrointestinal tract, but the cause for this remains poorly understood. At endoscopy, the appearance is that of an acute gastritis. Dyspepsia and mild gastritis may progress acutely to radiation induced ulceration and even perforation in severe cases, these effects becoming manifest within 1–4 months of the completion of the treatment [10]. Gastric motility and emptying are reduced during radiotherapy, which may exacerbate the clinical symptoms [11].

Radiotherapy was used reasonably successfully in the 1930s to heal gastric ulcers albeit with a high recurrence rate [12]. Gastric acid formation is significantly suppressed by irradiation of corpus or the pylorus of the stomach and significant reductions in gastric acid production are seen with doses as low as 20 Gy. The acute mucosal reaction in such patients was been studied by serial biopsy [13]. After 8 daily fractions of 1.6 Gy pyknosis was observed in the base of the glandular tubules in both the parietal and the chief cells, and the pits deepen as the treatment is prolonged. The damaged cells are repaired by the neck cells growing down into the tubules. As treatment is continued, the whole mucosal architecture becomes disorganised, with loss and distortion of the glandular structure, and a chronic interstitial inflammatory cell infiltrate appears.

2.2 Late effects of radiation on the stomach

The relatively severe late effects of radiation at even modest doses was well described many years ago by the experience at the Walter Reed Hospital [10]. These results clearly established the difficulties of delivering radiotherapy to the stomach, and since that time, relatively little information has been available on the long term pathological changes appearing after higher doses of radiation. The information available is mostly limited to post operative specimens where operation has been performed for chronic radiation injury.

At doses of more than 40 Gy delivered in 2 Gy fractions there is likely to be persisting ulceration. The suppressed gastric acid secretion does not appear to assist in the healing of the ulcers, which characteristically persist for many months. The radiological appearance of radiation induced ulcers is very similar of that of benign ulceration, usually on the dorsal wall of the antrum. They may be extremely reluctant to heal [13] and may show progressive deformities. Gastric acid production may not be restored, and chronic anaemia may ensue through blood loss.

There are a few reports of the histopathological appearances of chronic radiation injury to the stomach, derived from the gastrectomy specimens of patients having surgery for persistent radiation ulcer (e.g. Ref. [14]. Macroscopically, the stomach is oedematous with a rigid thickened wall, and pale probably due to a decreased vascularity. Microscopically, the mucosa is atrophic with a marked inflammatory cell infiltrate. Parietal cells and to a lesser extent chief cells are markedly reduced in number. The chronic phase of injury bears similarities to those seen in the small bowel, where most of the changes are mediated by vascular injury and consequent secondary atrophy. The submucosa is oedematous with the typical vascular changes of telangiectasis, and hyalinized arterioles. The resulting fibrosis and distortion of the muscularis mucosae and propria may lead to long term dysfunction of gastric motility and emptying [14].

Chronic atrophic gastritis has been observed after radiation to the stomach, but unlike autoimmune chronic atrophic gastritis, vitamin B12 deficiency and pernicious anaemia has not been found to be a problem in clinical practice [15].

2.3 Management of gastric radiation injury

Despite superficial resemblance to a peptic ulcer, radiation induced gastric ulcers and duodenitis do not respond to medical therapy in the same way. Paradoxically, the suppression of gastric acid secretion caused by radiation does not appear to prevent these injuries, although the degree of suppression is highly variable and often transient [12]. Initial therapy with H2-blockers, omeprazole and sucralfate may be of help. If serious radiation injury is suspected acutely, careful follow up and observation with early surgical intervention may help to reduce the mortality [10].

2.4 Effects of alterations of time, dose and fractionation upon gastric radiation injury

The long-term tolerance of the stomach to fractionated radiotherapy is low in comparison with other parts of the gastrointestinal tract. Most series would suggest that serious late morbidity is unlikely at doses of less than 40 Gy delivered in 2 Gy fractions daily. The Walter Reed Hospital data [10] is widely quoted, but it must be remembered that the radiation was delivered using a parallel opposed pair of 1 MV photon fields, with fraction sizes of 3 Gy or more, treating only one field per day. At a dose of 45–55 Gy they found an approximately 20% incidence of persistent ulceration. At a dose of 60 Gy the incidence of ulceration and perforation rose to 50%, most of them being serious.

Regarding more standard radiotherapy techniques using high energy linear accelerators at energies of 4–20 MV and fraction sizes of 2 Gy, there is approximately a 5% risk of long-term complications at a dose (to include the whole stomach) of 45–50 Gy delivered in 2 Gy fractions [13]. These dose levels appear relatively safe even with the addition of chemotherapy [16].

These comparative clinical data are suggestive of considerable fractionation effect, but there are little experimental data available. A study has been performed comparing a hyperfractionated chemo-radiotherapy (two fractions daily of 150 cGy with 5-fluorouracil) with standard once daily 180 cGy fractions [18], and have found the toxicity of the hyperfractionated regimen intolerable.

3. EFFECTS OF RADIATION UPON THE INTESTINES

3.1 Differences between the acute response of small and large bowel

The intestinal mucosa is a tissue in a state of continuous self renewal in a steady state fashion, with cells dividing in the crypts, migrating along the villi and finally being shed into the gut lumen. The cycling times of the different portions of the gut have been estimated by in vivo tritiated thymidine techniques. The cell cycle in human small and large bowel is likely to be about 30–36 h for the former and about 40–48 h for the rectum [18,19] and the mucosal turnover time and has been found to be approximately 5–6 days in the small intestine, rather longer but more variable in the rectum, and difficult to estimate in the stomach [20]. These parameters are rather longer than in most laboratory experimental animals.

The acute radiation reaction depends upon the interruption cellular proliferation in the crypts, as it is the function of the dividing cells which are most affected. As the cells of the villus are shed and not replaced, mucosal denudation will take place after a few days. There will therefore be a delay of onset of clinically apparent effects which is usually greater in the large bowel because of less rapid turnover time. The different radiosensitivities of the various parts of the gut in humans may also be related to the differing turnover or cycling times.

3.2 Acute effects of radiation upon the small bowel

Radiation enteritis may occur if the small bowel is irradiated even to low doses. The diarrhoea is loose and watery, and cramping abdominal pain is characteristic. The acute enteritis is however self limiting in general [21]. The time of onset of the diarrhoea depends on the dose and fractionation of the treatment, but using traditional fractionated radiotherapy with 2–3.5 Gy fractions it normally appears in the second week. This may be accompanied by cramps or pain. Serious morbidity at this time is extremely rare, but perforation has been reported with concomitant chemotherapy [22].

The human small bowel is rarely biopsied during radiotherapy, however the changes seen on pathological examination are broadly similar to those seen in animals except that the time course is different. Macroscopically, there is an inflammatory change, with oedema, a fibrinous peritonitis [8]. At the cellular level, with one dose, pyknosis is seen within 12–24 hours, mainly in the proliferating areas of the crypts. The epithelium becomes denuded within about a week, caused by not only the depression of mitotic activity, but also by the loss of postmitotic mucosal cells. Villous atrophy occurs in around 3 weeks, the lining surface cells become flat and focally ulcerated.

Serial jejunal biopsy studies [5] in patients having fractionated radiotherapy for carcinoma of the stomach have assessed the degree of damage by counting the number of crypt cells remaining in each crypt. Radiation was delivered 3 fractions of 3.5 Gy each week. The number of crypt cells had decreased by half by 7 days. At a total dose of 40 Gy, there was total disorganisation of the crypts and villi. As soon as the radiotherapy was stopped, there was a rapid and overshooting regeneration, showing that the regeneration process is largely inhibited by the radiotherapy. This was demonstrated by frequent mitoses, broad and irregular villi, and branched and irregular crypts. This hyperplastic response persisted for many months after the completion of treatment in some cases. Where radiotherapy is given in 2 Gy fractions, a steady state appears to be reached at about 40 Gy [11].

The vascular and connective tissue changes are dominated by oedema, with haemorrhage inflammation and vascular spasm [23], including large vessel endothelial damage within 49 hours of completion of fractionated radiotherapy. These changes peaked 1–3 weeks after radiotherapy and were nearly completely gone by 4 months. Frank ulceration is relatively rare, since the mucosa has a very high capacity for regeneration.

3.3 Acute reaction in the large bowel and the rectum

The majority of patients receiving radiotherapy to the pelvis undergo acute proctocolitis. After a single dose, this occurs between 4 and 7 days after the treatment. During a fractionated course of treatment, the symptoms develop during the second week of treatment. The symptoms are frequent loose and watery stools, which may be worse in patients who are having post operative radiotherapy after a low anterior resection as the rectal vault capacity is much diminished. Sigmoidoscopy during treatment simply reveals an inflamed oedematous mucosa. Serial biopsies studies at doses up to 20 Gy show, as in the small bowel, oedema and an inflammatory cell infiltrate, and the lymphatic tissue disappears [9]. There are also characteristic small abscesses containing eosinophilic granulocytes, the changes resolving by one month after treatment.

3.4 Clinical features of chronic radiation induced damage and its aetiology

While the incidence of serious morbidity following radiotherapy is relatively low, this is simply a consequence of a titration of dose against complications. The radiotherapist will frequently give the highest dose that is possible with a 2–5% incidence of complications. Many, if not the majority of patients following, for example pelvic radiotherapy will suffer from increase in stool frequency, or a permanent change in bowel habit, which persists long after the acute bowel reaction has passed [24]. Moreover, in the majority of patients, the site of damage will never be determined.

The commonest clinical manifestation of serious chronic radiation injury to the small bowel is obstruction, which may be preceded by episodes of colicky abdominal pain. The obstruction is rarely complete, radiological appearance. Some radiological surveys show partial obstruction and persisting stenosis. Other problems include fistulas, ulcerations and perforations. The most frequent site of fistula formation is the rectum. The symptoms of tenesmus, bleeding cramps and diarrhoea and rectal urgency are only too well known, and may require surgical intervention. A clinical syndrome, where the pelvic tissues become firmly indurated is not uncommon, and may be difficult to differentiate from recurrent tumour.

The median onset of clinically apparent injury to the intestines is about 1–5 years, and occasionally may be as long as 20 years: rectal bleeding may be apparent during the first year, whereas fistulas and strictures are rare before 2 years [25]. The onset of late effects may be hastened by the addition of chemotherapy.

There are also a number of well known risk factors, for example previous chemotherapy [22] diabetes mellitus, arteriosclerosis., hypertension, and previous pelvic surgery [26]. Many of these conditions predispose to a vascular narrowing, hence radiation damage may be more likely to produce clinical manifestations.

3.5 Pathology of chronic radiation injury to the small intestine (see Fig. 1)

The acute oedema and fibrinous peritonitis of the acute reaction usually settles after a number of weeks, but occasionally may be persistent many months after treatment and hence cause peritoneal adhesions. However it is fibrotic and hyaline changes which predominate [14]. The fatty coating of the peritoneal surface is lost, and the bowel wall becomes thickened and indurated. There are characteristic vascular changes, the most common being intimal fibrosis in the medium sized arterioles, with telangiectases in the capillaries of the lamina propria and sub mucosa in a background of hyaline change. As with vascular damage elsewhere, the overall picture is one where there are fewer vessels in total, but the ones remaining are dilated and tortuous [14]. Mesenteric angiography shows vessel crowding, with tortuosity angulations and narrowing in the mid arterial phase while the late arterial phase may reveal a vascular blush the affected small bowel wall. Studies performed with intravascular contrast medium on resected sections of bowel confirm this pattern [27].

3.6 Pathology and radiology of chronic radiation injury to the large intestine

The pathological features are well known due to the large number of specimens resected for radiation injury [28]. The predominant feature is an ischaemic, fibrotic process, with thickened,congested portions of bowel. The mucosa is atrophic, often oedematous and sometimes has a cobblestone appearance. Microscopically, the mucosa is regenerated, but the eosinophilic infiltrate seen in the acute phase persists. The crypts tend to be distorted. The lamina propria has the typical changes of hyaline fibrosis, telangiectasia and dilated lymph vessels with grossly abnormal endothelial cells. A characteristic, but rather uncommon feature is and infiltration of the mucosa in to the muscular layer, forming glandular structures covered by Paneth cells, which is termed 'colitis cystica profunda'. The normal appearance of the mucosal cells should not cause confusion with carcinoma.

When routine radiological investigation is performed after irradiation of the pelvis, a surprising number of patients have occult strictures, although even in the absence of stricture formation patients can be debilitated by mucosal damage [29]. The typical radiological appearance is a smooth elongated narrowing, where the segments of damaged bowel are often straightened and

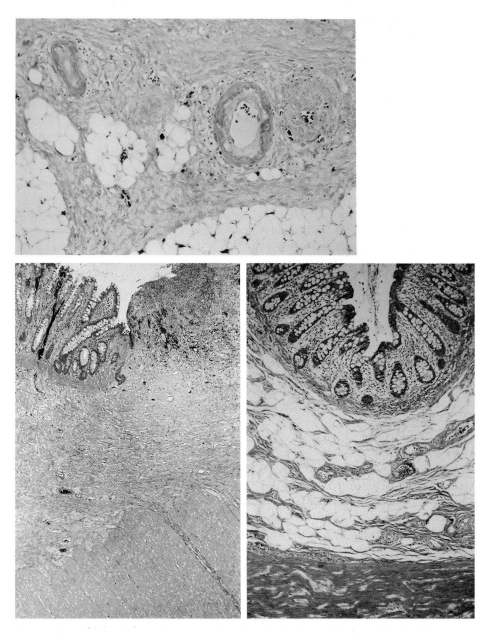

Fig. 1. Section of normal human bowel (top panel), and irradiated human bowel at 1 year after radiotherapy (bottom 2 panels). The irradiated samples show features of radiation colitis, namely ulceration, submucosal fibrosis, and atypical fibroblasts. Also apparent are vascular changes in the serosal blood vessels. There is marked myointimal thickening with narrowing of the lumina (courtesy of Dr. S. Banerjee, Department of Pathology, Christie Hospital). (See also colour plate on p. xvi.)

elevated out of the pelvis because of thickening of the both the bowel wall and the pelvic tissues. Sometimes there are also mucosal abnormalities, with a nodular or thumbprinting pattern. The ulceration may be superficial or deep, simulating either diverticulitis, or if the ulcer is sharply demarcated, it may be difficult to distinguish from a carcinoma [30].

3.7 Functional changes and malabsorption in the small intestine

Malabsorption in the acute phase is probably more common than is probably realised. Clinically, it may be important since it may be a cause for patients to lose weight, although it is rarely analysed in a systematic fashion in clinical practice. The acute effects on malabsorption have been systematically studied [11]. A dose of 50 Gy in five weeks in 2 Gy fractions using a parallel opposed pair of fields with a cobalt unit was delivered to the abdomen, and the absorption of carbohydrate, fat, and vitamin B12 were assessed mid way through and at the completion of the treatment. These parameters showed a 25–30% reduction as compared to controls. There was somewhat less of an effect on the absorption of amino acids — about 5–10% — which may not be clinically significant. However, during an acute radiation reaction, the most important clinical effect is the depletion of water and electrolytes. This may become an important factor in the gastrointestinal syndrome (see the section on total body irradiation).

A surprisingly high level of persisting minor gastrointestinal symptoms after radiotherapy has been recorded in several recent series [24,31]. The mechanism by which this occurs is not clear, but it may be due directly to the changes in transit time, and/or the malabsorption syndrome. There are numerous mechanisms by which the malabsorption injury may be produced, including alterations in bile acid formation and changes in the intestinal microflora.

Detailed analysis of long-term gastrointestinal function has been performed on a series of patients who have received radical radiotherapy for carcinoma of the cervix [32]. Absorption of bile acid, fat and vitamin B12, small bowel transit time and intestinal permeability were correlated with the presence of gastrointestinal symptoms. Over half the patients reported a permanent increase in frequency of bowel action after radiotherapy. All the patients had at least one abnormal test, the most frequently abnormal being that of bile acid malabsorption in over 50% of the patients. Vitamin B12 absorption is a measure of the function of the terminal ileum, but this although being abnormal initially (as found by Becciolini in the study on acute reaction) was more likely to normalise as time elapsed from the time of radiotherapy.

The enterohepatic circulation of bile salts may be interrupted by alterations in microflora, blind loops or disturbances of active transport systems, and may be important in generating some of the clinical abnormalities. The small intestine is normally sterile, and the bile salts should be reabsorbed in the terminal ileum without being deconjugated by bacteria. Assessment of this cycle is performed by a simple non-invasive test cholyl-glycocholic-^{14}C breath test. A small series of women tested in this way a year or more following radiation [24] nearly all showed marked abnormalities of this test, and about 60% of them also had frequency of bowel action.

3.8 Late functional changes in the rectum

The symptoms of radiation damage to the rectum include frequency and urgency of bowel action, and sometimes urge incontinence. These changes may be partly caused by the disturbance of the ability of the rectum to act as a dynamic reservoir. Its function relies critically on perception of filling and contractile properties. Intrarectal pressure is probably monitored by proprioceptive in the perirectal tissues. The mechanisms of tissue injury and their functional importance has been investigated by performing manometric studies on men with radiation proctitis [33]. The rectal volumes and the compliance was assessed in a series of men who had received radiotherapy for carcinoma of the prostate five years earlier, along with age and sex matched controls. The volume of the rectum and sensory threshold was reliably reduced, as was the compliance. Histological studies of samples from similar subjects showed smooth muscle hypertrophy and myenteric plexus damage, with degeneration of ganglion cells and hypertrophy of the nerve fibres. Such neurological change is not found in patients with similar symptoms who are suffering from ulcerative colitis, leading to speculation that it is the neurological damage which makes this type of injury refractory to treatment.

3.9 Medical and surgical management of radiation bowel disease

Although acute bowel reactions are traditionally managed symptomatically, with stool bulking agents, and occasionally loperamide and codeine, there have been surprisingly few formal studies to assess their efficacy. For acute radiation proctocolitis, steroid enemas and suppositories have been used in an analogous way to acute colitis, with no particular scientific evidence that they work. The sulphonamide–salicylate combination, salazopyrine, is widely used to prevent relapses in ulcerative colitis; however a recent randomised study failed to show any significant benefit in a randomised study in reducing the degree of the acute radiation induced bowel reaction, and indeed made it significantly worse in some cases [34].

Studies in the control of nausea and vomiting following abdominal radiotherapy have been limited. Even with the use of antiemetics such as metoclopramide a large proportion of patients continue to have symptoms [35]. A recent study comparing oral prochlorperazine with the 5-HT3 antagonist ondansetron [36] showed a significant improvement in the control of emesis with ondansetron, but little difference in the incidence and severity of nausea itself.

Most of the chronic reactions are self limiting, with for example minor rectal bleeding settling within 18 months in most cases [37]. Occasionally, small intestinal bacterial overgrowth may occur due to stenosis causing diarrhoea due a malabsorption syndrome. In these cases, treatment with appropriate antibiotics, cholestyramine for bile salt malabsorption and vitamin B12 injections may provide improvement [38]. One simple measure may be a trial of avoiding lactose containing products and milk — as there is a demonstrably high prevalence of lactose malabsorption due to lactase deficiency.

In general, surgical salvage of these radiation induced problems requires treatment in a specialist unit. The problems of operating in a field containing radiation induced damage in combination with a poorly nourished patient can result in a large number of complications. Surgical management comprises simply bypass or resection of the diseased area. Some suggest that bypass procedures may allow the bowel to heal, and that they may subsequently be reanastomosed [39]. Others have observed radiation induced bowel disease to be progressive even if defunctioning has been performed and radical excision of diseased bowel probably improves the overall outcome and survival [40]. The subject has been extensively reviewed [25].

3.10 Methods to reduce the radiotherapy dose to small bowel during clinical radiotherapy

During radiotherapy exposures, the small bowel is ideally continuously mobile, and hence may be moving in and out of the treatment volume, particularly for pelvic treatment. This movement is thought to be important in preventing serious small bowel morbidity. During the planning of radiotherapy treatments, simultaneous small bowel contrast radiography has been combined with X-ray simulation of the radiation fields, allowing a semi-quantitative method of assessing the volume of small bowel irradiated [41].

Many pelvic radiotherapy treatment, particularly when performed post operatively, are directed predominantly towards the pelvic lymph nodes. Unfortunately, following surgery such as antero-posterior resection the small bowel tends to prolapse into the pelvis. The situation may be exacerbated by post operative adhesions which will tend to immobilise loops of small bowel within the pelvic radiotherapy fields. There are various methods which have been applied to reduce the quantity of small bowel in the pelvis. Treating the patient prone rather than supine may reduce the amount of small bowel in the pelvis by as much as 15% [41]. Treatment with a full bladder can also reduce the small bowel exposure. most interest lies today in a variety of surgical devices which can be employed at the time of resection for reperitonalsing the pelvic floor. These range from merely suturing an omental pedicle flap in the pelvis, or the use of a prosthetic flap [41]. The technique of choice now would be the use of a polyglycolic mesh, which can suspend the intestine out of the pelvis [42]. This mesh is hydrolysed approximately three to six months after operation, and appears to be successful in excluding the small bowel in 80% of cases.

3.11 Time dose and fractionation effects on the intestine — theoretical considerations

Standard radiobiological theory can be applied to the human gut. α/β ratios are not precisely known for human tissues. Indeed, the small bowel is composed of sub-populations of cells, all having different α/β ratios. The acute effects are modulated mainly by the rapidly proliferating mucosa, and the late effects by the more slowly dividing interstitial tissues and vascular supply. Therefore, one would expect that extended radiotherapy regimens using small doses per fraction would spare the late responding tissues more than the acutely responding tissues. On the other hand, protracted regimens over a long overall time will allow repopulation of the acutely responding tissues to occur during treatment, sparing the acute rather than the late responding tissues. To a clinician the acutely responding tissues do not represent a serious problem, since they are essentially self limiting, and the treatment can be stopped if the toxicity becomes too much for the patient. The late morbidity on the other hand tends to be irreversible and causes serious morbidity and mortality.

3.12 Clinical experience in fractionation using external beam radiotherapy

There is general agreement that the late small bowel tolerance is increased by employing a smaller dose per fraction where tumour control is approximately equivalent. Much of these data is derived from comparing different fractionation regimens employed in treatment of the whole abdomen for carcinoma of the ovary, although such treatments are rarely employed today with the development of effective chemotherapy schedules. An overview of these data [43] suggested that serious late morbidity could be reduced from 8% to 3% by reducing the fraction size from 2 Gy to about 1.5 Gy (the same overall dose of 45–50 Gy applying in each case). A pattern of care study examining wide field abdominal radiation [44] reported an actuarial 3 year bowel complication rate of 2% for fraction sizes of 2 Gy or less compared with 5% for fraction sizes of greater than 2 Gy. Clearly, such data are very difficult to interpret. Shorter fractionation schedules typically employ a lower total dose, and it is not usually known whether the same degree of tumour control is achieved in all the series. In addition, the frequency with which bowel complications are recorded, particularly in retrospective series is likely to vary greatly.

Unfortunately, prospective studies which compare different fractionation schedules comparing, say treatment given in 15–20 fractions as compared to 30 fractions, and that achieve the same level of tumour control, have not been performed.

3.13 Hypofractionation studies

In certain circumstances, it might be particularly desirable to perform treatment only once weekly, for example in rural areas of India where the village women have a very long way to travel to the hospital. A study performed in India [46] compared treatment given once weekly with standard daily radiotherapy, the weekly dose being calculated from the TDF tables of Orton and Ellis. The standard dose was 40 Gy given in 20 daily fractions to a diamond shaped field, with anterior-posterior cobalt-60 fields, with a 40 Gy boost to the cervix via an Ernst applicator. The weekly arm consisted of 29 Gy in 5 high dose weekly fractions, with the same dose of 40 Gy to the cervix via intracavitary treatment. With this regimen the early reactions from the treatment were quite acceptable, indicating that it was indeed a similar dose according to early reactions. However, all the patients receiving this regimen suffered serious late morbidity from rectal complications which started about 7 months after the treatment was completed, and several of these patients died from the complications of the radiotherapy. This suggests that the α/β ratio for these late effects is relatively low. This study is at one extreme of the spectrum of regimens usually employed, and is clearly not recommended.

3.14 Hyperfractionation

The biological effects of reducing fraction sizes to less than 2 Gy, and treating the patient more than once per day are as yet far from clear. Indeed, the CHART (Continuous, hyperfractionated accelerated radiation therapy) data has shown some unexpected spinal cord toxicity in their series [46]. A study performed during radiotherapy for bladder cancer [47] compared 84 Gy in 1 Gy fractions three times daily against 64 Gy in 2 Gy fractions twice daily. Both treatments entailed a two week rest in the middle of the treatment. Local control was improved in the group receiving the hyperfractionated treatment with no increased complications.

The morbidity experienced in these studies is evidence that hyperfractionation can reduce late complications, but it is at the extreme end of the fractionation spectrum. There will continue to be controversy regarding the optimum regimens for fraction sizes, currently there being little evidence that reducing fraction sizes much below 2 Gy will reduce the small bowel complication rate still further.

3.15 Dose rate and brachytherapy in carcinoma of the cervix

There are very large amounts of clinical data available in this area. This is because carcinoma of the cervix is a frequently radiocurable condition often with a combination of external high energy photon beam treatment and brachytherapy. The patients are often relatively young and may live a long time following their treatment, hence data on long term effects of radiation will be obtained. In the treatment of carcinoma of the cervix, the cervix and paracervical tissues are often treated to a high dose using intracavitary applicators, where there is a high dose gradient. These tissues have intrinsically a low responsiveness to radiation. However, the small bowel may lie near the applicators, and the terminal ileum is most likely to be affected, particularly if a segment of small bowel is adherent to the uterus. In addition, the rectum lies just beneath the applicators, and is a frequent site of injury.

Most centres delivering radical radiotherapy for carcinoma of the cervix uterus utilise a combination of external beam radiation delivered in discrete fractions, and a radioactive implant in the form of an intracavitary applicator, which delivers radiation at a constant, but much slower dose rate. Some centres treat early FIGO stage 1 tumours with the intracavitary treatment alone, which makes the results easier to interpret. It is very difficult to compare results from different centres due to the variation in dose rate, fraction size, and the differing contribution from the external beam and intracavitary components. A system has therefore been devised to allow some degree of comparison between schedules. The ICRU 'reference volume' [48] is defined as the volume which is enclosed by the 60 Gy isodose line when the contributions from external beam and intracavitary radiation are added up. The volume thus specified is used as a guide to the overall dose.

3.16 Dose rate and remote afterloading

Where intracavitary treatment is used exclusively to treat early stage disease, there are several dose response curves available showing the overall dose correction according to the dose rate [49,50]. On the other hand, experience from Villejuif [51] suggested that there was no need to make any correction for change in dose rate when up to 80 Gy was delivered continuously in an overall time of between 3 and 7 days. Traditional Manchester brachytherapy techniques have delivered a dose to 'point A' — defined as 2 cm lateral to and 2 cm above the cervical os in the plane of the uterus of around 75 Gy over 10 days, given in two insertions with radium or caesium sources, at a dose rate of approximately 53 cGy per hour. In recent years, because of radiation protection problems, it has become necessary to introduce remote after loading systems, which require the patient to be connected to a machine throughout the treatment. Consequently a reduction in the treatment time was proposed when the systems were first introduced and the dose rate was increased to about 150 cGy per hour, or by about a factor of three. At the Christie Hospital, the new system was introduced with patients randomised between two doses — an unchanged dose of 75 Gy and a lower dose of 70 Gy [52]. It was found that there were considerably increased degrees of small bowel injury in the arm receiving the 75 Gy, and a dose reduction of 10% has been recommended (a total dose of 67.5 Gy in two fractions over 8 days). It was felt, however, that some of the complications in this series, particularly the high level of small bowel morbidity were due to the more rigid applicators and differences in the techniques used to perform the implants. In 1994 the dose reduction has been increased yet further to 15% (R.D. Hunter, pers. comm.).

More recent data from Villejuif [31] has shown a dose rate effect in patients receiving combined intracavitary and external bean treatment. A randomized study examined the effect of two low dose rates — 73 or 38 cGy per hour in 200 patients with carcinoma of the cervix up to stage 11. Complications were recorded as recommended by the Franco Italian glossary [53]. The overall level of complications was about 70%, a level which reflects the systematic recording of all complications. Late complications were more frequent in the high dose rate group, although statistical significance was only reached for the minor complications. There was no effect of the dose rate upon early reactions.

It is important to separate these low and medium dose rate studies from the 'high dose rate' afterloading systems, where the dose rate is more than 1 Gy per minute. There is unlikely to be significant repair of sublethal damage during the treatment, which will only last a number of minutes for each dose. If this type of system is adopted, then it is essential to fractionate the treatment in the same way as external beam treatment. A randomized trial has been performed [54] comparing high and low dose rate systems, where there was both higher local control and a higher complication rate in the high dose rate group. In this case, it would appear that there was considerable scope for a dose reduction in the high dose rate arm, and most other studies have found acceptable results by both increasing the number of fractions and reducing the overall dose by 30–40%. In a study comparing high dose rate with 'medium' dose rate, total of 42 Gy delivered in 6 fractions at 1 Gy/min gave fewer complications than 60 Gy in 3 fractions at 3 Gy per hour [55].

4. ANUS

4.1 Clinical features of delivering radiotherapy to the anus

In recent years it has become realised that tumours of the anus are radiosensitive, and that the results from radiotherapy are as good or better than those of AP resection. However, anal tumours are quite rare; more frequently the low rectal/anal region is treated with radiotherapy during treatment for carcinoma of the prostate.

Nearly all patients having radiotherapy to the anus will experience an acute, but self limiting perineal skin reaction. At doses of 40 Gy given in 2 Gy fractions five days per week with parallel opposed fields to the whole area, moist desquamation is common after about three weeks. It is thought that the toxicity from combining chemotherapy with the radiotherapy does not result in a vastly increased rate of complications [56]. Probably the most common reason for anal cancers to heal inadequately after radiation is that the resulting tissue defect following regression of the tumour is so large. At the Christie Hospital, doses of 55–60 Gy over 7 days resulted in a large number of necroses and about 6% of the patients required AP resection [57].

Ulceration in the anal canal may occur and cause pain, sometimes only on defecation, but in others it is persistent [25]. The onset of radiation necrosis is heralded by the development of intense pain. Conservative measures usually fail and antero-posterior resection of the rectum may eventually be required.

5. ACCIDENTAL AND WHOLE BODY EXPOSURE — THE GASTROINTESTINAL SYNDROME

5.1 Whole body radiation — overview

Gastrointestinal tract damage may cause death when the whole body is exposed to large doses of radiation. Mammals exposed to large single doses of radiation exhibit three peaks of death at differing time intervals following the radiation, and this has lead to the classification of three syndromes: the cerebrovascular syndrome, the gastrointestinal syndrome and the haemopoeitic syndrome. Although this is well established in experimental animals, human data at higher doses are sparse [58]. The differing time courses of these syndromes reflects the differing cycling times of the renewing tissues of the gut and the bone marrow.

5.2 Availability of data

There is a considerable amount of data available now from both therapeutic and accidental sources [1]: the atomic bomb survivors of world war two, the Japanese fishermen who were irradiated during the tests at Bikini Atoll, and more recently those surviving the nuclear accident at Chernobyl. In addition, total body irradiation is now routine in preparing patients for bone marrow transplants, be they allografts or autologous transplants.

The doses received in nuclear accidents, or in the atomic bomb survivors, differ considerably from those in clinical radiotherapy, since they may be highly non uniform, and may also be from a combination of different kinds of radiation of differing LET. In preparation for bone marrow transplant radiotherapy may be given either as a single fraction at low dose rate (e.g., 0.15 Gy/min, total dose 7.5 Gy mid plane dose or as a fractionated regimen, e.g., 12 Gy in 6 fractions over three days) [59]. However, the doses used in preparation for bone marrow transplant are well below the level that will cause a significant gastrointestinal syndrome, although some degree of mucositis and diarrhoea is to be expected.

5.3 Prodromal syndrome

The initial response is the prodromal radiation syndrome which occurs within a few minutes of exposure. This is of significance only at doses likely to cause death. At about a 50% lethal dose ($LD_{50/30}$), extreme fatigue, nausea , anorexia and vomiting are likely. After a supralethal dose there is likely to be fever, hypotension, and immediate diarrhoea. At supralethal doses, the effect is probably mediated through the autonomic nervous system and provokes the gastrointestinal and neuromuscular syndrome respectively. The symptoms are nausea, vomiting, diarrhoea, and cramps initially and these are followed by fatigue, apathy, listlessness, sweating, and finally hypotension and shock. Clinically half body irradiation at doses between 3 and 10 Gy can produce a milder version of the same syndrome [60]. The radiation induced vomiting may be partly caused by the effect of radiation on the chemoreceptor trigger zone and the vomiting centre, and partly by a direct effect on the stomach [61].

5.4 Gastrointestinal syndrome

The gastrointestinal syndrome occurs in animals at single doses of between 10 and 50 Gy [63] and the symptoms merge with that of the prodromal phase. These include anorexia, lethargy, diarrhoea, infection and loss of fluids and electrolytes. It is exacerbated by the decrease in the leukocyte count with haemorrhages and bacteraemia. The clinical effects of the syndrome are, however, rather difficult to dissect from the effects on the other organs.

Post mortem examination of the gut of some of the Japanese atomic bomb victims [63] showed an oedematous mucosa, with atypical epithelial cells, and a tendency to ulceration after one week. The villus system becomes depleted with the loss of reproductive capacity of the clonogenic cells in the crypts. These finding are similar to those expected after radiotherapy to the gut alone (see Sections 3.2 and 3.3). Along with these pathological changes are clinical effects, most significantly fluid and protein loss into the bowel lumen. The patient may then develop liquid stools with bleeding, followed by circulatory collapse and death.

Clearly the time course of the gastrointestinal toxicity depends on the transit time from the crypts to the tip of the villus where the cells are shed and within the dose range of 10–50 Gy appears to be more or less independent of dose. There are two peaks in time of death after the atomic bomb explosion [63], the first peak at 6–9 days corresponding to the gastrointestinal syndrome, and the second peak at 20–30 days corresponding to bone marrow death. I

In animals it has been shown that it is possible to delay these early deaths with best supportive care, although this has not been shown conclusively in humans even after the experience at Chernobyl.

5.5 Time dose and fractionation

Dose–response curves together with some information on fractionation are available for the prodromal responses to whole body irradiation. This prodromal syndrome has been shown to demonstrate a pronounced fractionation effect. A retrospective study [64] of patients receiving total body irradiation showed little in the way of symptoms either at very low dose rate (less than 30 cGy per day) or at doses per fraction of less than 20 cGy.

Some experience in clinical radiotherapy is available, but as previously mentioned, the gastrointestinal tract is not the dose limiting system, and it is the risk of pulmonary fibrosis which is the most feared late complication. The generally accepted tolerance dose is about 12 Gy delivered in six 2 Gy fractions, often over a time period of 3 days.

5.6 Experience from the Chernobyl accident

Prior to the Chernobyl experience, there was only one case of human gastrointestinal death reported in the literature [58]. Further experience has been gained from the Chernobyl accident and this has been reported to the United Nations [65].

At Chernobyl, workers in the plant were exposed to short-term external radiation from the gas emission cloud, radiation from the fragments of damaged reactor core scattered over the industrial site, inhalation of gases and aerosol dust particles and deposits on the skin. The most significant factor was a relatively uniform whole body irradiation (gamma) and beta radiation of body surfaces.

Diagnosis of radiation sickness was made by observation for the prodromal syndrome of nausea and vomiting and observing for skin erythema and a drop in the lymphocyte count. In all cases radionuclide ingestion was below the level which could be expected to give radiation syndrome. The dose calculations could now be made according to the number of chromosome abberations in a blood lymphocytes culture, using a dose response curve derived from patients receiving TBI for acute leukaemia.

In 10 of the patients, diarrhoea was observed from day 4–8. This suggested that the total gamma dose had been 10 Gy or above, and in fact all these patients subsequently died in the three weeks following irradiation. Other persons developing diarrhoea after eight days were supported with protein, fluids and electrolytes, and probably did not die from the gastrointestinal system. Patients who were suffering from acute radiation induced enteritis responded well to total parenteral nutrition.

6. CONCLUSIONS

The human gastrointestinal tract is a self renewing tissue in a steady state of self replacement. The acute responses to radiation are a result of a disturbance of this balance, with the production of new cells interrupted. This response varies throughout the gastrointestinal tract according to the renewal times of the mucosa. The late responses to radiation also vary throughout the gut, and are dependant upon the responses of the supportive and connective tissues. The tolerances doses of radiation are greatest in the rectum, are rather less in the small bowel, and least in the stomach. This has had wide implications for clinical radiotherapy, and critically limits the use of radiotherapy in the upper abdomen.

References

1.   United Nations Scientific Committee on the Effects of Atomic Radiation (1988) Sources, effects and risks of ionizing radiation, Report to the General Assembly.

United Nations Publication.

2. Barry, R. (1974) Malignancy, weight loss and the small intestinal mucosa. Gut 15, 562–570.
3. Harig, J., Soergel, K., et al. (1989) Treatment of diversion colitis with short chain fatty acid irrigation. New Engl. J. Med. 320, 23–28.
4. Goldgraber, M., et al. (1954) The early gastric response to irradiation — a serial biopsy study. Gastroenterology 27, 1–20.
5. Wiernik, G. and Plant, M. (1970) Radiation effects on the human intestinal mucosa. Curr. Top. Rad. Res. 38, 598–613.
6. Wiernik, G. (1966) Radiation damage and repair in the human jejunal mucosa. J. Pathol. 91, 499–513.
7. Tarpila, S. (1971) Morphological and functional response of the human small intestinal mucosa to ionizing radiation. Scand. J. Gastroenterol. 6, 1.
8. Trier, J. and Browing, T. (1966) Morphologic response of the mucosa of human small intestine to X ray exposure. J. Clin. Invest. 45, 194–204.
9. Gelfand, M.D., Tepper, M. et al. (1968) Acute irradiation proctitis in man. Gastroenterology 54, 401–411.
10. Hamilton, F.E. (1947) Gastric ulcer following irradiation. Arch. Surg. 55, 394–399.
11. Becciolini, A. (1987) Relative radiosensitivities of the small and large intestine. Adv. Radiat. Biol. 12, 83–121.
12. Ricketts, W.E. et al. (1948) Radiation therapy of peptic ulcer. Gastroenterology 11, 789–806.
13. Rodgers, L. and Goldstein, H. (1977) Roentgen manifestations of radiation injury to the gastrointestinal tract. Gastrointestinal Radiol. 2, 281–291.
14. Berthroung, M. and Farjardo, L. (1981) Radiation injury in surgical pathology, 11: Alimentary tract. Am. J. Surg. Pathol. 5, 153–178.
15. Rubin, P. and Casarett, G.W. (1968) Clinical Radiation Pathology. Saunders, Philadelphia, PA.
16. Gunderson, L. and Martenson, J. (1989) Gastrointestinal tract tolerance. Front. Radiat. Ther. Oncol. 23, 277–298.
17. O'Connel, M.J., Gunderson, L.L. et al. (1985) A pilot study to determine clinical tolerability of intensive combined modality therapy for locally unresectable gastric cancer. Int. J. Radiat. Oncol. Biol. Phys. 11, 1827–1831.
18. Wright, N.A. and Alison, M. (1984) The Biology of Epithelial Cell Populations. Clarendon Press, Oxford, pp. 634–672.
19. Kellett, M., Potten, C.S. and Rew, D.A. (1992) A comparison of *in vivo* cell proliferation measurements in the intestine of mouse and man. Epith. Cell Biol. 1, 147–155.
20. Macdonald, W., Trier, J. et al. (1963) Cell proliferation and migration in the stomach, duodenum and rectum of man: radioautographic studies. Gastroenterology 46, 405–417.
21. Smith, D.H. and DeCosse, J.J. (1986) Radiation damage to the small intestine. World J. Surg. 10, 189–194.
22. Danjoux, C.E. and Catton, G.E. (1979) Delayed complications in colorectal carcinoma treated by combination radiotherapy and 5FU ECOG study. Int. J. Radiat. Oncol. Biol. Phys. 5, 331–316.
23. Fonkalsud, E., Sanchez, M. et al. (1977) Serial changes in arterial structure following radiation therapy. Surgery Gynaecol. Obstetr. 145, 395–400.
24. Newman, A. et al. (1973) Small intestinal injury in women who have had pelvic

radiotherapy. Lancet ii, 1471–1473.

25. Schofield, P.F. (1989) Treatment of radiation induced bowel disease. In: P.F. Schofield and E. Lupton (Eds.), The Causation and Clinical Management of Pelvic Radiation Disease. Springer Verlag.

26. DeCosse, J., Rhodes, R. et al. (1969) The natural history and management of radiation induced injury of the gastrointestinal tract. Ann. Surg. 170, 369–384.

27. Carr, N.D. and Holden, D. (1989) Experimental findings in radiation bowel disease. In: P.F. Schofield and E. Lupton (Eds.), The Causation and Clinical Management of Pelvic Radiation Disease. Springer Verlag.

28. Haboubi, N.Y., Schofield, P.F. and Rowland, P. (1988) The light and electron microscopic features of early and late phase radiation induced proctitis. Am. J. Gastroenterol. 3, 1140–1144.

29. Mendelson, R.M. and Nolan, D.J. (1985) The radiological features of chronic radiation enteritis. Clin. Radiol. 36, 141–148.

30. Taylor, P.M., Johson, R.J. and Eddleson, B. (1989) Radiology of radiation injury. In: P.F. Schofield and E. Lupton (Eds.), The Causation and Clinical Management of Pelvic Radiation Disease. Springer Verlag.

31. Lambin, P. et al. (1993) Phase 111 trial comparing two low dose rates in brachytherapy of cervix carcinoma. Int. J. Radiat. Oncol. Biol. Phys. 25, 405–412.

32. Yeoh, E., Horowitz, M. et al. (1993) A retrospective study of the effects of pelvic irradiation for carcinoma of the cervix on gastrointestinal function. Int. J. Radiat. Oncol. Biol. Phys. 26, 229–237.

33. Varma, J.S. et al. (1985) Correlation of clinical and manometric abnormalities of rectal function following chronic radiation injury. Br. J. Surg. 72, 875–878.

34. Baughan, C., Canney, P. et al. (1993) A randomized trial to assess the efficacy of 5-aminosalicylic acid for the prevention of radiation enteritis. Clin. Oncol. 5, 19–24.

35. Priestman, S., Priestman, T. and Canney, P. (1987) A double blind randomised cross over comparison of nabilone and metoclopramide in the control of radiation induced nausea. Clin. Rad. 38, 543–4.

36. Priestman, T., Roberts, J. and Upadhyaya, B.K. (1993) A prospective randomized double blind trial comparing ondansetron versus porochlorperazine for the prevention of nausea and vomiting in patients undergoing fractionated radiotherapy. Clin. Oncol. 5, 358–363.

37. Gilinsky. N., Burns, D. et al. (1983) The natural history of radiation induced proctosigmoiditis. Q. J. Med. 52, 40–53.

38. Beer, W.H., Fan, A. et al. (1985) Clinical and nutritional implications of radiation enteritis. Am. J. Clin. Nutrition 41, 85–91.

39. Wobbes, T. et al. (1984) Surgical aspects of radiation enteritis of the small bowel. Dis. Colon Rectum 27, 89–92.

40. Rubin, P. (1984) Late effects of chemotherapy and radiation therapy. Int. J. Radiat. Oncol. Biol. Phys. 10, 5–34.

41. Green, N. (1983) The avoidance of small intestine injury in gynaecologic cancer. Int. J. Radiat. Oncol. Biol. Phys. 9, 1385–1390.

42. Devereux, D.F., Thompson, D. et al. (1986) Protection from radiation enteritis by an absorbable polyglycolic acid mesh sling. Surgery 101, 123–129.

43. Smalley, S.R. and Evans, R.G. (1991) Radiation morbidity to the gastrointestinal tract and liver. In: P.N. Plowman (Ed.), Complications of Radiation Therapy. Butterworth Heinemann, Oxford

44. Coia, L. and Hanks, G. (1988) Complications from large field intermediate dose

infradiaphragmatic radiation, an analysis of the patterns of care outcome studies for Hodgkin's disease and seminoma. Int. J. Radiat. Oncol. Biol. Phys. 15, 29–35.

45. Singh, K. (1978) Two regimens with the same TDF but differing morbidity used in the treatment of stage 111 carcinoma of the cervix. Br. J. Radiol. 51, 357–362.

46. Pigott, K., Dische, S. and Saunders, M. (1993) The long term outcome after radical radiotherapy for advanced head and neck cancer (continuous hyperfractionated accelerated radiotherapy). Clin. Oncol. 5, 343–349.

47. Edsmyr, F., Anderson, L., Esposti, P. et al. (1985) Irradiation therapy with multiple small fractions per day in urinary bladder cancer. Radiother. Oncol. 4, 197–203.

48. International Committee on Radiation Units and Measurements (1985) Dose and volume specification for reporting intracavitary therapy in gynaecology. ICRU Report No. 38, Bethesda, MD.

49. Paterson, R. (1963) Treatment of Malignant Disease by Radiotherapy. Williams and Wilkins Co., Baltimore, MD.

50. Ellis, F. (1968) Dose time and fractionation in radiotherapy. In: M. Elbert and A. Howard (Eds.), Current Topics in Radiation Research 4, Elsevier, pp. 359–397.

51. Pierquin, B. (1970) L'effet differentiel de l'irradiation continué a faible debit des carcinomas epidermoides. J. Rad. Electrol. 51, 533–53649.

52. Sherrah Davies, E. (1985) Morbidity following low dose rate selectron therapy for carcinoma of the cervix. Clin. Radiol. 36, 131–139.

53. Chassagne, D. Sismondi, P., Horiot, J.C. et al. (1988) A Glossary for Reporting Treatment Complication in Gynaecological Cancers. ESTRO 7th Annual Meeting, The Hague, Sept. 5–8, 1988.

54. Shigematsu, Y., Nishiyama, K., Masaki, N. et al. (1983) Treatment of carcinoma of the uterine cervix by remotely controlled afterloading intracavitary radiotherapy with a high dose rate. Int. J. Radiat. Oncol. Biol. Phys. 9, 351.

55. Glaser, F.H. (1988) Comparison of HDR afterloading with 192 Ir vs conventional radium therapy in cervix cancer, 5 year results and complications. In: H. Vahrson and G. Rauthe (Eds.), High Dose Rate Afterloading in the Treatment of the Cancer of the Uterus, Breast and Rectum. Urban and Schwarzenberg, Munich.

56. United Kingdom Council for Coordination of Cancer Research (1994) Preliminary results of a randomised trial comparing radiotherapy with chemoradiotherapy in carcinoma of the anus. Medical Research Council Cancer Trials Office Newsletter, Cambridge.

57. James, R.D., Pointon, R.C.S. and Martin, S. (1985) Local radiotherapy in the management of squamous cell carcinoma of the anus. Br. J. Surg. 72, 282–285.

58. Hall, E. (1994) Radiobiology for the Radiologist, 4th ed. Lippincott.

59. Quast, U. (1987) Total body irradiation, review of treatment techniques in Europe. Radiother. Oncol. 9, 91–106.

60. Salazar, O.M., Rubin, B., Kelloer, B. et al. (1978) Systematic half body radiation therapy — response and toxicity. Int. J. Radiat. Oncol. Biol. Phys. 4, 937–950.

61. Harding, R.K. and Davis, C.J. (1986) Progress in the elucidation of the mechanisms of radiation induced vomiting. Int. J. Radiat. Oncol. Biol. Phys. 50, 947–950.

62. Bond, V.P. and Fliedner (1965) Mammalian Radiation Lethality — A Disturbance in Cellular Kinetics. Academic Press, New York.

63. Oughterson, A.W. and Warren, S. (1956) Medical Effects of the Atomic Bomb in Japan. McGraw-Hill, New York.

64. Lushbaugh, C. (1982) The impact of estimates of human radiation tolerance upon radiation emergency management. In: The Control of Exposure of the Public to

Ionizing Radiation in the Event of Accident or Attack, Proceedings of a Symposium held in April 1981, NCRP.

65. Guskova, A.K. (Ed.) (1988) Acute radiation effects in victims of the Chernobyl nuclear power plant accident. Appendix, United Nations Scientific Committee on the Effects of Atomic Radiation Sources, effects and risks of ionizing radiation, Report to the General Assembly. United Nations Publication.

C.S. Potten and J.H. Hendry (Eds.), *Radiation and Gut*
1995 Elsevier Science B.V.

CHAPTER 9

Ingested Radionuclides

J.D. Harrison

National Radiological Protection Board, Chilton, Didcot, Oxon. OX11 0RQ, UK

1. INTRODUCTION

This chapter provides a review of the behaviour of ingested radionuclides, their absorption from the gastrointestinal (GI) tract and distribution and retention in other tissues. Doses to the GI tract are compared with doses to other tissues and contributions to total cancer risk assessed. The limited available data on effects of ingested radionuclides are discussed.

Doses to the GI tract from an ingested radionuclide will depend on the type and energy of emissions, radioactive half-life, the proportion absorbed and the route of excretion from the systemic circulation. In addition, transit times will vary between individuals and with age, and retention of nuclides in the wall of the GI tract may be important, particularly in newborn infants. The absorption of radionuclides from the GI tract will depend on the chemical nature of the element concerned and the chemical form in which it is ingested. The distribution and retention of the proportion absorbed will again depend on the chemical nature of the element and its similarity to elements that have a functional role in the body. For example, strontium and radium are chemically similar to calcium and behave qualitatively in the same way; that is, their main site of deposition is bone mineral. Both absorption and the subsequent distribution and retention of radionuclides may be affected by the age of the individual. In general, absorption is greatest in infants and loss from tissues and excretion may be more rapid in children than in adults.

The International Commission on Radiological Protection (ICRP) have recently published revised estimates of radiation risks, based largely on reassessments of the incidence of cancer in the survivors of the atomic bombs at Hiroshima and Nagasaki [1]. Specific risk estimates for cancer of the oesophagus, stomach and colon are now included and the overall estimate of fatal cancer risk has increased from 0.0125 Sv^{-1} in the 1977 recommendations [2] to 0.05 Sv^{-1} for the general public in the 1990 recommendations [1]. This new risk estimate means that, for example, if 2000 people were all exposed to 0.01 Sv, one additional cancer would be expected compared to a similar unexposed group.

Doses from intakes of radionuclides are the subject of a number of ICRP publications. Publication 30 [3–6] is concerned with doses from occupational exposures by either inhalation or ingestion. An ICRP Task Group is currently considering doses to members of the public including children; doses from the ingestion of radionuclides are addressed in Publications 56 [7], 67 [8] and 69 [9]. Publication 30 [3] includes a dosimetric model of the GI tract in which doses are calculated for the stomach, small intestine, upper large intestine and lower large intestine. Revisions to the model have been suggested on the basis of more recent data on transit times and the behaviour of different phases in the GI tract [10]. It is likely that ICRP will publish a revised model of the GI tract which will include doses to the oesophagus and the colon.

In the following sections, the ICRP model of the GI tract together with suggested revisions are discussed. General information is given on the absorption, distribution and retention of radionuclides and the ICRP terms, equivalent and effective dose are outlined. Elements with important radioisotopes are then considered separately: hydrogen (H), cobalt (Co), strontium (Sr), zirconium (Zr), niobium (Nb), ruthenium (Ru), iodine (I), caesium (Cs), cerium (Ce), lead (Pb), polonium (Po), radium (Ra), thorium (Th), uranium (U), neptunium (Np), plutonium (Pu) and americium (Am). In each case, the distribution of dose between tissues is considered and, in particular, the dose to the GI tract. On this basis, the relative risk of GI tract cancer for the different radionuclides is assessed. Finally, the available data on effects of ingested radionuclides are discussed; these studies have provided information on acute effects for different radiation types but no useful data on cancer induction.

2. DOSIMETRIC MODELS OF THE GI TRACT

In 1966, Eve [11] reviewed data on the transit of materials through the GI tract and other parameters necessary to calculate doses. Transit times were based largely on information from clinical studies using barium meals but also included reference to studies using materials labelled with iron-59 or lanthanum-140. These data provided the basis for the dosimetric model of the GI tract in ICRP Publication [3]. It is a catenary model with four compartments: the stomach, small intestine, upper large intestine and lower large intestine (Fig. 1). The model allows for time-varying input to the stomach and one-way intercompartmental transfer with first order kinetics. The absorption of materials to blood is taken to occur in the small intestine. The transfer rate coefficients for movement of intestinal contents are equal to the reciprocal of the mean residence times, taken to be 1 h for the stomach, 4 h for the small intestine, 13 h for the upper large intestine and 24 h for the lower large intestine (Table 1) on the basis of observed ranges of 25–120 min, 1–7 h, 6–22 h and 15–72 h, respectively.

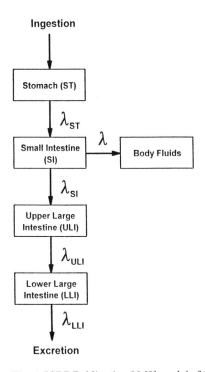

Ingestion

Excretion

Fig. 1. ICRP Publication 30 [3] model of the GI tract.

TABLE 1

Parameters for ICRP Publication 30 model of the GI tract

Section of GI tract	Mass of walls (g)	Mass of contents (g)	Mean residence time (day)	Transfer rate (day^{-1})
Stomach	150	250	1/24	24
Small intestine (SI)	640	400	4/24	6
Upper large intestine	210	220	13/24	1.8
Lower large intestine	160	135	24/24	1

Doses are calculated separately for the mucosal layer of each region of the GI tract. For penetrating radiations, the average dose to the wall of each region is used as a measure of the dose to the mucosal layer. For non-penetrating radiations, the fraction absorbed by the mucosal layer is taken to be equal to $0.5 \, v/M$ where M is the mass of the contents of that section of the GI tract and v is a factor between 0 and 1 representing the proportion of energy reaching

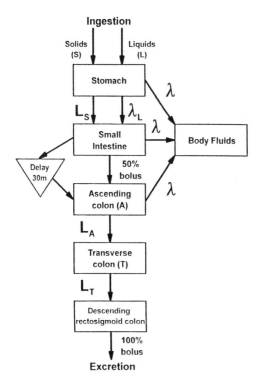

Fig. 2. Stubbs [10] model of the GI tract.

sensitive cells. The factor of 0.5 is introduced because the dose at the surface of the contents will be approximately half that within the contents for non-penetrating radiations. For β particles, v is taken to be 1. For α particles, a value of 0.01 is used. This value of 0.01 is arbitrary, the experimental evidence that it is warranted being from an acute toxicity study in rats in which LD_{50} for ingested yttrium-91 was estimated as about 12 Gy while a dose to the mucosal surface of more than 100 times greater from [239]Pu had no effect [12].

Recently, a revised GI transit model has been developed (Fig. 2) on the basis of a substantial body of new data obtained by non-invasive scintigraphic procedures [10]. These techniques have the advantage of avoiding any possible disturbance of normal GI motility. Currently, transit through the oesophagus is not included but this will be considered in developing the model for ICRP [10]. Removal from the stomach to the small intestine is described by a combination of zero and first order kinetics. Because liquid emptying is a first order process, the gastric emptying of liquids is best modelled by an exponential function of time. In contrast, the emptying of solids is thought to be a linear or zero-order process. Gastric emptying half-times were found to vary over a wide range; the values adopted in the model are 30 min for liquids and 60 min for solids. Transit through the small intestine is taken to be independent of the gastric emptying rates. A transit time of 4 h is assumed. Upon filling of the terminal ileum, (gastric emptying time plus SI transit time of 4 h) the model assumes that 50% of the activity is transferred to the ascending colon in a single bolus and that the remaining activity is transferred 30 min later as a bolus. The model partitions the large intestine into the ascending colon (AC), transverse colon (TC) and the descending/rectosigmoid colon (DRC). The activity transferred to the AC is assumed to be instantaneously uniformly distributed and completely retained during a 30 min cecal filling time interval. The transit times through the AC and TC are taken to be 8.4 h and 7.3 h, respectively. Elimination of activity from the GI tract is assumed to occur at 15.9 h after complete emptying of the transverse colonic contents to the descending colon. The model allows for absorption to blood from the stomach, small intestine and ascending colon.

The differences between the ICRP [3] model of the GI tract and the Stubbs [10] model have not yet been fully assessed. However, it would appear that the effect on mean residence times and doses to the different regions will not be large. For the example of the radionuclide, ^{99m}Tc, ingested in a non-absorbable form such as sulphur colloid, the largest differences in residence time would be for the small intestine with a 44% increase in the revised model.

Sex and age differences in transit times have been reported. There is a growing body of data that suggest that there is slowing of colonic transit in women during different stages of the menstrual cycle. Rao et al. [13] described a 78% increase in total colonic transit times for women in the follicular phase compared with normal males. Arhau et al. [14] reported that both segmental and total colonic transit times are shorter (26%) in children under 15 years of age relative to normal males.

3. GASTROINTESTINAL ABSORPTION

In the ICRP [3] model of the GI tract, the absorption of radionuclides is assumed to occur instantaneously from the small intestine. The level of absorption varies widely between different elements, depending on their chemical nature, with virtually complete absorption of iodine and caesium, for example, and less than 0.1% for the actinide elements, plutonium and americium. The chemical form of an ingested element might affect the absorption of some elements with the general observation that incorporation into food may lead to greater absorption than ingestion of inorganic forms of an element. There is good evidence from animal experiments, with supporting human data for some elements, that the absorption of a large number of elements is greater in newborn mammals than in adults.

ICRP Publication 30 [3–6] recommended values for the fractional absorption (f_1 values) of elements and their radioisotopes, specifically applying to occupational exposure of workers. An Expert Group set up by the Committee on Radiation Protection and Public Health of the Nuclear Energy Agency (NEA),

Organisation for Economic Cooperation and Development, reviewed data on the absorption of elements with radioisotopes considered important in the context of environmental exposures of members of the public [15]. They proposed the use of values greater than the ICRP Publication 30 values for a number of elements ingested in food and also proposed values for absorption in the first year of life.

Greater intestinal permeability in the immediate postnatal period is considered to be a general phenomenon, with information showing greater absorption for 18 of the 31 elements considered by the NEA Expert Group [15]. A number of factors, including the milk diet, may contribute to this increased availability of elements for absorption but the pinocytotic activity associated with the uptake of intact gamma globulins from milk [16,17] is thought to have an important role [18–21]. The acquisition of passive immunity by this process occurs in many mammalian species including mice, rats, hamsters, dogs and cattle. However, prenatal transfer of antibodies, through the yolk sac or placenta, also occurs in some species and is the predominant, or only, mechanism in man and other primates, rabbits and guinea pigs. Nevertheless, it would appear that the GI tract of these species, while being impermeable to gamma globulin molecules, is not fully mature and does allow the passage of other large molecules and polymers [22–24].

A general approach to the choice of infant f_1 values was proposed by NEA [15]. For absorption values between 0.01 and 0.5 in the adult, an increase by a factor of two was applied as an average for the first year. For values in the adult of 0.001 or less, an increase by a factor of ten was assumed. Adult values of between 0.001 and 0.01 were rounded to 0.01 by NEA [15]. An f_1 value of 0.1, for example, means that a fraction of 0.1 (10%) of the total ingested is absorbed from the GI tract to blood while the remaining fraction of 0.9 (90%) passes on unabsorbed through the GI tract to be eliminated from the body in the faeces.

Table 2 shows the elements considered by NEA [15] and the f_1 values proposed for adult members of the public and for infants. The adult values were taken to be applicable to children from one year of age. The infant values were proposed as averages for the first year of life although it is likely that their application to absorption in weaned children towards the end of the first year will be conservative. For Fe, Co, Sr and Pb, although it was recognised that absorption might exceed adult values at some periods during childhood, the adult value of 0.3 was considered to be sufficiently conservative to allow for these changes.

An ICRP Task Group is currently considering the biokinetics and dosimetry of intakes of radionuclides by members of the public. In Part 1, ICRP Publication 56 [7], data were published for H, C, I, Cs, Ru, Zr, Nb, Ce, Np, Pu and Am. For Part 2, ICRP Publication 67 [8] the elements considered were Co, Te, Ni, Ag, Po, Zn, Tc, S, Mo, Pb, Ra, Ba and Sr. For Part 3, ICRP Publication 69 [9], the elements are Fe, Se, Sb, Th and U. Table 3 summarises the f_1 values adopted. In general, the NEA [15] approach has been adopted to obtain f_1 values for infants in the first year of life. Unlike NEA [15], ICRP [7–9] have specified

TABLE 2

NEA f_1 values for members of the public

Element	Adult	Infant
I, Cs	1	1
Se, Tc	0.8	0.8
Fe, Co, Sr, Pb, Po	0.3	0.6
Ra	0.2	0.4
Sb, Ba	0.1	0.2
Ru, U	0.05	0.1
Sn	0.02	0.04
Zr, Nb, Pa	0.01	0.02
Y, La, Th, Np, Pu, Am, Cm	0.001	0.01

f_1 is the fraction of the total ingested that is absorbed to blood.

TABLE 3

ICRP f_1 values for members of the public

Element	Adult	Infant
H, C, I, Cs, S, Mo	1	1
Se	0.8	1
Zn, Tc, Po	0.5	1
Te, Sr*	0.3	0.6
Ba*, Ra*, Pb*	0.2	0.6
Co*, Fe*	0.1	0.6
Sb	0.1	0.2
Ru, Ni, Ag	0.05	0.1
U	0.02	0.04
Zr, Nb	0.01	0.02
Ce, Th, Np, Pu, Am	0.0005	0.005

*Intermediate values for 1, 5, 10, 15 year old children: Sr, Pb, 0.4; Co, Ra, Ba, 0.3; Fe, 0.2.
f_1 is the fraction of the total ingested that is absorbed to blood.

intermediate values for children for a number of elements (Co, Fe, Sr, Ba, Ra and Pb).

The increased absorption of elements observed in the immediate postnatal period is associated with high levels of intestinal retention in some mammalian species [7,15,18]. The levels of intestinal retention in different species appear to be related to the extent of pinocytotic activity. Table 4 compares the retention of [238]Pu in the small intestine of rats and guinea pigs [24]. Autoradiographic

TABLE 4

Intestinal retention of ^{238}Pu in newborn animals

Species	Age at ingestion (d)	Time after ingestion (d)	% Ingested activity in		
			1*	2*	3*
Rat	6	5	0.03	5.5	16.7
	12	5	0.01	4.6	36.3
Guinea pig	6	5	0.006	0.007	0.009
	12	5	0.008	0.009	0.009

*1, 2 and 3 refer to three equal lengths of small intestine.

studies show that for rats (Fig. 3A), as for pigs, the high levels of retention are confined mainly to the epithelial cells [7,18]. The kinetics of loss have been considered as a dynamic process involving the normal migration and sloughing of epithelial cells from the tips of villi. In guinea pigs (Fig. 3B), baboons and macaca, low levels of Pu are retained mainly in macrophages in the lacteal region in the tips of the villi [7,18]. It seems reasonable on current evidence to assume that retention in newborn children is most likely to resemble that in primates and guinea pigs.

4. DISTRIBUTION TO TISSUES AND EXCRETION

Radionuclides absorbed from the GI tract into body fluids, and circulated in blood, are then transferred to body tissues depending on their chemical nature. While this process is taking place, the radionuclides are regarded as being in the "transfer compartment" and are assumed by ICRP to be distributed uniformly throughout the whole body [3,7]. Distribution and retention in body tissues may be age-dependent and in general retention half-times tend to be shorter at younger ages. For those radionuclides where sufficient data are available, this age dependence has been taken into account in ICRP models as well as the smaller masses of body tissues and organs [3,7]. If insufficient age-specific data are available adult biokinetic parameters are adopted for all ages. The age groups considered by ICRP are 3 month-old infants, 1 year, 5 year, 10 year and 15 year-old children, and adults.

Estimates of the overall proportions of urinary and faecal excretion are also given in the most recent ICRP models for most elements [7–9]. This ratio is not intended for the interpretation of bioassay measurements but is necessary for dose calculations because the cancer risk from irradiation of the urinary bladder and the colon are considered explicitly in the new ICRP recommendations [1]. Age-

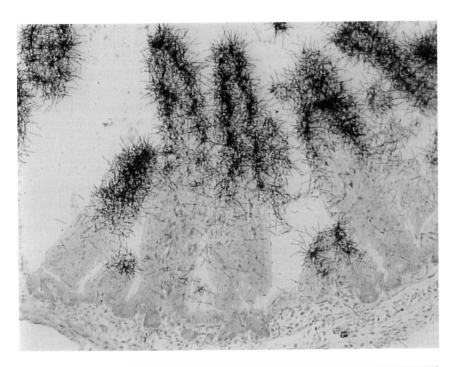

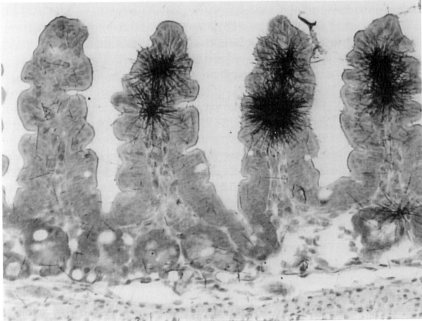

Fig. 3. Autoradiographs showing the retention of ^{238}Pu in the villi of the small intestine of newborn rats (A) and guinea pigs (B).

specific parameters for urine flow rates and the size of the bladder are used to calculate doses [8]. The fraction excreted in the faeces is assumed to pass through the large intestine. For the alkaline earths and actinide elements, dynamic models have been introduced which consider the time course of urinary and faecal excretion [8].

If a radionuclide has radioactive decay products, the contribution to dose from their build-up in the body is considered by ICRP [7–9]. However, specific biokinetic data are given for these only when experimental evidence is available on their biological behaviour (e.g. iodine daughters of tellurium). In all other cases the biokinetic behaviour of the radioactive decay products is assumed to be the same as that of the parent radionuclide taken into the body.

Doses within the skeleton are calculated taking account of the distribution of radionuclides and sensitive cells. The radiation-sensitive parts of the skeleton are taken to be the red bone marrow and a layer of cells in the inner bone surface (endosteal cells) [3]. In adults, red bone marrow is contained exclusively in the trabecular or "spongy" bone which constitutes, for example, the vertebrae and the ends of the long bones. Cortical or compact bone, which constitutes the shafts of the long bones, contains only inactive fatty marrow in the adult. Radionuclides are classified as bone-surface or bone-volume seekers and they are respectively assumed to remain on endosteal surfaces or be distributed uniformly throughout bone mineral for the duration of their retention. Clearly, this will affect the doses received by the two target tissues, particularly for alpha and beta particle irradiation.

The assumptions of either surface or volume distribution of radionuclides in bone takes no account of their movement between different skeletal components as a result of bone turnover and growth. In addition, the distribution of red marrow in bone changes with age, completely filling marrow spaces in young children and subsequently being progressively lost from cortical regions. Dynamic models for the skeleton developed by Leggett and his colleagues [25–28] have been adopted by ICRP [7–9] for the main groups of bone-seeking radionuclides, those of the alkaline earth elements, barium, radium and strontium, and the actinides, plutonium, americium, neptunium, thorium and uranium. The alkaline earth model is also used for lead. These models take account of the burial of surface deposits, transfer of activity to marrow and recycling to the circulation and between organs.

5. EQUIVALENT AND EFFECTIVE DOSE

When the distribution of activity in different organs or tissues is known, the resulting distribution of the absorbed energy and absorbed dose, defined as absorbed energy per unit mass, can be calculated. For non-penetrating radiations, energy will in most cases be deposited largely in the tissue in which the radionuclide is deposited. For penetrating radiations, however, it is necessary to take account of cross-fire between tissues. This is done using a "mathematical phantom" which describes the geometric relationship between the different tissues and organs of the body (i.e. a phantom which can be described with simple mathematical equations). Such phantoms have been developed for different ages [29]. Different mathematical methods, including Monte Carlo techniques, may then be used to calculate the absorbed dose in a given organ from decays taking place in the same or another organ, making the assumption that the radionuclides in the source regions is homogeneously distributed. The values obtained are referred to as specific effective energy (SEE(TS S)) for a particular radionuclide [7], expressing the energy absorbed in the tissue T per transformation in the source organ S [7,29].

To provide a tool for the interpretation of absorbed dose in different organs in terms of the total risk of cancer and hereditary effects, ICRP use the concepts of equivalent dose and effective dose [1,2]. Radiation weighting factors take account of the relative biological effectiveness of different radiation types in causing malignancy or genetic damage. Thus the absorbed dose in Gy (Joules kg^{-1}) is multiplied by a radiation weighting factor of 20 for alpha irradiation and 1 for beta and gamma radiations to give the equivalent dose in Sv. Tissue doses are commonly integrated over a 50-year period for adults or to age 70 years for children and the resulting values are referred to as committed equivalent doses. Tissue weighting factors are attributed to different tissues and organs, taking account of the incidence of fatal cancer and hereditary effects, weighted for the incidence of non-fatal disease and years of life lost [1]. The committed effective dose is then the sum of all committed equivalent doses multiplied by the appropriate tissue weighting factors. The committed effective dose can be interpreted in terms of risk estimates for whole body exposure.

TABLE 5

ICRP Tissue Weighting Factors, W_T

Organ/Tissue	Publication 60	Publication 26
Skin	0.01	
Bone surfaces	0.01	0.03
Thyroid	0.05	0.03
Liver	0.05	
Oesophagus	0.05	
Breast	0.05	0.15
Bladder	0.05	
Remainder	0.05	0.3
Lung	0.12	0.12
Red bone marrow	0.12	0.12
Stomach	0.12	
Colon	0.12	
Gonads	0.2	
Total	1	1

Committed effective dose is applicable to workers and members of the public including children.

The tissue weighting factors (W_T) specified by ICRP in their 1990 recommendations [1] are given in Table 5. These are rounded values, corresponding to overall estimates of the risk of fatal cancer in the population of 0.05 Sv^{-1} and an estimate of total aggregated detriment of about 0.07 Sv^{-1}. It should be noted that the oesophagus and colon are assigned weighting factors although the current dosimetric model for the gastrointestinal tract does not include doses to these regions. As an approximation, therefore, doses to the oesophagus are taken to be the same as to the thymus and the colon is taken to be equivalent to the mass weighted average of doses to the upper and lower large intestine as defined in the dosimetric model of the GI tract. Also shown in Table 5 are the weighting factors used previously by ICRP in 1977 [2] when cancer risk estimates were available for fewer organs with none specified for regions of the GI tract. The earlier weighting factors corresponded to an estimated total risk of fatal cancer or serious hereditary disease in the first two generations of 0.0125 Sv^{-1}.

6. BIOKINETIC DATA AND DOSES

6.1 Hydrogen (H)

Experiments with humans have shown that hydrogen in the form of deuterium oxide or tritiated water is rapidly and virtually completely absorbed from the GI tract [30,31]. For organically-bound forms of tritium, absorption may be less than complete, but in the absence of specific information, complete absorption is assumed. Absorption and mixing with body water are assumed to be instantaneous so that concentrations in all body fluids are the same at all times following ingestion. ICRP [3,7] recommend an f_1 of 1 for all chemical forms.

For ^{3}H entering body fluids as tritiated water, doses to tissues are calculated by ICRP [7] assuming that 97% equilibrates with body water and is retained with a half-time of 10 days in adults (range 4–18 days). On the basis of animal data, the remaining 3% is assumed to be incorporated into organic molecules and retained with a half-time of 40 days. For ^{3}H absorbed following ingestion of organically-bound tritium, the assumption made based on the available animal data is that 50% will be readily exchangeable with hydrogen from the body water pool and will therefore be retained with a half-time of 10 days in the adult. A half-time of 40 days is applied to the remaining 50%. On the basis of these assumptions and uniform distribution of retained ^{3}H, the equivalent dose to all body tissues from absorbed ^{3}H is the same and is about 2.5 times greater for organically-bound tritium than tritiated water. The concentration of tritium in urine is assumed to be the same as in total body water and urinary excretion is not assumed to result in a significant additional dose to the bladder wall.

For children, half-times of retention lower than in adults have been calculated which take account of their smaller mass of total body water together with values for daily water balance based on their energy expenditure and, for the organically bound component, of carbon content and balance. For example, for a 3-month-old-infant, half-times of 3 and 8 days are applied to the same fractions as for adults. Despite the more rapid loss of ^{3}H from the body of children, doses are greater than for adults because the effect of smaller body mass dominates. For example, the committed effective dose to a one-year-old from the ingestion of tritiated water is estimated to be about 3 times greater than the value for adults.

6.2 Cobalt (Co)

Human volunteer studies with ^{60}Co chloride [32,33] showed that when the cobalt was present in trace quantities (less than 1 µg Co), fractional absorption (f_1) was 0.05 or less but when stable cobalt was administered (1–12 mg), absorption was 0.1–0.3. A higher value of 0.44 (from 1.2 mg Co) was recorded by Valberg et al. [34], and this was increased to 0.7 when volunteers suffering from iron deficiency were studied. Ramsden (AEA Winfrith; personal communication) measured the absorption of ^{60}Co from crab meat by volunteers and obtained a value of 0.05. Evidence obtained from the inhalation of cobalt oxide suggested minimal absorption of this compound from the gastrointestinal tract [35].

In Publication 30 [3], an f_1 for occupational exposure of 0.3 was recommended for all organically complexed compounds of cobalt and for all inorganic forms of the element, except oxides and hydroxides, in the presence of carrier material. For oxides, hydroxides and all inorganic compounds of cobalt ingested in tracer quantities, the recommended f_1 was 0.05. In Publication 67 [8], a value of 0.1 was adopted for adult members of the public on the basis that the range of results from human studies suggested that absorption of trace quantities is usually less than 0.1. For children from 1 to 15 years of age, an f_1 value of 0.3 was adopted, with a value of 0.6 for infants in the first year of life.

Following the entry of cobalt into the blood, a large fraction is rapidly excreted. Based on two studies of retention in humans, ICRP [3] recommended a model in which 50% of cobalt reaching the circulation is rapidly excreted with a half-time of 0.5 days, 5% is taken up by the liver and 45% is uniformly distributed in all other tissues. Fractions of 0.6, 0.2 and 0.2 are assumed to be lost from the liver and other tissues with biological half-times of 6, 60 and 800 days, respectively. Limited animal data on the effect of age on cobalt distribution and retention, reviewed by ICRP [8], show no age-dependence. The adult values have therefore been assumed to be valid for all ages. A urinary to faecal excretion ratio of 6:1 is assumed for cobalt that has entered the circulation.

Because of low absorption from the GI tract and rapid excretion of a large proportion after absorption, equivalent doses from ingested ^{60}Co in adults are greatest for the colon, resulting mostly from unabsorbed material. In children, because of greater absorption, doses to the colon are similar to doses to the liver.

For the infant, the dose to the colon is less than the dose to the liver. The committed effective dose is about 16 times greater for the 3-month-old infant than for adults.

6.3 Strontium (Sr)

Strontium is the second member of the alkaline earth metal series but, unlike Ca, it has no known physiological function. Due to the presence of Sr isotopes in fall-out material from nuclear weapons tests and its long-term retention in bone as a Ca analogue, the metabolism of strontium has been the subject of a number of human volunteer studies. Similar absorption values were obtained from experiments where known quantities of radiostrontium incorporated in food were ingested [36,37] and from those where radiostrontium tracers were administered orally in solution [38–40]. In each case, mean values of fractional absorption (f_1) were between 0.1 and 0.3. Results from animal studies are generally similar [41]. A number of factors have been found to increase absorption, including fasting and low dietary levels of Ca, Mg and P; milk diets and vitamin D may also increase absorption. Spencer et al. [38] showed that overnight fasting increased absorption from about 0.25 to 0.55. A decrease in Ca content of the diet from 30–40 to 0–10 mg d^{-1} kg^{-1} increased Sr absorption from an average of 0.2 to 0.4 [40]. Results for the absorption of Sr administered as the titanate ($SrTiO_3$) to rats show low levels of absorption [42].

In Publication 30 [3], the recommended f_1 values for occupational exposure were 0.01 for $SrTiO_3$ and 0.3 for all other compounds. An f_1 value of 0.3 is assumed for strontium ingested in food by adults [7,8]. An f_1 value of 0.6, twice the adult value, is used for children in the first year of life, consistent with the NEA [15] approach and available data. For ages 1–15 years an intermediate value of 0.4 is assumed.

For strontium absorbed to body fluids, the age-dependent model for alkaline earth elements developed by Leggett [28] has been adopted by ICRP [8]. This model describes in detail the kinetics of alkaline earth elements in bone, the rapid loss of activity from bone surfaces to blood as well as the slow loss of strontium from bone surfaces to bone volume as a result of bone remodelling. The model also takes account of recycling of strontium from soft tissues and from bone volume to body fluids. Age-dependent parameters take account of greater uptake and retention during periods of rapid skeletal growth.

The committed effective dose for long-lived strontium isotopes like ^{90}Sr is dominated by the contributions from the equivalent doses to bone surfaces and red bone marrow. Doses are greatest for 3-month-old infants (about 8 times the adult value) and 1-year-old children because of their lower skeletal mass and high ^{90}Sr uptake during rapid bone growth. Doses are lower in older children and adults but a peak value at 15 years of age similar to the dose for a one-year-old corresponds to a renewal of rapid bone growth during adolescence. For ^{89}Sr, because of its shorter half-life (50.5 days cf 29 years for ^{90}Sr) the committed effective dose has a larger contribution from the equivalent dose to the colon and is relatively insensitive to changes in bone remodelling rates.

6.4 Zirconium (Zr)

No human data on absorption are available. Fletcher [43] obtained f_1 values ranging from 3×10^{-4} to 0.002 for absorption in rats given [95]Zr in a number of chemical forms including the chloride and sulphate and organic complexes with lactate and oxalate; similar values were obtained for [95]Nb. The results of Shiraishi and Ichikawa [44] for [95]Zr/[95]Nb retention in rats after administration as the oxalate suggest absorption of less than 0.001 for [95]Zr. In ICRP Publication 30 [3], an f_1 value of 0.002 was recommended for occupational exposures. In Publication 56 [7], a value of 0.01 was adopted, as for Nb, for adult members of the public, and a value of 0.02 for infants in the first year of life.

It is assumed by ICRP [7] that 50% of systemic zirconium is retained in the skeleton with a half-time in the adult of 10,000 days, and that the other 50% is distributed throughout all other tissues and is retained with a biological half-time of 7 days. Zirconium is considered to be distributed uniformly over bone surfaces. Retention in the skeleton is taken to be related to the rate of bone remodelling with shorter half-times in children (1000 days for 10-year-olds, 100 days for 3-month-old). A urinary to faecal excretion ratio of 5:1 is assumed for systemic zirconium.

Committed effective doses for ingestion of [95]Zr are greatest for infants with values about 9 times greater than in adults. Because of the low absorption of ingested Zr, the greatest equivalent doses are to the colon from unabsorbed material.

6.5 Niobium (Nb)

Urinary excretion data produced by Schroeder and Balassa [45] suggested that fractional niobium absorption from the human gastrointestinal tract was at least 0.6. However, animal data show considerably lower values of absorption and the human data are considered unreliable.

Furchner and Drake [46] measured whole body retention of [95]Nb, by external counting after gavage as the oxalate and estimated fractional absorption as about 0.02 in mice, 0.08 in rats, 0.09 in monkeys and 0.02 in dogs. Because the retention of [95]Nb rapidly fell to less than detection limits, these values may overestimate the true absorption. Thomas et al. [47] estimated absorption to be between 0.01 and 0.05 for [95]Nb administered as oxalate. Mraz and Eisele [48] reported absorption of about 0.001 for [95]Nb oxalate in rats, similar to the value obtained by Fletcher [43] who quoted a range of 4×10^{-4} to 0.002 for [95]Nb administered to rats in different chemical form. Harrison et al. [49] measured absorption of 0.008 for [95]Nb administered as the citrate to normally fed guinea pigs and 0.014 for animals fasted 24 h before and 2 h after administration.

ICRP [3,7] recommended an f_1 value of 0.01 for occupational exposures and for adult members of the public. This value is also applied to children of 1 year and older, while for a 3-month old infant, an f_1 value of 0.02 is adopted.

On the basis of the available animal data, the deposition fractions for systemic niobium assumed for adults are 0.4 for mineral bone, 0.2 for liver, 0.03 for kidneys, and 0.37 for all other tissues [7]. The deposition fraction in the skeleton is increased for infants and children to 0.6 (3-month-old infants) and 0.5 (1-year-old and 5-year-old children). The distribution in the remaining tissues is similar to that in adults. The retention is described by a two-component exponential function for all tissues and organs, with biological half-times of 6 days (0.5) and 200 days (0.5). Niobium-95 in the skeleton is assumed to be distributed over bone surfaces. A urinary to faecal excretion ratio of 5:1 is assumed for niobium that has entered the transfer compartment [8].

Committed effective doses from ingested [95]Nb are about 8 times greater for 3-month-old infants than for adults. Because of its low absorption and relatively short physical half-life (35 d), the greatest equivalent doses are to the colon from unabsorbed [95]Nb.

6.6 Ruthenium (Ru)

Measurements of the absorption of Ru from contaminated clams in a male volunteer gave a value of about 0.01; similar values were obtained after ingestion of chloro-complexes of Ru(III) and Ru(IV) but values for nitrosyl Ru(III) were about three times greater [50].

Results from a number of studies of the absorption of [106]Ru administered as the chloride to mice, rats, rabbits, guinea pigs, chickens, cats, dogs and monkeys, including values for fasted animals, were in the range of 0.03–0.06 [51–55]. Values for [106]Ru administered as the oxide to rats and rabbits were in the range of 0.003–0.03. Bruce and Carr [54,56] measured the absorption of Ru administered in the form of nitrosyl derivatives. Both nitrate and nitro-complexes of nitrosyl Ru are formed during dissolution in nitric acid in the reprocessing of U fuels. The nitro-complexes are probably more important because they are more resistant to hydrolysis in neutral and alkaline conditions. Results obtained for the nitrate-nitrosyl complex in rats and rabbits were 0.06 and 0.13, respectively. A value of 0.04 was reported for the absorption of Ru administered to rats as a nitro-nitrosyl.

An f_1 value of 0.05 is considered appropriate for occupational exposures to Ru compounds and for ruthenium incorporated in food and drinking water by adults and children from one year of age [4,7]. For infants in the first year of life, a value of 0.1 is adopted [7].

For ruthenium absorbed to body fluids, animal data have shown that the subsequent tissue distribution is fairly uniform. Biological half-times of 8 days (35%), 35 days (30%), and 1000 days (20%) have been derived from these data for adult animals, with 15% of systemic activity being assumed to be excreted directly with a biological half-time of 0.3 days. A urinary to faecal excretion ratio of 4:1 is assumed for systemic ruthenium.

In the absence of information on the effect of age on tissue distribution and retention, greater committed effective doses for ingestion of [103]Ru or [106]Ru by younger children are due solely to their lower body mass. The value of committed effective dose for the 3-month-old infant also takes into account the increased gut transfer. However, the increase in f_1 from 0.05 to 0.1 results in only a small increase in committed effective dose because about 70–80% in each case is due to equivalent doses to the colon from unabsorbed [103]Ru and [106]Ru.

6.7 Iodine (I)

The absorption of dietary iodine or iodide from the gastrointestinal tract of humans is rapid and virtually complete, as demonstrated in a number of human volunteer studies reviewed by Wayne et al. [57] and Underwood [58]. An f_1 value of 1 is applied to all intakes of iodine at all ages [3,7].

The biokinetic model for the uptake of iodine by the thyroid and its subsequent distribution and retention is that adopted by the ICRP [3] with parameters recommended in ICRP Publication 56 [7]. It is assumed that of iodine reaching blood a fraction of 0.3 is accumulated in the thyroid gland and 0.7 is excreted directly in the urine with a half-time of 0.25 days. Iodide incorporated into thyroid hormones leaves the gland with a half-time of about 80 days in the adult and enters other tissues. Most iodide (80%) is subsequently released with a half-time of 12 days and is available in the circulation for uptake by the gland and urinary excretion; the remainder (20%) is excreted in the faeces in organic form. Information on age-related changes in the retention of radioiodine in the thyroid and in the other tissues is taken into account. The limited data available indicate that the turnover of iodine decreases with increasing age. Shorter biological half-times in the thyroid and in other tissues have therefore been adopted for children and infants.

The dose from isotopes of iodine is delivered very largely to the thyroid with much lower doses to other tissues (differences up to 4 orders of magnitude). For the long-lived isotope, [129]I (half-life of $1.6 \cdot 10^7$ years), the reduction in dose at younger ages due to shorter biological half-times counteracts the effect of smaller thyroid mass which leads to similar committed effective doses for 3-month-old infants and 1-, 5- and 10-year-old children, with slightly lower values for 15-year-old children and adults. For ^{131}I, because of its shorter half-life (8 days), the effect of changes in retention times is reduced and the dominant factor determining the age-dependence of doses is the thyroid mass. Doses therefore show a progressive increase with decreasing age, with about an order of magnitude difference between adults and 3-month-old infants.

There is a great variation in different regions in the uptake of iodine by the thyroid gland, according to the availability of stable iodine in the diet. However, because reduced intake results in a compensatory increase in the mass of the thyroid, the effect on the concentration of [129]I or ^{131}I in the thyroid and the committed equivalent dose to the thyroid is not very large. The uptake of radioactive iodine by the thyroid can be reduced to a large extent by administration of stable iodine.

6.8 Caesium (Cs)

Caesium is the fifth member of the alkali metal group and virtually complete absorption would be expected. This has been confirmed by human volunteer studies using ^{137}Cs in soluble inorganic form [59–62]. Thus, for example, Rundo et al. [60] measured an average fractional absorption (f_1) of 0.99 for 10 normal subjects following the ingestion of [137]CsCl.

Measurements of uptake of ^{137}Cs from meat (venison, mutton, caribou) in human volunteers after contamination following the Chernobyl accident have given f_1 values in the range 0.6–0.99 [63,64].

Studies have shown that ^{137}Cs incorporated into insoluble particles may be less available for absorption. Talbot [65] measured absorption of ^{137}Cs from irradiated reactor fuel particles (2–10 μm) in adult rats to be less than 0.1. Le Roy et al. [62] reported values of less than 0.1 for the uptake of ^{137}Cs from real and simulated fall-out in a large study on 102 volunteers. In contrast, Fujita et al. [66] studied the absorption of ^{137}Cs from fall-out in five volunteers and obtained results consistent with virtually complete absorption.

An f_1 value of 1 was recommended by ICRP for all intakes of caesium at all ages [3,7]. It is recognised, though, that absorption may not be complete in particular circumstances, particularly for insoluble particulate materials.

Caesium is distributed uniformly throughout all body tissues and retained there with biological half-times of 2 days (0.1) and 110 days (0.9), respectively [3,7]. The biological half-time for females, however, are significantly smaller than those for males here (less than 70 days instead of 110 days). There is also evidence that in some countries the mean biological half-time of caesium in adult males is shorter than 110 days [61,67,68]. Thus the use of a value of 110 days for the biological half-time in adults will result in conservative estimates of effective dose. There is good evidence that the rates of loss of caesium from the body is greater in children than adults, and shorter biological half-times have therefore been used for children [69]. A urinary to faecal excretion ratio of 4:1 is assumed.

Because of the uniform distribution of caesium in the body, equivalent doses to all tissues after ingestion of ^{137}Cs are very similar. In general, the shorter biological half-times at younger ages counteract the effect of lower body mass, resulting in values of dose that are largely independent of age; only doses for the 3-month-old infant are increased significantly, by about a factor of two, with the use of a biological half-time of 16 days compared with 13 days for the 1-year-old child.

6.9 Cerium (Ce)

Cerium is a member of the elements known as the Rare Earth or Lanthanide series. They are characterised by a relatively small ionic radius and high ionic charge. In solution, in the absence of binding ligands, they exhibit a strong tendency to hydrolyse to form insoluble hydroxy species, poorly available for intestinal absorption. These chemical characteristics are similar to those of the trivalent actinide series elements.

The accidental exposure of a radiation worker to a cerium-containing dust indicated very little uptake from the gastro-intestinal tract [70]. The fractional absorption (f_1) of Ce in rats has been reported as less than 0.001.

In ICRP Publication 30 [3], an f_1 of 3×10^{-4} was recommended for all compounds of cerium. In ICRP Publication 56 [7], a value of 0.001 was adopted for adult members of the public by analogy with trivalent actinides. However, the f_1 value for trivalent actinides has since been changed to 5×10^{-4} and this value is also applied to Ce and all other lanthanides [71]. For infants in the first year of life, a value of 5×10^{-3} is adopted, taking account of measurements of increased absorption in rats, mice and pigs.

On the basis of measurements of the distribution of cerium in rats and dogs, it is assumed that of cerium entering the circulation in adults, fractions of 0.3, 0.5 and 0.2 are taken up by the skeleton, liver, and other tissues, respectively, and retained in each case with a biological half-time of 3500 days. It appears that skeletal uptake is greater in younger animals. Thus, the initial distribution to skeleton and liver is taken to be 0.7 and 0.1, respectively, in 3-month-old infants, 0.5 and 0.3, respectively, in 1- and 5-year-old children and 0.4 in both tissues for 10- and 15-year-old children. A urinary to faecal excretion ratio of 1:9 is assumed for cerium that has entered the circulation for all ages.

For ingestion of ^{144}Ce the equivalent doses to the colon are highest for all ages, contributing about 90% or more to the committed effective dose. The committed effective dose for the 3-month-old infant is about 13 times greater than for the adult.

6.10 Lead (Pb)

Lead absorption has been studied extensively in man and animals [72,73]. Factors shown to affect absorption of Pb include ingestion of milk, calcium and iron status, and fasting. Of these, fasting causes the greatest variation in uptake. For example, James et al. [74] measured fractional absorption in volunteers given Pb acetate in water to be about 0.65 after a 12 h fast compared with about 0.04 when taken with a meal. At 3 h after a meal, absorption averaged about 0.16 with a range of 0.05 to 0.5, and after 5 h the average was about 0.45 with a range of 0.3 to 0.65. Individual variation was also shown by Blake [75] who measured absorption ranging from 0.1 to 0.7 in ten volunteers given Pb chloride. Heard and Chamberlain [76] showed that fasting values of about 0.4 to 0.5 were reduced to 0.1 to 0.2 by giving Pb in tea, coffee or beer rather than distilled water. Incorporation of Pb into liver or kidney or into spinach reduced uptake to about 0.03–0.06.

An f_1 value of 0.2 is assumed for occupational exposure and intakes of lead in food by adults [4,8]. Greater values are recommended for infants and children on the basis of human and animal data; 0.6 for a 3-month-old infant, and 0.4 for 1- to 15-year-old children.

To model the biokinetics of lead, a modification of the age-dependent alkaline earth model of Leggett [28] has been used. In this modification, red blood cells are considered as a separate compartment, excretion via sweat and hair are considered explicitly, the liver is assumed to consist of two compartments, and the kidneys are considered explicitly with two compartments. This model takes account of the considerable differences in the time-dependent distribution of lead and the alkaline earth elements.

Radioisotopes of bismuth and polonium formed as progeny of lead radioisotopes produced in bone mineral are assumed to follow the behaviour of the parent radionuclide until removed from the bone. Outside bone volume the isotopes of bismuth and polonium are assumed to follow their own specific behaviour.

The greatest equivalent doses to tissues for ingestion of ^{210}Pb are to bone surfaces, kidneys and liver. The committed effective dose for the 3-month-old is about 12 times greater than that for adults.

6.11 Polonium (Po)

Fink [77] measured polonium uptake in a patient being treated for chronic myeloid leukaemia. Blood concentrations and urinary excretion after oral administration of [210]Po chloride were about one-tenth of corresponding values obtained in other subjects after intravénous injection of polonium chloride, suggesting an f_1 of 0.1. Data from humans consuming meat from reindeer exposed to [210]Po indicated f_1 values of about 0.3–0.5 [78–80]. In a recent study of the absorption of [210]Po from crabmeat, Hunt et al. [81] estimated absorption to be about 0.8.

The absorption of [210]Po in rats has been reported as 0.03–0.06 for an unspecified chemical form [82] and 0.06 for the chloride [83]. Haines et al. [84] obtained f_1 values for rats of 0.05 for [210]Po as the nitrate and 0.13 for [210]Po incorporated into liver. For [210]Po administered as the citrate, absorption was reported as 0.07–0.09 in rats and guinea pigs.

In ICRP Publication 30 [3], an f_1 value of 0.1 was recommended for inorganic forms of Po. In ICRP Publication 67 [8], a value of 0.5 was adopted for uptake from food. A factor of two increase to 1 is recommended for the first year of life.

Based on human and animal data, it is assumed that of polonium entering the circulation, fractions of 0.3, 0.1, 0.05, 0.1, and 0.445 are taken up by liver, kidneys, spleen, red bone marrow, and all other tissues and retained in all tissues with a biological half-time of 50 days. A urinary to faecal excretion ratio of 1:2 is assumed for polonium that has entered the circulation.

The greatest equivalent doses to tissues from ingestion of [210]Po are to the kidneys, spleen and liver. The committed effective dose for the 3-month-old infant is about 18 times that for the adult.

6.12 Radium (Ra)

Data from balance studies reviewed by the ICRP Task Group on Alkaline Earth Metabolism in Adult Man [85] indicated the fraction of radium absorbed from food or drinking water to be between 0.15 and 0.21. Results from a study of a single human volunteer who ingested a known quantity of radium suggested a higher f_1 value of around 0.5 [86]. Normal elderly subjects ingesting mock radium dial paint containing $^{224}RaSO_4$ absorbed an average of about 0.2 [87,88]. The ICRP Publication 30 [3] f_1 value of 0.2 for occupational exposure was adopted in ICRP Publication 67 [8] for adult members of the public. Greater values are assumed for infants and children: 0.6 for 3-month-old infants, and 0.4 for 1- to 15-year-old children.

Radium absorbed to the circulation, like strontium and barium, behaves qualitatively in the same way as calcium. The biokinetic model used for strontium [8] is applied to the other alkaline earth elements, using element-specific parameters for uptake and retention in bone and other tissues. Isotopes of other elements produced in the body by the decay of radium isotopes are considered to have their own biokinetic behaviour depending on the site where they have been produced.

The committed effective dose for ingestion of ^{226}Ra, as for ^{90}Sr, is dominated by the contribution from the equivalent doses to bone surfaces and red bone marrow. Doses are greatest for 3-month-old infants (17 times the adult value) and 1-year-old children because of their lower skeletal mass and high ^{226}Ra uptake during rapid bone growth. Doses are lower in older children and adults but a peak value at 15 years of age, similar to the dose for a one-year-old, corresponds to a renewal of rapid bone growth during adolescence.

6.13 Thorium (Th)

Maletskos et al. [88] measured the absorption of ^{234}Th ingested as the sulphate in a mock "dial" paint by six 63 to 83 year-old humans. The f_1 values obtained were in the range 10^{-4} to 6×10^{-4} with a mean of 2×10^{-4}. Estimates of Th absorption have also been derived from data on skeletal content, dietary intake, estimated inhalation rates and excretion data, giving f_1 values of less than 0.001–0.01 [89,90]. However, these estimates of absorption are uncertain because they are based on balance studies involving disparate data sources. There have been several reports of Th absorption in rats and mice, with f_1 values of 5×10^{-5} to 0.006 for rats [91,92], about 6×10^{-4} for mice [92,93] and 0.001 for fasted mice [94].

In ICRP Publication 30 [3], an f_1 value of 2×10^{-4} was recommended. For adult members of the public, a value of 5×10^{-4} is used for Th and other actinides other than U [8,9]. This value is applied, in the absence of specific information, to children from one year of age. For infants in the first year of life, a value of 5×10^{-3} is used.

For thorium absorbed to body fluids, as for plutonium, the main sites of deposition are the liver and skeleton. As discussed for plutonium (see below, p. 276), an actinide model is used which takes account of the redistribution of elements between and within tissues, particularly bone, and loss by excretion. The model uses element-specific data for transfer rates.

The committed effective dose from ingestion of ^{230}Th or ^{232}Th is due largely to doses received by bone surfaces, red bone marrow, liver, kidneys and gonads. For infants, the greater f_1 value of 5×10^{-3} results in a proportional increase in doses. The committed effective dose for the 3-month-old infant is about 15 times greater than that for the adult. Committed effective doses for intakes by children of one year of age and older differ by less than a factor of two because greater doses due to lower skeletal mass at younger ages are counteracted by shorter retention half-times. For ^{228}Th, because of its relatively short half-life (1.9 years), the effect of changes of retention half-time with age is less important and committed effective dose for the one-year-old is about 5 times greater than adult values.

6.14 Uranium (U)

Data on the absorption of U have been reviewed by Wrenn et al. [95], Harrison [96], Leggett and Harrison [97] and in ICRP Publication 69 [9].

In the first controlled human study involving more than one subject, Hursh et al. [98] administered uranyl nitrate to 4 hospital patients. The data obtained were taken to suggest fractional absorption (f_1) in the range 0.005–0.05. Leggett and Harrison [97] have interpreted the data as suggesting absorption of 0.004, 0.01, 0.02 and 0.06 for the 4 subjects. Wrenn et al. [99] estimated absorption in 12 normal healthy adult volunteers given drinking water high in U. On the basis that 40–60% of absorbed U was excreted in the urine in the first three days, rather than the authors assumption of 79%, Leggett and Harrison [97] concluded that mean absorption was 0.006–0.015, maximum absorption was in the range 0.02–0.04, and that five or six subjects absorbed less than 0.003. Recently, Harduin et al. [100] reported results for the absorption of U from drinking water either administered on one day or over 15 days. The data for acute administration suggested fractional absorption of 0.005–0.05 with an average f_1 value of 0.015–0.02. The data for 15-day administration suggested absorption of 0.003–0.02 and average absorption of 0.01–0.015.

A number of dietary balance studies have indicated mean absorption values in the range 0.004–0.04 (97,99,101,102]．

Measurements of U absorption have been made in rats, hamsters, rabbits, dogs and baboons [reviewed 95–97]. A number of studies have shown that absorption is substantially greater in fasted than fed animals. For example, Bhattacharyya et al. [103] found that uptake was increased by an order of magnitude in mice and baboons deprived of food for 24 h prior to U administration. Animal studies provide the only quantitative information on the relative uptake of U ingested in different chemical forms. Absorption appears to be greatest for U ingested as $UO_2(NO_3)_26H_2O$, UO_2F_2 or $Na_2U_2O_7$, roughly half as great for UO_4 or UO_3, and 1–2 orders of magnitude lower for UCl_4, U_3O_8, UO_2 and UF_4.

In ICRP Publication 30 [3], an f_1 of 0.05 was recommended for water soluble inorganic forms of U(VI) and a value of 0.002 for U(IV) in relatively insoluble compounds such as UF_4, UO_2 and U_3O_8. For dietary intakes of uranium by adults, ICRP [9] have adopted an f_1 of 0.02 on the basis of more recent data as reviewed by Wrenn et al. [95], Harrison [96] and Leggett and Harrison [97]. This value is also applied to children from one year of age and a value of 0.04 is applied to infants.

The principal site of retention of uranium in the body is the skeleton. Because uranium tends to follow the qualitative behaviour of calcium to a large extent with regard to its behaviour in bone, the model used for the alkaline earth elements is applied to uranium, using data for transfer rates specific for uranium (see strontium, p. 266).

The greatest equivalent doses to tissues for ingestion of ^{234}U, ^{235}U or ^{238}U are for the bone surfaces, red bone marrow, kidneys and liver. The committed effective dose for the 3-month-old infant is about 7 times greater than that for the adult.

6.15 Neptunium (Np)

Popplewell et al. [104] have measured the absorption of ^{239}Np and ^{242}Cm in five adult male volunteers by comparing urinary excretion after oral and intravenous administration. In each case the elements were administered as the citrate complexes; the solutions were ingested with a mid-day meal. The mean f_1 value obtained was 2×10^{-4} for both Np(V) and Cm(III) with a range of 10^{-4} to 3×10^{-4} in both cases.

Animal data on the absorption of Np have been reviewed in ICRP Publication 48 [105] and by Harrison [96]. The first measurements of Np absorption involved administration of mg quantities of ^{237}Np to rats and f_1 values of about 0.01 were obtained [106–108]. Subsequent experiments established that absorption at low concentrations in a number of animal species was an order of magnitude or more lower. Metivier et al. [109,110] obtained similar results in rats and baboons; fractional absorption was about 0.001 in two baboons given 11 ng ^{239}Np as the nitrate and about 0.01 at a dose of 5 mg ^{237}Np. Harrison et al. [111] reported f_1 values of 0.003 for a 0.5 mg dose of ^{237}Np as the nitrate and 3×10^{-4} for 0.5 ng of ^{239}Np. Metivier et al. [110] studied the effect of dietary changes on Np absorption in baboons. A milk-supplemented diet reduced absorption by a factor of five to $1–2\times10^{-4}$, while a potato diet increased absorption by a similar factor.

In ICRP Publication 30 [4], f_1 was taken to be 0.01 based on measurements on rats given high masses of ^{237}Np. In Publication 48 [105], the effect of mass was discussed and a general value for actinides of 0.001 was applied to Np. This value was also adopted for adult members of the public in ICRP Publication 56 [7]. However, subsequently in ICRP Publication 67 [8], the recent human data for Np, Pu, Am and Cm were summarised and the conclusion was reached that, together with human data for Th and available animal data, these provided a sufficient basis for the use of a value of 5×10^{-4}. This value is applied, in the absence of specific information, to children from one year of age. For infants in the first year of life, a value of 5×10^{-3} is used.

For neptunium absorbed to body fluids, as for plutonium, the main sites of deposition are the liver and skeleton. As discussed for plutonium, an actinide model is used which takes account of the redistribution of elements between and within tissues, particularly bone, and loss by excretion. The model uses element-specific data for transfer rates.

The committed effective dose from ingestion of ^{237}Np is due largely to doses received by bone surfaces, red bone marrow, liver and gonads. For infants, the greater f_1 value of 5×10^{-3} results in a proportional increase in doses. The committed effective dose for the 3-month-old infant is about 15 times greater than that for the adult. Committed effective doses for intakes by children of one year of age and older differ by less than a factor of two because greater doses due to lower skeletal mass at younger ages are counteracted by shorter retention half-times.

6.16 Plutonium (Pu)

Hunt et al. [112,113] have carried out two studies of the absorption of plutonium and americium by volunteers eating winkles collected on the Cumbrian coast near to the nuclear-fuel reprocessing plant at Sellafield. The overall f_1 value obtained for Pu was 2×10^{-4} with a range of 2×10^{-5} to 5×10^{-4}. The absorption of fallout Pu from reindeer meat was estimated by Mussalo-Rauhamaa et al. [114]. An f_1 of 8×10^{-4} was obtained by comparing the ratio of body content to dietary intake of $^{239/240}$Pu in persons who had lived in Lappland or the urban areas of southern Finland. Large uncertainties were associated with this estimate of absorption.

Animal data on the absorption of Pu in species including rodents, pigs, dogs and primates were extensively reviewed in Publication 48 [105] and by Harrison [96]. Studies have shown the effect of chemical form with absorption being generally greater for organic complexes and Pu incorporated into food materials than for inorganic forms. Fasting has also been shown to increase absorption by up to an order of magnitude. Studies in which pure oxides have been administered indicate that absorption was more than an order of magnitude lower than for other compounds. In general, ingested mass and valence are not considered important factors affecting absorption. However, at high masses of Pu(V), absorption may be increased by an order of magnitude [115].

In ICRP Publication 30 [3], the recommended f_1 values were 10^{-5} for oxides and hydroxides and 10^{-4} for all other inorganic forms. In ICRP Publication 48

[105], f_1 values of 10^{-5} for oxides and hydroxides and 10^{-4} for nitrates were recommended. In addition, on the basis of animal data, an f_1 of 0.001 was recommended for all other forms of Pu and was taken to apply as a general value for all actinides other than U. This value was also adopted for adult members of the public in ICRP Publication 56 [7]. However, subsequently in ICRP Publication 67 [8], the recent human data for Np, Pu, Am and Cm were summarised and the conclusion was reached that, together with human data for Th and available animal data, these provided a sufficient basis for the use of a value of 5×10^{-4} for intakes of plutonium in food by adults [8]. This value is applied, in the absence of specific information, to children from one year of age. For infants in the first year of life, a value of 5×10^{-3} is used.

For plutonium absorbed to body fluids, the main sites of deposition are the liver and skeleton. Leggett and his colleagues have developed an actinide model which take into account bone remodelling and recycling of elements from the skeleton and soft tissues to body fluids [25,27]. Movement of plutonium and other actinides within the skeleton is modelled, taking account of burial of initial surface deposits on and transfer from surfaces and bone volume to the marrow. The model also applies to children, taking into account greater initial deposition on bone surfaces and greater bone turnover.

The committed effective dose from ingestion of ^{239}Pu is due largely to doses received by bone surfaces, red bone marrow, liver and gonads. The dose for infants takes account of greater gut transfer of 5×10^{-3} compared with 5×10^{-4} for children of one year of age and older. This results in a proportional increase in the doses to the skeleton, liver and gonads. The committed effective dose for the 3-month-old infant is about 17 times greater than that for the adult. Committed effective doses for intakes by children of one year of age and older differ by less than a factor of two.

6.17 Americium (Am)

Hunt et al. [112,113] have carried out two studies of the absorption of plutonium and americium by volunteers eating winkles collected on the Cumbrian coast near to the nuclear-fuel reprocessing plant at Sellafield. The overall f_1 value obtained for americium was 1×10^{-4} with a range of 4×10^{-5} to 3×10^{-4}.

Animal data on the absorption of Am was reviewed in Publication 48 [105] and by Harrison [96]. Results for rodents and primates suggest that the absorption of Am, unlike Pu, is not increased by binding to organic ligands. Limited data for different chemical forms of Am do not indicate large differences between the absorption of the oxides and other inorganic forms.

In ICRP Publication 30 [3], an f_1 value of 5×10^{-4} was recommended. In ICRP Publication 48 [105], a general value of 0.001 for actinides was used. This value was also adopted in Publication 56 [7] for adult members of the public. However, in ICRP Publication 67 [8], the recent human data for Np, Pu, Am and Cm were summarised and the conclusion was reached that, together with human data for Th and available animal data, these provided a sufficient basis for the use of a value of 5×10^{-4}. This value is applied, in the absence of specific information, to children from one year of age. For infants in the first year of life, a value of 5×10^{-3} is used.

For americium absorbed to body fluids, as for plutonium, the main sites of deposition are the liver and skeleton. As discussed for plutonium, an actinide model is used which takes account of the redistribution of elements between and within tissues, particularly bone, and loss by excretion. The model uses element-specific data for transfer rates.

The committed effective dose from ingestion of ^{241}Am, as for ^{239}Pu, is due largely to doses received by bone surfaces, red bone marrow, liver and gonads. For infants, the greater f_1 value of 5×10^{-3} results in a proportional increase in doses. The committed effective dose for the 3-month-old infant is about 18 times greater than that for the adult. Committed effective doses for intakes by children of one year of age and older differ by less than a factor of two because greater doses due to lower skeletal mass at younger ages are counteracted by shorter retention half-times.

7. OBSERVED EFFECTS OF INGESTED RADIONUCLIDES

Animals receiving acute doses to the gastrointestinal tract of between about 10 Gy and 50 Gy die with signs of the gastrointestinal syndrome [116,117]. The symptoms in man follow those of the prodromal phase which includes anorexia, increased lethargy, diarrhoea, infection and loss of fluids and electrolytes. Other signs include weight loss, reduced food and water intake, gastric retention and decreased intestinal absorption. There may be haemorrhages and bacteraemia which aggravate injury and contribute to death. In various species of animal, the mean time to death after doses of the order of 50 Gy is from about 4–10 days.

The results of bone marrow transplantation studies in humans indicate that, when therapy is sufficient to compensate for haematological complications, the total-body dose for intestinal death is above 10 Gy [118]. Data obtained from studies in which the GI tract of rats was exposed to X-irradiation, either in situ or surgically exteriorised, indicated an LD_{50} of about 15 Gy for acute exposure [119]. Based on these data, a dose-response relationship with a LD_{50} of 15 Gy, an LD_{10} of 10 Gy and an LD_{90} of 20 Gy would apply to acute exposures to the gut occurring within about 6 hours.

In practice, death from irradiation of the gut is likely to be important, in comparison with death from irradiation of the bone marrow, only in situations involving ingested radioactivity delivering large internal doses. Because of the normal clearance times through the GI tract, the dose would be delivered in a few days. Severe acute injury to the intestinal mucosa has not been reported for ingested radionuclides in man although many cases of accidental intakes have been published [120]. Haemopoietic injury was observed after ingestion of 37 MBq ^{241}Am reported to deliver 5.5 Gy to the skeleton over 5 years [121] and after ingestion of Ra giving 2 Gy over six weeks and more than 50 Gy over three years [122].

Dose–effect relationships for intestinal damage have been obtained from animal data; this is considered reasonable because different mammals respond in a similar way to irradiation of the gut [123,124]. Values of LD_{50} of about 33 Gy for rats (25–41 Gy) and 40 Gy for dogs (20–52 Gy) were obtained in experiments in which rats ingested either ^{106}Ru/^{106}Rh (average 1.4 MeV beta) or ^{147}Pm (average 0.06 MeV beta) and dogs were given ^{106}Ru/^{106}Rh [125,126]. The estimated dose to crypt cells in rats was the same for both ^{106}Ru/^{106}Rh and ^{147}Pm, about 35 Gy, although the dose to the mucosal surface was about 35 times greater for ^{147}Pm than for ^{106}Ru/^{106}Rh. This dose is comparable to a dose of about 13 Gy of external irradiation delivered acutely and is consistent with an expected reduction in effect at lower dose rate. Death was due to damage to the large intestine in both rats and dogs. Based on these data, an LD_{50} of 35 Gy has been suggested, with a simple linear function with a LD_0 of 20 Gy and an LD_{100} of 50 Gy [127]. This is consistent with the approach taken by Scott and Hahn [128] for assessing the consequences of reactor accidents.

Comparisons of the toxicity of ^{106}Ru/^{106}Rh in rats of different ages showed sensitivity in the order: newborn > adults > weanlings [129]. The reason for the sensitivity of the newborn is the uptake and retention of radionuclides in the mucosal cells of the intestine, particularly the proximal small intestine. This non-specific uptake of radionuclides, discussed above and illustrated for ^{239}Pu (Fig. 3), occurs to a decreasing extent over the suckling period and distinct species differences have been observed. It would appear that at the high levels of retention observed in rats, doses of up to 100 Gy d^{-1} may be received by cells towards the tips of the villi without evidence of mucosal injury [129]. The greater sensitivity of adults than weanlings to the effect of ^{106}Ru/^{106}Rh was probably a reflection of greater transit times in the adult.

Only very limited information is available on cancer induction in the GI tract by ingested radionuclides. Tumours induced by internal irradiation have been observed in the gastrointestinal tract of rodents after parental administration of ^{137}Cs, ^{95}Nb and ^{144}Ce and after oral administration of ^{90}Y, ^{144}Ce, ^{106}Ru and ^{137}Cs [130]. Intestinal polyps in dogs and rats fed ^{210}Po or ^{144}Ce were also reported, mostly occurring in the large intestine with a tendency to malignant change and showing different latencies in the two species [131].

8. RELATIVE TOXICITY OF RADIONUCLIDES

The relative toxicity of radionuclides in terms of cancer induction and hereditary effects can be predicted using the biokinetic and dosimetric models discussed above. Table 6 gives values of committed effective dose for the radionuclides included in this chapter for the examples of ingestion by adults (20 y) and infants (3 months).

TABLE 6

Committed effective doses from ingestion of radionuclides by adults and infants (Sv Bq^{-1})

Nuclide	Principal emissions	Half-life (d/year)	Committed effective dose (Sv Bq^{-1})	
			Adult	Infant
^{3}H	β	12.3 y	1.8×10^{-11}	6.3×10^{-11}
^{60}Co	β,γ	5.3 y	3.4×10^{-9}	5.4×10^{-8}
^{90}Sr	β	28.5 y	2.8×10^{-8}	2.3×10^{-7}
^{95}Zr	β,γ	64 d	9.6×10^{-10}	8.5×10^{-9}
^{95}Nb	β,γ	35 d	5.9×10^{-10}	4.6×10^{-9}
^{106}Ru	β	368 d	7.0×10^{-9}	8.4×10^{-8}
^{131}I	β,γ	8 d	2.2×10^{-8}	1.8×10^{-7}
^{137}Cs	β	30 y	1.4×10^{-8}	2.1×10^{-8}
^{144}Ce	β	285 d	5.2×10^{-9}	6.6×10^{-8}
^{210}Pb	β	22 y	7.0×10^{-7}	8.1×10^{-6}
^{210}Po	α	138 d	1.2×10^{-6}	2.1×10^{-5}
^{226}Ra	α	1600 y	2.8×10^{-7}	4.7×10^{-6}
^{232}Th	α	1.4×10^{10} y	1.1×10^{-6}	1.4×10^{-5}
^{238}U	α	4.5×10^{9} y	4.5×10^{-8}	3.3×10^{-7}
^{237}Np	α	2.1×10^{6} y	1.1×10^{-7}	2.0×10^{-6}
^{239}Pu	α	2.4×10^{4} y	2.5×10^{-7}	4.2×10^{-6}
^{241}Am	α	433 y	2.1×10^{-7}	3.7×10^{-6}

The least toxic radionuclide, because of its weak β emissions and short biological half-times, is ^{3}H ingested as ^{3}H$_2$O for which an intake of 56 MBq by an adult is equivalent to an external whole body dose of 1 mSv. (1.8×10^{-11} Sv Bq^{-1}; Table 6). The probability of different cancer types would be the same for ^{3}H as for external irradiation because of the uniform distribution of ^{3}H in the body. As shown in Table 7, the combined dose to the stomach and colon from ^{3}H accounts for 24% of the committed effective dose, corresponding to the use of tissue weighting factors of 0.12 for each of these regions of the GI tract (Table 5).

The most toxic radionuclide considered is the α emitter ^{210}Po for which ingestion by an adult of 0.8 MBq is equivalent to an external whole body dose of 1 mSv in terms of total estimated risk. However, the probability of different cancer types would be different. For ^{210}Po, doses to the liver and red bone marrow contribute 25–30% each to the committed effective dose compared with 5% and 12%, respectively, for uniform irradiation. As shown in Table 7, contributions to the committed effective dose from irradiation of the GI tract are smaller than from uniform whole body irradiation.

Estimates of doses from ^{210}Po have increased recently with the use of an f_1 value of 0.5 rather than 0.1 (ICRP 1979, 1993) and the inclusion in the model of specific uptake in bone marrow (ICRP 1993). These changes also affect

TABLE 7

Committed equivalent doses to stomach and colon from ingestion of radionuclides by adults and infants

Nuclide	Committed equivalent dose (Sv Bq^{-1})				Total % of committed effective dose	
	Stomach		Colon			
	Adult	Infant	Adult	Infant	Adult	Infant
^{3}H	1.8×10^{-11}	6.3×10^{-11}	1.8×10^{-11}	6.3×10^{-11}	24	24
^{60}Co	2.6×10^{-9}	5.1×10^{-8}	8.9×10^{-9}	7.7×10^{-8}	42	29
^{90}Sr	9.1×10^{-10}	1.5×10^{-8}	1.3×10^{-8}	1.2×10^{-8}	6	1
^{95}Zr	3.9×10^{-10}	3.5×10^{-9}	5.1×10^{-9}	5.1×10^{-8}	69	76
^{95}Nb	2.9×10^{-10}	2.4×10^{-9}	2.7×10^{-9}	2.4×10^{-8}	61	68
^{106}Ru	3.2×10^{-9}	4.4×10^{-8}	4.6×10^{-8}	5.1×10^{-7}	84	79
^{131}I	3.1×10^{-10}	3.5×10^{-9}	1.2×10^{-10}	2.6×10^{-9}	0.2	0.4
^{137}Cs	1.3×10^{-8}	2.2×10^{-8}	1.5×10^{-8}	3.7×10^{-8}	24	34
^{144}Ce	1.1×10^{-9}	1.4×10^{-8}	4.2×10^{-8}	4.8×10^{-8}	98	89
^{210}Pb	9.1×10^{-8}	2.1×10^{-6}	9.7×10^{-8}	2.2×10^{-6}	3	6
^{210}Po	2.8×10^{-7}	4.6×10^{-6}	3.0×10^{-7}	4.8×10^{-6}	6	5
^{226}Ra	4.1×10^{-8}	5.4×10^{-7}	1.0×10^{-7}	1.2×10^{-6}	6	4
^{232}Th	6.1×10^{-8}	1.7×10^{-6}	8.6×10^{-8}	2.0×10^{-6}	2	3
^{238}U	2.6×10^{-8}	1.3×10^{-7}	5.2×10^{-8}	4.3×10^{-7}	21	20
^{237}Np	8.4×10^{-9}	3.1×10^{-7}	4.0×10^{-8}	6.8×10^{-7}	5	6
^{239}Pu	1.6×10^{-8}	5.6×10^{-7}	4.8×10^{-8}	9.5×10^{-7}	3	2
^{241}Am	1.7×10^{-8}	4.4×10^{-7}	5.3×10^{-8}	8.5×10^{-7}	4	4

estimates of dose from intakes of ^{210}Pb for which a large proportion of the dose is due to the daughter ^{210}Po (intermediate ^{210}Bi, half-life 5d).

The long-lived α emitting actinide nuclides, ^{232}Th, ^{239}Pu and ^{241}Am also have relatively high toxicities. Despite their low absorption from the GI tract (f_1 = 5×10^{-4} in adults, 5×10^{-3} in infants; Table 3), the committed effective doses from these nuclides are dominated by doses to the bone surfaces, red bone marrow and liver. Because of their long retention times in these tissues, doses are delivered over an individuals life-time.

As shown in Table 7, examples of radionuclides for which doses to the GI tract contribute a large proportion to the committed effective dose are ^{95}Zr, ^{95}Nb, ^{106}Ru and ^{144}Ce. The importance of doses to the GI tract in these cases is due to a combination of factors. They are all β emitters with short physical half-lives and their absorption from the GI tract is low, particularly for ^{144}Ce (f_1 = 5×10^{-4} in adults, 5×10^{-3} in infants; Table 3). For ^{95}Zr, ^{95}Nb and ^{106}Ru, a large fraction of the absorbed nuclide has a short half-time of retention in the body.

9. CONCLUSION

Limited information is available on early and late radiation effects in the GI tract from ingested radionuclides. However, estimates of dose and risk can be made using the comprehensive biokinetic and dosimetric models developed by ICRP [3–9]. As shown in this chapter, radionuclides differ considerably in the dose delivered per unit of ingested activity and in the proportion of the dose delivered to the GI tract.

An important development will be the revision of the dosimetric model of the GI tract to take account of more recent information on transit times and include age-dependent data. Further work is required to determine the extent to which radionuclides, particularly α emitters, in gut contents irradiate stem cells in the crypts. It may be necessary to include irradiation of sensitive cells from nuclides in transit through mucosal cells during absorption in some cases.

At NRPB, studies are planned to compare the induction of intestinal tumours in mice following ingestion of nuclides emitting different radiations or after external irradiation. It is intended to use mice with a predisposition to the development of intestinal adenomas due to a germ-line mutation in the homologue of the human APC gene [132,133]. In humans, mutations of the APC gene are responsible for familial adenomatous polyposis, an autosomal dominantly inherited disease. Patients with this disease develop multiple benign colorectal tumours. The mouse model should provide information on doses to target cells from different radiation types and allow studies of the molecular changes involved in cancer induction and progression.

References

1. International Commission on Radiological Protection (1991) 1990 Recommendations of the International Commission on Radiological Protection. ICRP Publication 60. Pergamon Press, Oxford. Ann. ICRP 21, (1–3).
2. International Commission on Radiological Protection (1977) Recommendations of the International Commission on Radiological Protection. ICRP Publication 26. Pergamon Press, Oxford. Ann. ICRP 1, (3).
3. International Commission on Radiological Protection (1979) Limits on Intakes of Radionuclides for Workers. ICRP Publication 30, Pt.1. Pergamon Press, Oxford. Ann. ICRP 2, (3/4).
4. International Commission on Radiological Protection (1980) Limits on Intakes of Radionuclides for Workers. ICRP Publication 30, Pt.2. Pergamon Press, Oxford. Ann. ICRP 4, (3/4).
5. International Commission on Radiological Protection (1981) Limits on Intakes of Radionuclides for Workers. ICRP Publication 30, Pt.3. Pergamon Press, Oxford. Ann. ICRP 6, (2/3).
6. International Commission on Radiological Protection (1988) Limits on Intakes of Radionuclides for Workers. ICRP Publication 30, Pt.4. Pergamon Press, Oxford. Ann. ICRP 19, (4).

7. International Commission on Radiological Protection (1989) Age-dependent Doses to Members of the Public from Intake of Radionuclides. Pt.1. ICRP Publication 56. Pergamon Press, Oxford. Ann. ICRP 20, (2).

8. International Commission on Radiological Protection (1993) Age-dependent Doses to Members of the Public from Intake of Radionuclides. Pt.2, Ingestion Dose Coefficients. ICRP Publication 67. Pergamon Press, Oxford. Ann. ICRP 23, (3/4).

9. International Commission on Radiological Protection. Age-dependent Doses to Members of the Public from Intake of Radionuclides. Pt.3, Ingestion Dose Coefficients. ICRP Publication 69. Pergamon Press, Oxford. Ann. ICRP (in press).

10. Stubbs, J.B. (1992) Results from a new mathematical model of gastrointestinal transit that incorporates age and gender-dependent physiological parameters. In: D.M. Taylor, G.B. Gerber and J.W. Stather (Eds.), Age-dependent Factors in the Biokinetics and Dosimetry of Radionuclides. Radiat. Prot. Dosim. 41 (2/4), 63–69.

11. Eve, I.S. (1966) A review of the physiology of the gastrointestinal tract in relation to radiation doses from radioactive materials. Health Phys. 12, 131–161.

12. Sullivan, M.F., Hackett, P.L., George, L.A. and Thompson, R.C. (1960) Irradiation of the intestine by radioisotopes. Radiat. Res. 13, 343–355.

13. Rao, S.S.C., Read, N.W., Brown, C., Bruce, C. and Holdsworth, C.D. (1987) Studies on the mechanism of bowel disturbance in ulcerative colitis. Gastroenterology 93, 934–940.

14. Arhau, P., Devroede, G., Jehannin, B., Lanza, M., Faverdin, C., Persoz, B., Terreault, L., Perey, B. and Pellerin, D. Segmental colonic transit time. Dis. Colon Rectum 24, 625–629.

15. Committee on Radiation Protection and Public Health, NEA, OECD (1988) Gastrointestinal absorption of selected radionuclides — A report by an NEA Expert Group. NEA, Paris.

16. Brambell, F.M.R. (1970) Transmission of passive immunity from mother to young. Frontiers in Biology 18, North Holland, Amsterdam.

17. Clarke, R.M. and Hardy, R.N. (1971) Structural changes and the uptake of polyvinyl pyrrolidone in the small intestine. J. Anat. 108, 79–87.

18. Fritsch, P., Moutairou, K., Lataillade, G., Beauvallet, M., L'Hullier, I., Lepage, M., Metivier, H. and Masse, R. (1988) Localisation of plutonium retention in the small intestine of the neonatal rat, guinea pig, baboon and macaca after Pu-citrate ingestion. Int. J. Radiat. Biol. 54, 537–543.

19. Sullivan, M.F. (1980) Absorption of actinide elements form the gastrointestinal tract of neonatal animals. Health Phys. 38, 173–185.

20. Sullivan, M.F. and Gorham, L.S. (1982) Further studies on the absorption of actinide elements from the gastrointestinal tract of neonatal animals. Health Phys. 43, 509–519.

21. Harrison, J.D., Bomford, J.A. and David, A.J. (1987) The gastrointestinal absorption of plutonium and americium in neonatal mammals. In: G.B. Gerber, H. Metivier and H. Smith (Eds.), Age-related Factors in Radionuclide Metabolism. Martinus Nijhoff, Lancaster. pp. 27–34.

22. Walker, W.A. and Isselbacher, K.J. (1974) Uptake and transport of macromolecules by the intestine. Possible role in clinical disorders. Gastroenterology 67, 531–550.

23. Udall, J.N., Pang, K., Fritze, L., Kleinman, R. and Walker, W.A. Development of gastrointestinal mucosal barrier: I. The effect of age on intestinal permeability to macromolecules. Pediatr. Res. 15, 241–244.

24. Harrison, J.D. and Fritsch, P. (1992) The effect of age on the absorption and intestinal retention of ingested radionuclides. In: D.M. Taylor, G.B. Gerber and J.W. Stather (Eds.), Age-dependent Factors in the Biokinetics and Dosimetry of Radionuclides. Radiat. Prot. Dosim. 41 (2/4), 71–76.

25. Leggett, R.W. and Eckerman, K.F. (1984) A model for the age-dependent skeletal retention of plutonium. In: A. Kaul, R. Neider, J. Pensko, F.-E. Stieve and H. Brunner (Eds.), Radiation Risk Protection. Vol. 1, Fachverband fur Strahlenschutz e.V., Berlin. pp. 454–457.

26. Leggett, R.W., Eckerman, K.F. and Williams, L.R. (1982) Strontium-90 in bone: a case study in age-dependent dosimetric modelling. Health Phys. 43, 307–322.

27. Leggett, R.W. (1985) A model for the retention, translocation and excretion of systemic plutonium. Health Phys. 49, 1115–1137.

28. Leggett, R.W. (1992) A generic age-specific biokinetic model for calcium-like elements. In: D.M. Taylor, G.B. Gerber and J.W. Stather (Eds.), Age-dependent Factors in the Biokinetics and Dosimetry of Radionuclides. Radiat. Prot. Dosim. 41 (2/4), 183–198.

29. Cristy, M. and Eckerman, K.F. (1987) Specific Absorbed Fractions of energy at various ages from internal photon sources. ORNL/TM-8381/V1-7. Oak Ridge National Laboratory, Oak Ridge.

30. Pinson, E.A. and Langham, W H. (1957) Physiology and toxicology of tritium in man. J. Applied Physiol. 10, 108–126.

31. Wiseman, G. (1964). Absorption from the Intestine. Academic Press, New York.

32. Paley, K. and Sussman, E. (1963) Absorption of radioactive colbaltous chloride in human subjects. Metabolism 12, 975–982.

33. Smith, T., Edmonds, C. and Barnaby, C. (1972) Absorption and retention of cobalt in man by whole body counting. Health Phys. 22, 359–367.

34. Valberg, L., Ludwig, J. and Olatunbosun, D. (1969) Alteration in colbalt absorption in patients with disorders of iron metabolism. Gastroenterology 56, 241–251.

35. Sill, C., Anderson, J. and Percival, D. (1964) Comparison of excretion analysis with whole body counting for assessment for internal radioactive contaminants. In: Assessment of Radioactivity in Man. Vol.1, IAEA, Vienna. pp. 217–229.

36. Fujita, M., Yabe, A., Akaishi, J. and Ohtani, S. (1966) Relationship between ingestion, excretion and accumulation of fallout caesium-137 in man on a long term scale. Health Phys. 12, 1649–1653.

37. Carr, T.E.I. (1967) An attempt to quantitate the short term movement of strontium in the human adult. In: J. Lenihan, J.F. Loutit and J.H. Martin (Eds.), Strontium Metabolism. Academic Press, London. pp. 139–148.

38. Spencer, H., Samachson, J. and Laszlo, D. (1960) Metabolism of strontium-85 and calcium-45 in man. Metab. Clin. Exp. 9, 916–925.

39. Suguri, S., Ohtani, S., Oshino, M. and Yanagidhita, K. (1963) The behaviour of strontium-85 in a normal man following a single ingestion — application of the whole body counter for the retention. Health Phys. 9, 529–535.

40. Shimmins, J., Smith, D.A., Nordin, B.E.C. and Burkinshaw, L.A. (1967) A comparison between calcium-45 and strontium-85 absorption, excretion and skeletal uptake. In: J. Lenihan, J.F. Loutit and J.H. Martin (Eds.), Stontium Metabolism. Academic Press, London. pp. 149–159.

41. Coughtrey, P.J. and Thorne, M.C. (1983) Radionuclide distribution and transport in terrestrial and aquatic ecosystems. Vol. 1. A.A. Balkema, Rotterdam. pp. 170–178.

42. McClellan, R.O. and Bustad, L.K. (1964) Gastrointestinal absorption of [85]Sr titanate. In: Hanford Biology Research Annual Report for 1963, Washington (HW 80500), pp. 100–101.

43. Fletcher, C.R. (1969) The radiological hazards of zirconium-95 and niobium-95. Health Phys. 16, 209–220.

44. Shiraishi, Y. and Ichikawa, R. (1972) Absorption and retention of [144]Ce and [95]Zr-[95]Nb in newborn, juvenile and adult rats. Health Phys. 22, 373–378.

45. Schroeder, H.A. and Balassa, J.J. (1965) Abnormal trace elements in man: niobium. J. Chron. Dis. 18, 229–241.

46. Furchner, J.E. and Drake, G.A. (1971) Comparative metabolism of radionuclides in mammals — VI. Retention of [95]Nb in the mouse, rat, monkey and dog. Health Phys. 21, 173–180.

47. Thomas,R.G., Walker, S.A. and McClellan, R.O. (1971) Relative hazards of inhaled [95]Zr and [95]Nb particles formed under various thermal conditions. Proc. Soc. Exp. Biol. Med. 138, 228–234.

48. Mraz, F.R. and Eisele, G.R. (1977) Gastrointestinal absorption of [95]Nb by rats of different ages. Radiat. Res. 69, 591–593.

49. Harrison, J.D., Haines, J.W. and Popplewell, D.S. (1990) The gastrointestinal absorption and retention of niobium in adult and newborn guinea pigs. Int. J. Radiat. Biol. 58, 177–186.

50. Yamagata, N., Iwashima, K., Iinuma, T.N., Watari, K. and Nagai, T. (1969) Uptake and retention experiments of radioruthenium in man — I. Health Phys. 16, 159–166.

51. Burykina, L.N. (1962) The metabolism of radioactive ruthenium in the organism of experimental animals. In: A.A. Letavel and E.P. Kurlyandsicaya (Eds.), The Toxicology of Radioactive Substances, Vol. 1. Pergamon Press, Oxford. pp. 60–76.

52. Thompson, R.C., Weeks, M.H., Hollis, L., Ballou, J.F. and Oakley, W.D. (1958) Metabolism of radioruthenium in the rat. Amer. J. Roentgen. 79, 1026–1044.

53. Furchner, J.E., Richmond, C.R., and Drake, G.A. (1971) Comparative metabolism of radionuclides in mammals, VII. Retention of 106-Ru in the mouse, rat, monkey and dog. Health Phys. 21, 355–365.

54. Bruce, R.S. and Carr, T.E.F. (1961) Studies in the metabolism of carrier-free radio-ruthenium — I. Preliminary investigations. Reactor Sci. Technol. (JNE Pts AB) 14, 9–17.

55. Stara, J.F., Nelson, N.S., Della Rosa, R.J. and Bustad, L.K. (1971) Comparative metabolism of radionuclides in mammals: a review. Health Phys. 20, 113–137.

56. Bruce, R.S. (1963) Some factors influencing the absorption, retention and elimination of radioruthenium. In: Diagnosis and Treatment of Radioactive Poisoning. IAEA, Vienna. pp. 207–224.

57. Wayne, E.J. Koutras, D.A. and Alexander, W.D. (1964) Clinical Aspects of Iodine Metabolism. Blackwell Scientific Publications, Oxford.

58. Underwood J. (1971). Iodine. In: Trace Elements in Human and Animal Nutrition. Academic Press, New York.

59. Rossof, B., Cohn, S.H., and Spencer, H. (1963) Caesium-137 metabolism in man. Radiat. Res. 19, 643–654.

60. Rundo, J., Mason, J.I., Newton, D. and Taylor, B.T. (1963) Biological half-life of caesium in man in acute and chronic exposure. Nature 200, 188–189.

61. Naverston, Y. and Liden, K. (1964) Half-life studies of radiocaesium in humans. In: Assessment of Radioactive Body Burden in Man. IAEA, Vienna. pp. 79–87.

62. LeRoy, G.V., Rust, J.H. and Hasterlik, R.J. (1966) The consequences of ingestion by man of real and simulated fall-out. Health Phys. 12, 449–473.

63. Henrichs, K., Paretzke, H.G., Voight, G. and Berg, D. (1989) Measurement of Cs absorption and retention in man. Health Phys. 57, 571–578.

64. Talbot, R.J., Newton, D., Warner, A.J., Walters, B. and Sherlock, J.C. (1993) Human uptake of ^{137}Cs in mutton. Health Phys. 64, 600–604.

65. Talbot, R.J. (1991) The gastrointestinal absorption of fission products. In: Radiological Protection Research 1991 Annual Report, AEA Environment and Energy, AEA Technology. p. 64.

66. Fujita, M., Yabe, A., Akaishi, J. and Ohtani, S. (1966) Relationship between ingestion, excretion and accumulation of fall-out caesium-137 in man on a long term scale. Health Phys. 12, 1649–1653.

67. Suomela, M. (1971) Elimination rate of ^{137}Cs in individuals and in the control group. In: Proc. Nordic Soc. Radiation Protection, Copenhagen. Institute of Radiation Hygiene, Copenhagen. pp. 285–298.

68. Hasanan, E. and Rahola, T. (1971) The biological half-life of ^{137}Cs and ^{24}Na in man. Ann. Clin. Res. 3, 236–240.

69. Leggett, R.W. (1986) Predicting the retention of Cs in individuals. Health Phys. 50, 747–759.

70. Sill, C.W., Voelz, G.L., Olson, D.G. and Anderson, J.I. (1969) Two studies of acute internal exposure to man involving cerium and tantalum radioisotopes. Health Phys. 16, 325–332.

71. International Commission on Radiological Protection. (1994) Dose Coefficients for Intakes of Radionuclides by Workers based on the 1990 Basic Recommendations and on the 1994 Respiratory Tract model: Revision of ICRP Publication 61. Publication 68. Pergamon Press, Oxford. Ann. ICRP 24, (4).

72. Chamberlain, A.C., Heard, M.J., Little, P., Newton, D., Wells, A.C. and Wiffen, R.D. (1978) Investigations into lead from motor vehicles. AERE-R 9198. Harwell: Environmental and Medical Sciences Division, AERE.

73. Wetherill, G.W., Rabinowitz, M. and Kopple, J.D. (1975) Sources and metabolic pathways of lead in normal humans. In: Recent advances in the assessment of the health effects of environmental pollution. CEC, Paris. pp. 847–860.

74. James, H.M., Hilburn, M.E. and Blair, J.A. (1985) Effects of meals and meal times on uptake of lead from the gastrointestinal tract in humans. Human Toxicol. 4, 401–407.

75. Blake, K.C.H. (1976) Absorption of ^{203}Pb from the gastrointestinal tract of man. Environ. Res. 11, 1–4.

76. Heard, M.J. and Chamberlain, A.C. (1982) Effects of minerals and food on uptake of lead from the gastrointestinal tract in humans. Human Toxicol. 1, 411–415.

77. Fink, R.M. (1950) Biological Studies with Polonium, Radium and Plutonium. McGraw-Hill, London.

78. Hill, C.R. (1965) ^{210}Po in man. Nature 208, 423–428.

79. Kauranen, P. and Miettinen, J.K. (1967) ^{210}Po and ^{210}Pb in environmental samples in Finland. In: B. Aberg and F.P. Hungate (Eds.), Radiological Concentration Processes. Pergamon Press, Oxford. pp. 275–280.

80. Landinskaya, L.S., Parfenov, Y.D., and Popov, D.K. (1973) Lead-210 and ^{210}Po content in air, water, foodstuffs and the human body. Arch. Environ. Health 27, 254–258.

81. Hunt, G.J. and Allington, D.J. (1993) Absorption of environmental ^{210}Po by the

human gut. J. Radiol. Prot. 13, 119–126.

82. Anthony, D.S., Davis, R.K., Cowden, R.N., and Jolley, W.P. (1956) Experimental data useful in establishing maximum single and multiple exposure to polonium. In: Proceedings of the International Conference on the Peaceful Uses of Atomic Energy, 13. United Nations, New York. pp. 215–218.

83. Della Rosa, J.R., Thomas, R.G. and Stannard, J.N. (1955) The acute toxicity and retention of orally administered polonium-210. University of Rochester, UR-392.

84. Haines, J.W., Naylor, G.P.L., Pottinger, H. and Harrison, J.D. (1993) Gastrointestinal absorption and retention of polonium in adult and newborn rats and guinea pigs. Int. J. Radiat. Biol. 64, 127–132.

85. International Commission on Radiological Protection (1973) Alkaline Earth Metabolism in Adult Man. ICRP Publication 20. Pergamon Press, Oxford.

86. Seil, H.A., Viol, C.H. and Gordon, M.A. (1915) The elimination of soluble radium salts taken intravenously and per os. New York Med. J. 5, 40–44.

87. Maletskos, C.J., Keane, A.T., Telles, N.C. and Evans, R.D. (1966) The metabolism of intravenously administered radium and thorium in human beings and the relative absorption from the human gastrointestinal tract of radium and thorium in simulated radium dial paints. In: Annual Report of Radioactivity Centre, Mass. Inst. of Technology, MIT-952-3, p.202.

88. Maletskos, C.J., Keane, A.T., Telles, N.C. and Evans, R.D. (1969) Retention and absorption of [224]Ra and [234]Th and some dosimetric considerations of [224]Ra in human beings. In: C.W. Mays, W.S.S. Jee, R.D. Lloyd, B.J. Stover, J.H. Dougherty and G.N. Taylor (Eds.), Delayed Effects of Bone-seeking Radionuclides. University of Utah Press, Salt Lake City. pp. 29–49.

89. Johnson, J.R. and Lamothe, E.S. (1989) A Review of the Dietary Uptake of Th. Health Phys. 56, 165–168.

90. Dang, H.S. and Sunta, C.M. (1990) Gastrointestinal absorption factor (f_1) for Th from diet. Health Phys. 58, 220–221.

91. Traikovich, M. (1970) Absorption, distribution and excretion of certain soluble compounds of natural thorium. In: A.A. Letavet and E.B. Kurlyandskaya (Eds.), Toxicology of Radioactive Substances, Vol. 4: Thorium-232 and Uranium-238. English Translation (G.W. Dolphin, Ed.). Pergamon Press, Oxford.

92. Sullivan, M.F. (1980) Absorption of actinide elements from the gastrointestinal tract of rats, guinea pigs, pigs and dogs. Health Phys. 38, 159–171.

93. Sullivan, M.F., Miller, B.M. and Ryan, J.L. (1983) Absorption of thorium and protactinium from the gastrointestinal tract in adult mice and rats and neonatal rats. Health Phys. 44, 425–428.

94. Larsen, R.P., Oldham, R.D., Bhattacharyya, M.H. and Moretti, E.S. (1984) Gastrointestinal absorption and distribution of thorium in the mouse. In: Environmental Research Division Annual Report, July 1982–June 1983; Argonne National Laboratory, ANL-83-100-Pt.2. pp. 65–68.

95. Wrenn, M.D., Durbin, P.W., Howard, B., Lipzstein, J., Rundo, J., Still, E.T. and Willis, D.L. (1985) Metabolism of ingested U and Ra. Health Phys. 48, 601–603.

96. Harrison, J.D. The gastrointestinal absorption of the actinide elements. Sci. Total Environment 100, 43–60.

97. Leggett, R.W. and Harrison, J.D. (1995) Fractional absorption of ingested U in humans. Health Phys. 68, 484–498.

98. Hursh, J.B., Neuman, W.R., Toribara, T., Wilson, H. and Waterhouse, C. (1969) Oral ingestion of uranium by man. Health Phys. 17, 619–621.

99. Wrenn, M.D., Singh, N.A., Ruth, H., Rallison, M.I. and Burleigh, D.P. (1989) Gastrointestinal absorption of soluble uranium from drinking water by man. Radiat. Prot. Dosim. 26, 119–122.

100. Harduin, J.C., Royer, Ph and Piechowski, J. (1994) Uptake and urinary excretion of uranium after oral administration in man. In: J.W. Stather and A. Karaoglou (Eds.), Intakes of Radionuclides. Radiat. Prot. Dosim. 53, 245–248.

101. Larsen, R.P. and Orlandini, K.A. (1984) Gastrointestinal absorption of uranium in man. In: Environmental Research Division Annual Report, July 1982–June 1983; Argonnne National Laboratory, ANL-83-100-Pt.2. pp. 46–50.

102. Spencer, H., Osis, D., Fisenne, I.M., Perry, P.M. and Harley, N.H. (1990) Measured intake and excretion patterns of naturally occurring ^{234}U, ^{238}U and calcium in humans. Radiat. Res. 124, 90–95.

103. Bhattacharyya, M.H., Larsen, R.P., Cohen, N., Ralston, L.G., Moretti, E.S., Oldham, R.D. and Ayres, L (1989) Gastrointestinal absorption of plutonium and uranium in fed and fasted adult baboons and mice: application to humans. Radiat. Prot. Dosim. 26, 159–165.

104. Popplewell, D.S., Harrison, J.D. and Ham, G.J. (1991) Gastrointestinal absorption of neptunium and curium in humans. Health Phys. 60, 797–805.

105. International Commission on Radiological Protection (1986) The Metabolism of Plutonium and Related Elements. ICRP Publication 48. Pergamon Press, Oxford. Ann. ICRP 16, (2/3).

106. Ballou, J.E., Bair, W.J., Case, A.C. and Thompson, R.C. (1962) Studies with neptunium in the rat. Health Phys. 8, 685–688.

107. Sullivan, M.F. and Crosby, A.L. (1975) Absorption of uranium-233, neptunium-237, plutonium-238, americium-241, curium-244, and einsteinium-253 from the gastrointestinal tract of newborn and adult rats. In: Pacific Northwest Laboratory Annual Report for 1974, Pt. 1. Biomedical Sciences. BNWL-1950, p. 105.

108. Sullivan, M.F. and Crosby, A.L. (1976) Absorption of transuranic elements from rat gut. In: Pacific Northwest Laboratory Annual Report for 1975, Pt. 1. Biomedical Sciences. BNWL-2000, p. 91.

109. Metivier, H., Masse, R. and Lafuma, J. (1983) Effect de la masse sur l'absorption intestinale du neptunium V chez le singe et le rat. Radioprot. 18, 13–17.

110. Metivier, H., Bourges, J., Fritsch, P., Nolibe, D. and Masse, R. (1986) Gastrointestinal absorption of neptunium in primates: Effect of ingested mass, diet and fasting. Radiat. Res. 106, 190–200.

111. Harrison, J.D., Popplewell, D.S. and David, A.J. (1984) The effect of concentration and chemical form on the gastrointestinal absorption of neptunium. Int. J. Radiat. Biol. 46, 269–277.

112. Hunt, G.J., Leonard, D.R.P., and Lovett, M.B. (1986) Transfer of environmental plutonium and americium across the human gut. Sci. Total Environ. 53, 89–109.

113. Hunt, G.J., Leonard, D.R.P., and Lovett, M.B. (1990) Transfer of environmental plutonium and americium across the human gut: A second study. Sci. Total Environ. 90, 273–282.

114. Mussalo-Rauhamaa, H., Jaakola, T., Mietttinen, J.K. and Laiho, K. (1984) Plutonium in Finish Lapps — An estimate of the gastrointestinal absorption of plutonium by man based on a comparison of the plutonium content of Lapps and southern Finns. Health Phys. 46, 549–556.

115. Metivier, H., Madic, C., Bourges, J. and Masse, R. (1985) Valency five, similarities between plutonium and neptunium in gastrointestinal uptake. In: R.A. Bulman

and J.R. Cooper (Eds.), Speciation of Fission and Activation Products in the Environment. Elsevier Applied Science Publishers, London. pp. 175–178.

116. United Nations Scientific Committee on the Effects of Atomic Radiation (1988) Sources, Effects and Risks of Ionising Radiation. Report to the General Assembly. United Nations, New York. p. 552.

117. Stather, J.W., Muirhead, C.R., Edwards, A.A., Harrison, J.D., Lloyd, D.C. and Wood, N.R. (1988) Health Effects Models Developed from the 1988 UNSCEAR Report. National Radiological Protection Board, NRPB-R226. HMSO, London. pp. 6–7.

118. Thomas, R.L., Storb, R. and Clift, R.A. (1975) Bone marrow transplantation. New Engl. J. Med. 292, 832–843.

119. Sullivan, M.F., Marks, S., Hackett, P.L. and Thompson, R.C. (1959) X-irradiation of the exteriorised or *in situ* intestine of the rat. Radiat. Res. 73, 11, 653–666.

120. Fry, S.A. and Sipe, A.H. (1986) The REAC/TS registries status. In: A. Kaul et al. (Eds.) Biological Indicators for Radiation Dose Assessment. MMV Medizin Verlag, Munich.

121. Thompson, R.C. (1978) Hanford americium exposure incident: overview and perspective. Health Phys. 45, 837–845.

122. Guskova, A.K. and Baisogolov, G.D. (1971) Radiation Sickness in Man. Meditsina Publishers, Moscow.

123. Bond, V.P., Fliedner, T.M. and Archambau, J.O. (1965) Mammalian Radiation Lethality. Academic Press, New York.

124. Maisin, J., Maisin, J.R. and Dunjic, A. (1971) The gastrointestinal tract. In: C.C. Berjis, (Eds.) Pathology of Irradiation. William and Wilkins, Baltimore. p. 296.

125. Sullivan, M.F., Ruemmler, P.S., Beamer, J.L., Mahoney, T.D. and Cross, F.T. (1978) Acute toxicity of beta-emitting radionuclides that may be released in a reactor accident and ingested. Radiat. Res. 73, 21–36.

126. Cross, F.T., Endres, G.W.R. and Sullivan, M.F. (1978) Dose to the GI tract from ingested insoluble beta emitters. Radiat. Res. 73, 37–50.

127. Pochin, E.E. (1988) Sizewell B Inquiry. The biological bases of the assumptions made by NRPB in the calculation of health effects. Proof of Evidence. Chilton, NRPB/P/2.

128. Scott, B.R. and Hahn, F.F. (1985) Early and continuing effects. In: J.S. Evans, J.W. Moeller, and D.W. Cooper (Eds.), Health Effects Model for Nuclear Power Plant Accident Consequence Analysis. USNRC, NUREG/CR 4214 (SAND 85-7185). NTIS, Springfield.

129. Sullivan, M.F., Cross, F.T. and Dagle, G.E. (1987) Dosimetry of the gastrointestinal tract. In: G.B. Gerber, H. Metivier and H. Smith (Eds.), Age-related Factors in Radionuclide Metabolism. Martinus Nijhoff, Lancaster. pp. 49–66.

130. Casarett, G.W. (1973) Pathogenesis of radionuclide-induced tumours. In: C.L. Sanders, R.H. Busch, J.E. Ballou and D.D. Mahlum (Eds.), Radionuclide Carcinogenesis. NTIS, Springfield. pp. 1–14.

131. Lebedeva, G.A. (1973) Intestinal polyps arising under the influence of various kinds of ionising radiations. Vop. Onkol. 19, 47–51.

132. Moser, A.R., Pitot, H.C. and Dove, W.F. (1990) A dominant mutation that predisposes to multiple intestinal neoplasia in the mouse. Science 247, 322–324.

133. Su, L-K., Kinzler, K.W., Vogelstein, B., Preisinger, A.C., Moser, A.R., Luongo, C., Gould, K.A. and Dove, W.F. (1992) Multiple intestinal neoplasia caused by a mutation in the murine homolog of the APC gene. Science 256, 668–670.

C.S. Potten and J.H. Hendry (Eds.), *Radiation and Gut*

CHAPTER 10

Radiation Carcinogenesis in the Gut

J.D. Boice Jr.[1] and R.J. Michael Fry[2]

[1]*National Cancer Institute and* [2]*Biology Division, Oak Ridge National Laboratory,*
P.O. Box 2009, Oak Ridge, TN 37831-8077, USA

1. INTRODUCTION

In England and Wales and in the USA, cancer of the oesophagus, stomach, small intestine, colon and rectum accounts for about 15–16% of the total cancer mortality. In contrast, cancer in these sites accounts for about 31% of the total cancer mortality in Japan. In the USA, colorectal cancers account for about 79% of the mortality from cancers of the gastrointestinal tract, whereas in Japan cancer of the stomach predominates.

The importance of radiation-induced cancer of the gut in the estimate of excess risk of all types of cancer after exposure to low doses of radiation is indicated by the fact that the risk of cancer of the oesophagus, stomach and colon accounts for about 45% of the estimate by the International Commission on Radiological Protection [1]. This estimate is based on the cancer mortality in the atomic bomb survivors and a transfer of the estimate to other populations. It is not clear how appropriate it is to base the risk of radiation-induced cancer for a population on the estimates of risk for a different population with substantially different background rates of cancer mortality for specific cancer sites, nor is it known how the risks should be transferred from one population to another.

In the case of experimental animals, the incidence of naturally occurring cancers of the gut is very low, and information about induction of cancer in the gut by radiation is sparse. The very low incidence of naturally occurring tumours and the low susceptibility for induction of cancer of the small intestine by radiation in both experimental animals and humans remain unexplained. In this chapter the evidence for induction of cancer of the gut in both humans and experimental animals by radiation is presented and the comparative aspects are discussed.

2. HUMAN EVIDENCE FOR RADIATION EFFECTS

Evidence that ionizing radiation causes cancer of the gut in humans comes from epidemiological studies of survivors of the atomic bombings in Japan [2,3], patients given radiotherapy for cervical cancer [4,5], and patients treated with radiation for benign conditions such as ankylosing spondylitis [6], gynaecological disorders [7,8], and peptic ulcer [9]. These analytical studies have applied sound methodology to determine cancer occurrence within defined populations. Further, comprehensive dosimetry programs were able to reconstruct radiation doses to specific organs, resulting in estimates of risk per Gy.

The studies of the atomic bomb survivors have followed subjects prospectively for nearly 40 years at the level of mortality [10,11] and most recently incidence [3]. The average whole-body dose was relatively low, about 0.23 Gy, but the distribution of doses ranged up to 4 Gy, permitting dose-response evaluations. This is the single most informative study on radiation risks, including exposures of both men and women, and children and adults. Its major limitation is that risks apply to acute brief radiation exposures and not necessarily to the chronic or periodic exposures experienced in daily life from environmental, occupational or medical sources.

Cervical cancer patients given radiotherapy provide a large experience of incident second cancers [4,5]. Although doses to the pelvic region were enormous, many tens of gray, doses outside the pelvis were much lower due to scatter or machine leakage. This study provides an opportunity to evaluate quantitatively the effects of high-dose partial-body irradiation. The dosimetry was based on existing medical records. The major limitations include the cell-killing effects of therapeutic radiation and the possible influence of the underlying cancer on the development of new cancers.

Ankylosing spondylitis patients treated with radiation have provided important information on radiation risks [6]. Mortality comparisons have been with general population rates. Prospective follow-up has occurred since the 1950s. The major limitations include the absence of individual dosimetry, except for leukaemia cases, which precludes a convincing evaluation of dose–response relationships for solid tumours. Further, the crippling condition being treated and subsequent therapies could have influenced cancer risk.

Women treated with radiation for benign gynaecological disorders, mainly uterine bleeding, have provided useful information on radiation risks [7,8]. The doses were a magnitude lower than those given to cancer patients, and survival was quite good. The major limitation is perhaps the small number of treated subjects, which can result in unstable risk estimates.

A new study is the one of peptic ulcer patients treated with about 16 Gy to the stomach to reduce acid secretion [9]. The doses could be computed accurately, but the uniformity of treatments limited dose–response evaluations. Further, peptic ulcer patients who undergo surgical procedures were known to be at high risk for stomach cancer.

One study of diagnostic radiation has provided information on radiation doses to organs in the trunk. Tuberculosis patients undergoing lung collapse had received up to several hundred chest fluoroscopies to monitor the extent of the collapse [11]. The exposures were fractionated over a period of several years. Organ doses could be estimated based on assumptions of patient orientation and time the fluoroscope was on.

In general, radiation risk estimates for cancers of the gut are much lower than for leukaemia and thyroid cancer, and somewhat lower than for cancers of the lung and breast. However, because cancers of the gut make up nearly 15–16% of all human cancers, whole-body exposures of sufficient dose can result in a large cancer burden; e.g., approximately 40% of the excess cancers among atomic bomb survivors are attributable to those arising in the gut.

Radiation risk can be measured in several ways. A relative risk (RR) is the ratio of observed (O) cancers in exposed persons over that expected (E) in the absence of radiation exposure. A relative risk is influenced by the baseline cancer incidence in the population being studied. Absolute excess risk can be defined as the observed minus expected cancers divided by the person-years (PY) of observation, i.e., (O – E)/PY. Radiation risk coefficients are usually normalized to a certain dose, such as 1 Gy for a specific period of observation. For example, the RR at 1 Gy for fatal oesophageal cancers among Japanese atomic bomb survivors is 1.59, indicating a 59% relative excess over expectation. The corresponding absolute excess risk is 0.44 per 10,000 per PY per Gy, i.e., in 100,000 persons exposed to 1 Gy between 4–5 extra deaths due to cancer of the oesophagus might be expected to occur each year after a minimum latency of 5–9 years had passed. Please note that this example is just for illustrative purposes since the actual estimate of risk for atomic bomb survivors was not statistically significant and chance might have been the reason for the suggested increase.

2.1 Oesophagus (Table 1)

Only one of the four population studies evaluating radiation-induced oesophageal cancer reports a significant excess. Studies of cervical cancer patients and Massachusetts tuberculosis patients were negative. The A-bomb series found modest increases that were not significant. Ankylosing spondylitis patients received the highest estimated dose, 4 Gy, and were at a significantly increased risk of mortality in comparison with the general population. Interestingly, the TB series reported a significant mortality risk when compared with general population rates, but when the comparison was made with a non-exposed TB population there was no excess in mortality from oesophageal cancer. The authors were able to evaluate smoking and alcohol as risk factors for oesophageal cancer. They concluded that the apparent excess when compared with the general population was because persons with TB drank and smoked cigarettes to a much greater extent. Conceivably the fractionated nature of the low-dose exposures, accumulating to over 1 Gy, could also have allowed cellular repair of radiation damage to occur.

TABLE 1

Human studies of radiation-induced cancer of the oesophagus

Study	Cancers		Mean dose (Gy)	Relative risk at 1 Gy	Absolute excess risk $(10^4 \text{ PY-Gy})^{-1}$ [a]
	Observed	Expected			
A-bomb survivors					
Mortality [2]	103	90.8	0.23	1.59	0.44
Incidence [3]	84	78.9	0.23	1.29	0.29
Cervical cancer [4]	12	11.0	0.35	1.26	0.16
Massachusetts TB fluoroscopy [11]	14	13.8	1.06	1.01	0.01
Ankylosing spondylitis [6]	28*	12.7	4.00	1.30	0.21

*Statistically significant excess.
[a]PY: person years.

2.2 Stomach (Table 2)

Stomach cancer is perhaps the most important radiation effect among A-bomb survivors, making up 30% of the total incident cancers and 16% of the excess attributable to radiation [3]. Significant excess has occurred in only 2 other series, cervical cancer patients (2 Gy) and peptic ulcer patients (16 Gy). Studies of patients irradiated for gynaecological conditions, spondylitis and hyperthyroidism were essentially negative.

TABLE 2

Human studies of radiation-induced cancer of the stomach

Study	Cancers		Mean dose (Gy)	Relative risk at 1 Gy	Absolute excess risk $(10^4 \text{ PY-Gy})^{-1}$
	Observed	Expected			
A-bomb survivors					
Mortality [2]	1163*	1108	0.23	1.22	2.02
Incidence [3]	1307*	1222	0.23	1.30	4.68
Cervical cancer [5]	348*	117.3	2.00	1.54	0.3
Ankylosing spondylitis [6]	55	54.3	1.65	1.01	0.03
Benign gynaecological disease [7]	23	21.8	0.20	1.28	0.78
Metropathia haemorrhagica [8]	33	26.8	0.23	1.01	5.72
Peptic ulcer [9]	40	17.4	14.8	1.09	0.43
Hyperthyroidism, ^{131}I [12]	92	87.6	0.25	1.20	1.35

*Statistically significant excess.

Radiotherapy and surgery have both been linked to excesses of stomach cancer in patients treated for peptic ulcer [9]. When given together, radiotherapy and surgery appeared to greatly enhance the development of stomach cancer, suggesting a complex carcinogenic process involving radiation damage of stem cells, extreme treatment-induced hypoacidity, and associated increased bacterial growth and exposure to N-nitroso compounds (or other promoting factors) of cells no longer protected by stomach mucosa.

The stomach plays a critical role in the risk estimates used for radiation protection purposes in that absolute risks from Japan are transported across the Pacific Ocean to Western countries to estimate the cancer burden for occupationally exposed groups [13]. The use of absolute risks appears reasonable for breast cancer since there are a number of irradiated populations in Western countries providing comparative information [14]. An analogy for stomach cancer, however, does not seem to hold up; i.e., relative and not absolute risks appear similar (Table 2). Why should this matter? Because the underlying rate of stomach cancer in Japan is so high in comparison with Western countries, equality in the relative risk estimates per unit dose implies a much larger absolute excess risk. Thus it may be that the practice of transporting absolute risks greatly overestimates the possible cancer hazard in Western populations. Females appear to be at higher radiation risk than males [3].

2.3 Colon (Table 3)

Colon cancer has occurred in excess in most irradiated populations with the notable exception of cervical cancer patients. Conceivably, the cytotoxic doses used to treat cancer of the uterine cervix resulted in cellular killing, overpowering any possible transforming effect that such high doses might have. As seen for radiogenic leukaemia, cells with high proliferative activity may be especially sensitive to the killing effects of therapeutic radiation [15]. For the studies reporting significant excess of colon cancer, the relative risk (RR) at 1 Gy ranges from 1.13 to 1.67 and the absolute risk per 10^4 PY-Gy from 0.45 to 2.81. In contrast to most other sites, exposures under the age of 20 carried a lower risk than those over age 20 [3].

2.4 Rectum (Table 4)

The only evidence that cancer of the rectum can be induced by radiation comes from the study of cervical cancer patients where the doses were enormous, ranging between 30 to 60 Gy. No other study finds excess, even from doses on the order of several Gy. The cellular destruction caused by massive deposition of radiation energy must be involved in a mechanism different from carcinogenic processes at lower doses. The possibility that the turnover of cells is lower in the rectum than in the colon might also account for the different patterns seen at high and low doses.

TABLE 3

Human studies of radiation-induced cancer of the colon

Study	Cancers		Mean dose (Gy)	Relative risk at 1 Gy	Absolute excess risk $(10^4 \text{ PY-Gy})^{-1}$
	Observed	Expected			
A-bomb survivors					
Mortality [2]	129*	116.5	0.23	1.47	0.45
Incidence [3]	223*	193.7	0.23	1.67	1.65
Cervical cancer [5]	409	409	24.0	1.00	0.00
Benign gynaecological disease [7]	75*	46.6	1.30	1.47	2.81
Metropathia haemorrhagica [8]	47*	33	3.20	1.13	0.93
Peptic ulcer [9]	25	20.6	6.00	1.04	0.07

*Statistically significant excess.

TABLE 4

Human studies of radiation-induced cancer of the rectum

Study	Cancers		Mean dose (Gy)	Relative risk at 1 Gy	Absolute excess risk $(10^4 \text{ PY-Gy})^{-1}$
	Observed	Expected			
A-bomb survivors					
Mortality [10]	216	219.5	0.23	0.93	−0 07
Incidence [3]	179	170.8	0.23	1.21	0.43
Cervical cancer [5]	488*	266.7	30–60	1.02	0.06
Benign gynaecological disease [7]	21	18.9	3.00	1.04	0.06
Metropathia haemorrhagica [8]	14	12.4	4.9	1.03	0.06

*Statistically significant excess.

2.5 Generalizations

1. Irradiation of the human gut can result in excess cancers. An overall RR at 1 Gy is about 1.4 and the excess absolute risk per 10^4 PY-Gy is about 10 among Japanese A-bomb survivors.

2. Not all organs comprising the gut are equally susceptible to the induction of cancer. No study finds excess risks for cancers of the small intestine, and only therapeutic doses appear to raise the risk of rectal cancer. Cancers of the stomach and colon carry the greatest risk of late radiation effects.

3. Cancers of the gut do not occur immediately after irradiation, and a minimum latent period of 5–9 years is required.

4. Cancers of the gut play a pivotal role in the total risk estimate used in radiation protection in that the method used to transport risks from the A-bomb study to Western countries determines substantially the predicted level of risk from occupational exposures. The current use of absolute risks, given the high natural occurrence of stomach cancer in Japanese populations, may overestimate radiation risks from occupational exposures.

3. EXPERIMENTAL ANIMALS

3.1 Mice

Naturally occurring tumours of the gastrointestinal tract of mice and rats are rare. Wells et al. [16] reported that in 142,000 autopsies of mice they found no tumours of the small intestine and only 19 tumours in the entire gastrointestinal tract. Eleven of the tumours were associated with prolapsed rectums. Several more recent reports confirmed the low incidence of intestinal tumours [17]. Rowlatt et al. [18] noted incidences of 10% benign tumours and 2% cancers in the small and large intestines in a study of almost 1000 old C57Bl mice. The incidences of tumours reported by these authors are higher than in other reports, suggesting that C57BL may be more susceptible than some other strains. Cosgrove et al. [19] examined two hybrids and one inbred strain. The incidence of naturally occurring tumours of the gastrointestinal tract obtained from the studies of Cosgrove et al. [19]; Nowell and Cole [20], and Watanabe et al. [21] are shown in Table 5.

Strain differences in susceptibility to chemical carcinogens have been noted [22–24]. For example, marked strain differences in susceptibility to the induction of colon cancer by 1–2 dimethylhydrazine (DMH), which requires metabolic activation, have been reported [25]. The studies of Deschner et al. [24] on hybrid

TABLE 5

Incidence of naturally occurring carcinomas in the gastrointestinal tract of various strains and hybrid mice

	Strain and hybrid mice				
	RF[a]	LAF1 [a]	IC3F[a]	LAF1 [b]	ICR-JCL[c]
Incidence (%) Mean±SE	0.0	0.6±0.4	0.5±0.3	0.2±0.3	0.0
Number of mice	2503	815	690	610	18

[a]From Ref. [19]; [b]from Ref. [20]; [c]from Ref. [21].

crosses between the AKR/J strain, which is resistant to induction of tumours of the colon by DMH, and SWR/J, a sensitive strain, suggested that the parental AKR/J strain contributed a repressor gene that influenced progression from dysplasia to neoplasia in the colon. While the number of germ-free mice that have been studied is small, no naturally occurring or radiation-induced tumours of the gut were found [19]. The role of the microflora of the gut in the metabolism of certain carcinogens to the proximate form has been demonstrated by the finding that germ-free mice do not develop tumours of the gut when treated with carcinogens such as cycasin that require metabolic activation [26].

On general principles strain-dependent differences in the susceptibility for the induction of intestinal tumours would be expected. However, there are no studies of radiation carcinogenesis in the gut in which different strains of mice were exposed to the same doses of radiation of the same quality.

4. RADIATION CARCINOGENESIS

In the early studies of the effects of X-rays and neutrons, the reported incidences of induced intestinal tumours were not in excess of 1%. The first report of high incidences of malignant tumours of the gut in mice was by Nowell et al. [27] and Nowell and Cole [20], who exposed C57L × LAF$_1$ mice to 250 kV X-rays and 2 MeV and 8 MeV neutrons generated by the 60-inch cyclotron at Berkeley. The doses ranged from 310–400 rad and 290–580 rad of 2 MeV and 8 MeV neutrons, respectively. The higher doses caused some acute deaths. The two dose groups of X-rays were in the lethal range, namely 800 R and 1000 to 1100 R. The mice in the 800 R group were protected against acute death by injection of isologous haematopoietic cells and the mice in the higher-dose groups by shielding the marrow in one limb. Less than a third of the irradiated mice in this higher-dose group survived. The findings were as follows:

(1) There was no sex-dependent difference in susceptibility for the induction of intestinal tumours.

(2) The data for the 2 and 8 MeV neutron groups were pooled and indicated that 41 of the 310 mice (13%) had adenocarcinomas of the small intestine and the caecum, the incidence being higher in the caecum. Lower incidences of gastric adenocarcinomas (4%) and squamous cell carcinomas (2%) were noted.

(3) There were not sufficient dose groups to determine the dose–response relationships, but no intestinal carcinomas were found in 70 mice exposed to doses of less than 350 rad of 8 MeV neutrons. In the case of the 2 MeV neutrons, adenocarcinomas were found at all doses: 310 to 400 rad.

(4) In the groups exposed to X-rays, 3% of the 285 mice that received 800 R and 22% of the 19 mice at risk after 1000–1100 R developed adenocarcinomas.

(5) The carcinomas were detected between 6 and 16 months after irradiation and did not appear to be dependent on the induction of precancerous lesions.

(6) Neutron irradiation was more effective than X-irradiation for the induction of intestinal carcinomas.

Hirose et al. [28] induced rectal carcinomas of ICR and CF$_1$ female mice with local X-irradiation to the pelvic region. To determine a dose-response relationship, various doses of X-rays were given at weekly intervals. In the ICR mice the incidence of carcinomas rose from zero after a single dose of 20 Gy to 42% after two such doses and 95% with three. After a single dose of 30 Gy the incidence was 31%, but only 6% after two doses of 15 Gy. The authors considered that the results indicated that the CF$_1$ mice were less susceptible. In a study by Rostom et al. [29] to investigate the effect of misonidazole on the induction of intestinal tumours by radiation, high doses, 16–24 Gy, were given by local irradiation of the lower abdomen of C57BL mice. The lowest part of the colon, the majority of the rectum, a small fraction of the small intestine, and in some cases the caecum were in the radiation field. In the mice that survived 50–240 days after 16 Gy, 18% had adenocarcinomas of the small and large intestine. In the mice pretreated with misonidazole, the incidence was 20%. While the number of mice per dose group was small, the incidence rose with dose, and if the data for all the dose groups are pooled, the incidences were 60% with irradiation alone and 68% in the group pretreated with misonidazole. The only significant difference between the irradiated controls and the group pretreated with misonidazole was that the incidence of multiple tumours was higher in the latter group.

4.1 Stomach

The induction of tumours of the stomach has been reported by several investigators [19,20]. Nowell and Cole [20], in the study of the effects of neutron and X-irradiation discussed above, found 11 adenocarcinomas (4%) and 5 squamous cell carcinomas (2%) in the 310 mice exposed to 290–580 rad neutrons, but after 800 R X-rays, the incidence of both types of gastric cancers was only 0.4%. Saxen [30] failed to induce gastric carcinomas in mice that were treated with 1000 R to the gastric region. The evidence, unsatisfactory as it is, suggests that high doses of low-LET radiation are required to induce tumours in the gastro-intestinal tract of mice.

4.2 Rats

An early demonstration of induction of intestinal tumours in the rat by radiation was by Bond et al. in 1952 [31]. These investigators used local irradiation with single equivalent doses of deuterons in the range of 1800–2800 rem. The large doses required to induce intestinal tumours makes it difficult to ensure survival for sufficient time for the development of the tumours, and various approaches have been used to circumvent the problem.

Brecher et al. [32] used parabiosis and pretreatment with para aminopropriohenome or glutathione to protect the animals from the early lethal effects of the radiation. Four carcinomas, three of the small intestine and one in the colon, were induced in the parabiosis group exposed to 700–1000 R within 11–16 months after irradiation.

Osborne and his colleagues have carried out extensive studies on induction of intestinal tumours in the rat by radiation. They exposed exteriorized jejunum and ileum of male Holtzman rats to 1000–2000 R of 250 kV X-rays [33]. In some groups the vascular supply to the intestine was clamped during irradiation, which resulted in a markedly higher survival rate. No tumours were found within 12 months in 70 unirradiated controls or in 25 rats that received 1200 R or less and that survived more than 30 days. Fifty-four tumours were found in 121 rats who received 1600–2500 R and in which the intestinal vessels had been clamped during most of the exposure period. In the 1400 R exposure group without the vessels clamped, 9 of the 14 animals survived more than 30 days, of which 5 developed tumours. The minimum latent period was surprisingly short, 55 days, and tumours continued to appear up to 255 days after irradiation. The histological appearance was considered to be that of adenocarcinoma.

Although metastases were found in two cases, the tumours were considered to be of low-grade malignancy. The results indicated that high doses of radiation were required to induce tumours in the small intestine of the rat. Marks and Sullivan [34] exposed the exteriorized intestine of Sprague-Dawley rats to X-rays. No cancers were produced in the 900–1300 R dose range but were induced by doses in the range of 1500–1900 R.

Denman et al. [35] induced adenocarcinomas with very large doses of X-rays (2500–6500 R). A technique in which the majority of the radiation to be localized to the colon of rats allowed the study of the carcinogenic effect of 2500–6500 R. There was a dose-dependent increase in the incidence of tumours of the colon to an apparent maximum of 47%. At the higher doses, survival was so compromised that the incidence decreased.

5. EXPERIMENTAL SYSTEMS AND THE STUDY OF MECHANISMS

Unfortunately, the studies of the molecular changes involved in the induction and development of intestinal cancers have been restricted, so far, to chemical carcinogenesis. Since the evidence suggests that unique mutations may be induced by specific carcinogens and furthermore may be species specific, it is impossible to predict what oncogenes or tumour suppressor genes may be involved in the radiation-induced cancers of the gut. Mutations in genes of the *ras* family have been detected in the early or even preneoplastic changes in various tissues. In the rat colon treated with chemical carcinogens such as azoxymethane [36], mutations in codons 12 and 13 in K-*ras* have been found. The number of samples with such mutations increased from 7% in aberrant crypt foci, which are thought to be the earliest stage in colon carcinogenesis. The frequency remained low in adenomatous polyps but increased to 37% in invasive adenocarcinomas.

The genetic basis of colon cancer in humans is being revealed with exciting findings [37–39], and recently a dominant mutation that predisposes to multiple intestinal neoplasia has been found in the mouse [40]. This germline mutation results in multiple tumours in the intestine of all carriers. The phenotypic expression is multiple adenomas in young mice, and the adenomas progress to cancers in old mice. Anaemia develops frequently and is thought to be secondary to the tumour. The mutant gene responsible for the multiple intestinal neoplasms has been called *Min* and is the homolog of adenomatous polyposis coli gene in humans [41]. It has been shown that a germ-line nonsense mutation in the *mApc* gene is responsible for the *Min* phenotype. The *Min* mouse appears to be a very good model for familial adenomatous polyposis in humans [42].

The *Min* mouse should provide a useful model for investigating the effect of radiation on progression of adenomas to carcinomas. This possibility has been increased by the development of Min/+ hybrids with AKR/J or MA/MyJ strains that live up to about 300 days and in which the adenomas that develop do so by 100 days [42]. Most recently, a gene, *Mom* 1, that influences the development of tumours of the colon in mice carrying *Min* 1 has been described [43]. *Mom* 1 appears to be a modifier gene that can reduce or suppress the tumours associated with *Min* 1, the homolog of the *Apc* gene in humans. Presumably it will not be long before *Mom* 1 is sequenced. While the initial events of the carcinogenesis process are essential, it is the factors that influence expression that result in overt cancer, and thus determine the incidence of cancers. This mouse model system should be very useful in elucidating the effects of radiation on progression.

6. SUSCEPTIBILITY FOR CANCER

For a long time there has been the question of why the small intestine, with a clonogenic cell population, estimated to be about 1×10^7 [44], has a low incidence of cancer in comparison to the large intestine. Furthermore, the small intestine appears to be resistant to the induction of cancer by chemical carcinogens. In the case of ionizing radiation, the human small intestine has a very low susceptibility, and in experimental animals relatively high doses are required to induce tumours. Over the years there has been speculation about the reasons for the apparent paradox of a tissue with a rapid cell renewal and large stem cell population having a low frequency of cancer as well as a low susceptibility for induction of tumours. The most recent suggestion is that stem cells in the large intestine that are damaged, and may have incurred a genetic change with the potential for malignant change, are not eliminated as efficiently as damaged stem cells in the ileum [45]. The suggestion is based on the fact that in the ileum apoptosis is seen at the same cell positions in the crypt that the presumptive stem cells are found. In contrast, in the colon apoptosis is noted at cell positions higher in the crypts than where the presumptive stem cells are found.

It is possible that in the large intestine various metabolites play a significant interactive role that does not occur in the small intestine. Whatever the reason, the difference in cancer and susceptibility for induction of tumours between the small and large intestine is independent of species.

7. CONCLUSION

The radiosensitivity for induction of cancer in the gut shows important similarities between humans and experimental animals, for example, (1) the differences in susceptibility between regions in the gut, (2) the fact that the small intestine is singularly resistant to cancer induction, and (3) that high doses are necessary to induce significant increases in the incidences of tumours of the gut in several species.

Cancer of the stomach is a major late effect in the atomic bomb survivors, and this high susceptibility appears to be related to the high background rate. Such a relationship suggests that the interaction between some dietary (or other) factors and radiation is multiplicative. In this Japanese population the colon, but not the rectum, is susceptible to the induction of cancer by radiation. The explanation of the marked differences in susceptibility between regions of the gut remains unclear. A difference in the ability to eliminate potential cancer cells and differences in the amounts of factors that influence tumour cell growth between the different regions of the gut may be important.

The discovery of two mutations in mice, one of which is a homolog of the gene associated with colon cancer in humans, promises well for future studies. Hopefully, the interaction of radiation and this germline mutation will be elucidated soon.

Acknowledgement

The research was sponsored by the Office of Health and Environmental Research and the Office of Epidemiology and Health Surveillance, US Department of Energy, under contract DE-AC05-84OR21400 with Martin Marietta Energy Systems, Inc. "Accordingly, the U.S. Government retains a nonexclusive, royalty-free license to publish or reproduce the published form of this contribution, or allow others to do so, for U.S. Government purposes."

It is a pleasure to acknowledge the help of Mrs. S. Allen.

Note added in proof

A comprehensive overview of all human radiation studies conducted through 1994 has recently been published by the United States Scientific Committee on the Effects of Atomic Radiation [46] and a new follow-up of the ankylosing spondylitis patients in the United Kingdom has been reported [47].

References

1. ICRP (1991) Recommendations of the International Commission on Radiological Protection, ICRP Publication 60, Pergamon Press, Oxford.
2. Ron, E., Preston, D.L., Mabuchi, K., et al. (1994) Cancer incidence in atomic bomb survivors. Part IV: Comparison of cancer incidence and mortality. Radiat. Res. 137, S98–S112.
3. Thompson, D.E., Mabuchi, K., Ron, E., et al. (1994) Cancer incidence in atomic bomb survivors. Part II: Solid tumors, 1958–1987. Radiat. Res. 137, S17–S67.
4. Boice, J.D., Day, N.E., Andersen, A., et al. (1985) Second cancers following radiation treatment for cervical cancer. An international collaboration among cancer registries. J. Natl. Cancer Inst. 74, 955–975.
5. Boice, J.D. Jr., Engholm, G., Kleinerman, R.A., et al. (1988) Radiation dose and second cancer risk in patients treated for cancer of the cervix. Radiat. Res. 116, 3–55.
6. Darby, S.C., Doll, R., Gill, S.K., et al. (1987) Long-term mortality after a single treatment course with X-rays in patients treated for ankylosing spondylitis. Br. J. Cancer 55, 179–190.
7. Inskip, P.D., Monson, R.R., Wagoner, J.K., et al. (1990) Cancer mortality following radium treatment for uterine bleeding. Radiat. Res. 123, 331–334.
8. Darby, S.C., Reeves, G., Key, T., Doll, R., and Stovall, M. (1994) Mortality in a cohort of women given X-ray therapy for metropathia haemorrhagica. Int. J. Cancer 56, 793–801.
9. Griem, M.L., Kleinerman, R.A., Boice, J.D. Jr., et al. (1994) Cancer following radiotherapy for peptic ulcer. J. Natl. Cancer Inst. 86, 842–849.
10. Shimizu, Y., Kato, H. and Schull, W.J. (1990) Studies of the mortality of A-bomb survivors. Part 9: Mortality, 1950–1985; Part 2: Cancer mortality based on the recently revised doses (DS86). Radiat. Res. 121, 120–141.
11. Davis, F.G., Boice, J.D. Jr., Hrubec, Z., et al. (1989) Cancer mortality in a radiation-exposed cohort of Massachusetts tuberculosis patients. Cancer Res. 49, 6130–6136.
12. Holm, L-E., Hall, P., Wiklund, K.E., et al. (1991) Cancer risk after iodine-131 therapy for hyperthyroidism. J. Natl Cancer Inst. 83, 1072–1077.
13. Land, C.E. and Sinclair, W.K. (1991) The relative contributions of different organ sites to the total cancer mortality associated with low-dose radiation exposure. In: Risks associated with ionizing radiation. Annals of the ICRP 22(1). Pergamon Press, Oxford, pp. 31–57.
14. Boice, J.D. Jr., Land, C.E., Shore, R.E., et al. (1979) Risk of breast cancer following low-dose radiation exposure. Radiology 131, 589–597.
15. Boice, J.D. Jr., Blettner, M., Kleinerman, R.A., et al. (1987) Radiation dose and leukemia risk in patients treated for cancer of the cervix. J. Natl. Cancer Inst. 79, 1295–1311.
16. Wells, H.G., Slye, M. and Holmes, H.F. (1938) Comparative pathology of cancer of the alimentary canal, with report on cases in mice. Am. J. Cancer 33, 223–238.
17. Rowlatt, C. and Chesterman, F.C. (1979) Tumors of the intestines and peritoneum. In: V.S. Turusov (Ed.), Pathology of Tumors in Laboratory Animals, Vol. II, Tumors of the Mouse. International Agency for Research on Cancer, Lyon, pp. 169–175.
18. Rowlatt, C., Franks, M.U. and Sheriff, F.C. (1969) Naturally occurring tumors and other lesions of the digestive tract in untreated C57BL mice. J. Natl. Cancer Inst. 43, 1353–1364.

19. Cosgrove, G.E., Walburg, H.E. and Upton, A.C. (1968) Gastrointestinal lesions in aged conventional and germfree mice exposed to radiation as young adults. In: M.E. Sullivan (Ed.), Gastrointestinal Injury. Monogr. Nucl. Med. Biol. Vol. 1, Excerpta Medica Foundation, Amsterdam, pp. 303–312.
20. Nowell, P.C. and Cole, L.G. (1959) Late effects of fast neutrons versus X rays in mice: Nephroscelerosis, tumors, longevity. Radiat. Res. 11, 545–556.
21. Watanabe, H., Akihiro, I. and Hirose, F. (1986) Experimental carcinogenesis in the digestive and genitourinary tracts. In: A.C. Upton, R.E. Albert, F.J. Burns and R.E. Shore (Eds.), Radiation Carcinogenesis. Elsevier, New York, pp. 232–244.
22. Stewart, H.L. (1953) Experimental cancer of the alimentary tract. In: F. Homburger and W.H. Fishman (Eds.), The Physiopathology of Cancer. Hoeber and London, Casell, New York, pp. 3–45.
23. Boffa, L.C., Dewar, B.A., Gruss, R. and Allfug, V.G. (1980) Differences in colonic nuclear proteins of two mouse stains with different susceptibilities to 1,2 dimethyl hydrazine-induced carcinogenesis. Cancer Res. 40, 1771–1780.
24. Deschner, E.D., Long, F.C. and Hakissian, M. (1988) Susceptibility to 1,2-dimethylhydrazine-induced colonic tumors and epithelial cell proliferative characteristics of F₁, F₂ and reciprocal backcrosses derived from SWR/J and AKR/J parental mouse strains. Cancer 61, 478–482.
25. Diwan, B.A., Meier, H. and Blackman, K.E. (1977) Genetic differences in the induction of colorectal tumors by 1,2-dimethylhydrazine in inbred mice. J. Natl. Cancer Inst. 59, 455–457.
26. Laqueur, G.L. (1964) Carcinogenic effects of cycad meal and cycasin, methylazoxymethanol glycoside, in rats and the effect of cycasin in germfree rats. Fed. Proc. 23, 1386–1388.
27. Nowell, P.C., Cole, L.J. and Ellis, M.F. (1956) Induction of intestinal carcinoma in the mouse by whole-body fast-neutron irradiation. Cancer Res. 16, 873–876.
28. Hirose, F., Fukazawa, K., Watanabe, H., Terada, Y., Fujii, I. and Ootuska, S. (1977) Induction of rectal carcinoma in mice by local x-irradiation. Gann. 68, 669–680.
29. Rostom, A.Y., Kauffman, S.L. and Steel, G.G. (1978) Influence of misonidazole on the incidence of radiation-induced intestinal tumors in mice. Br. J. Cancer 38, 530–536.
30. Sáxen, E.A. (1952) Squamous-cell carcinoma of the forestomach in x-irradiated mice fed 9,10-dimethyl-1,2-benzanthracene, with a note on failure to induce adenocarcinoma. J. Natl. Cancer Inst. 13, 491–453.
31. Bond, V.P., Swift, M.N., Tobias, C.A. and Brecher, G. (1952) Bowel lesions following single deuteron irradiation. Fed. Proc. 11, 408–409.
32. Brecher, G., Cronkite, E.P. and Peers, J.H. (1953) Neoplasms in rats protected against lethal doses of irradiation or para aminopropriophenome. J. Natl. Cancer Inst. 14, 159–175.
33. Osborne, J.W., Nicholson, D.P. and Prasad, K.N. (1963) Induction of intestinal carcinoma in the rat by x-irradiation of the small intestine. Radiat Res. 18, 76–85.
34. Marks, S. and Sullivan, M.F. (1960) Tumors of the small intestine in rats after intestinal X-irradiation. Nature 188, 953.
35. Denman, D.L., Kirchner, F.R. and Osborne, J.W. (1978) Induction of colonic adenocarcinoma in the rat by X-irradiation. Cancer Res. 38, 1899–1905.
36. Vivona, A.A., Shpitz, B., Medline, A., Bruce, W.R., May, K., Ward, M.A., Stern, H.S. and Gallinger, S. (1993) K-*ras* mutations in aberrant crypt foci, adenomas and adenocarcinomas during azoxymethane-induced colon carcinogenesis. Carcino-

genesis 14, 1777–1781.

37. Vogelstein, B.E., Fearon, E.R., Hamilton, S.R., Kerr, S.E., Preisinger, A.C., Lepper, T.M., Nakamura, K., White, R., Smits, A.M.M. and Bos, J.L. (1988) Genetic alterations during colorectal-tumor development. N. Eng. J. Med. 319, 525–532.

38. Fearon, E.R. and Vogelstein, B.E. (1990) A genetic model for colorectal tumorigenesis. Cell 61, 759–767.

39. Lynch, H.T., Smyrk, T.C., Watson, P., Larspa, S.J., Lynch, J.F., Lynch, P.M., Cavalieri, R.J. and Boland, C.R. (1993) Genetics natural history tumor spectrum and pathology of hereditary non polyposis colorectal cancer: an updated review. Gastroenterology 104, 1535–1549.

40. Moser, A.R., Pitot, H.C. and Dove, W.F. (1990) A dominant mutation that predisposes to multiple intestinal neoplasia in the mouse. Science 247, 322–324.

41. Su, L-K., Kinzler, K.W., Vogelstein, B., Preisinger, A.C., Moser, A.R., Luongo, C., Gould, K.A. and Dover, W.F. (1992) Multiple intestinal neoplasia caused by a mutation in the murine homolog of the APC gene. Science 256, 668–670.

42. Moser, A.R., Dove, W.F., Roth, A. and Gordon, J.I. (1992) The *Min* (Multiple Intestinal Neoplasia) mutation: Its effect on gut epithelial cell differentiation and interaction with a modifier system. J. Cell Biol. 116, 1517–1526.

43. Dietrich, W.F., Lander, E.S., Smith, J.S., Moser, A.R., Gould, K.A., Luongo, C., Borenstein, N. and Dove, W. (1993) Genetic identification of *Mom*-1, a major modifier locus affecting *Min*-induced intestinal neoplasia in the mouse. Cell 75, 631–639.

44. Potten, C.S., Hendry, J.H., Moore, J.V. and Chwalinski, S. (1983) Cytotoxic effects in gastro-intestinal epithelium (as exemplified by small intestine). In: C.S. Potten and J.H. Hendry (Eds.) Cytotoxic Insult to Tissue. Churchill Livingstone, Edinburgh, pp. 105–152.

45. Potten, C.S., Ly, Y.Q., O'Conner, P.J. and Winton, D.J. (1992) A possible explanation for the differential cancer incidence in the intestine, based on distribution of the cytotoxic effects of carcinogens in the murine large bowel. Carcinogenesis 13, 2305–2312.

46. United Nations Scientific Committee on the Effects of Atomic Radiation (1994) Sources and Effects of Ionizing Radiation. Publ. E.94 IX.11. United Nations, New York.

47. Weiss, H.A., Darby, S.C. and Doll, R. (1994) Cancer mortality following X-ray treatment for ankylosing spondylitis. Int. J. Cancer 59, 327–338.

Index